MANAGEMENT OF BENIGN PROSTATIC HYPERTROPHY

CURRENT CLINICAL UROLOGY

Eric A. Klein, SERIES EDITOR

Essential Urology: A Guide to Clinical Practice, edited by **Jeannette M. Potts,** 2004

Management of Benign Prostatic Hypertrophy, edited by **Kevin T. McVary,** 2004

Laparoscopic Urologic Oncology, edited by **Jeffrey A. Cadeddu,** 2004

Essential Urologic Laparoscopy: The Complete Clinical Guide, edited by **Stephen Y. Nakada,** 2003

Urologic Prostheses: The Complete Practical Guide to Devices, Their Implantation, and Patient Followup, edited by **Culley C. Carson, III,** 2002

Male Sexual Function: A Guide to Clinical Management, edited by **John J. Mulcahy,** 2001

Prostate Cancer Screening, edited by **Ian M. Thompson, Martin I. Resnick, and Eric A. Klein,** 2001

Bladder Cancer: Current Diagnosis and Treatment, edited by **Michael J. Droller,** 2001

Office Urology: The Clinician's Guide, edited by **Elroy D. Kursh and James C. Ulchaker,** 2001

Voiding Dysfunction: Diagnosis and Treatment, edited by **Rodney A. Appell,** 2000

Management of Prostate Cancer, edited by **Eric A. Klein,** 2000

MANAGEMENT OF BENIGN PROSTATIC HYPERTROPHY

Edited by

KEVIN T. MCVARY, MD

Northwestern University Feinberg School of Medicine, Chicago, IL

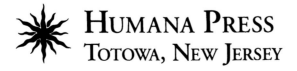

HUMANA PRESS
TOTOWA, NEW JERSEY

© 2004 Humana Press Inc.
Softcover reprint of the hardcover 1st edition 2004
999 Riverview Drive, Suite 208
Totowa, New Jersey 07512

www.humanapress.com

For additional copies, pricing for bulk purchases, and/or information about other Humana titles, contact Humana at the above address or at any of the following numbers: Tel.: 973-256-1699; Fax: 973-256-8341, E-mail: humana@humanapr.com; or visit our Website: http://humanapr.com

Production Editor: Mark J. Breaugh.

Cover design by Patricia F. Cleary.

This publication is printed on acid-free paper. ∞
ANSI Z39.48-1984 (American National Standards Institute) Permanence of Paper for Printed Library Materials.

E-ISBN: 1-59259-644-4

Library of Congress Cataloging-in-Publication Data

Management of benign prostatic hypertrophy / edited by Kevin T. McVary.
        p. ; cm. -- (Current clinical urology)
Includes bibliographical references and index.

Additional material to this book can be downloaded from http://extra.springer.com.

ISBN 978-1-4684-9806-6   ISBN 978-1-59259-644-7 (eBook)
DOI 10.1007/978-1-59259-644-7
1. Benign prostatic hyperplasia.
[DNLM: 1. Prostatic Hyperplasia--therapy. 2. Bladder
Diseases--etiology. 3. Prostatic Hyperplasia--complications. 4.
Prostatic Hyperplasia--diagnosis. WJ 752 M2673 2004] I. McVary, Kevin
T. II. Series.
RC899.M36 2004
616.6'5--dc21
                             2003007891

Preface

Benign prostatic hyperplasia (BPH) is the most common neoplastic condition afflicting men and constitutes a major health factor impacting patients in every part of the world. Bladder neck obstruction secondary to BPH can result in significant medical complications including renal failure, urinary retention, recurrent urinary tract infection, bladder stones, significant hematuria, and marked and disruptive bladder symptoms. Current studies estimate that upwards of 30% of males will require some type of surgical or other significant intervention to correct this problem sometime in their lives. Because there is a major restructuring of the treatment algorithms used to manage this important clinical problem and because of new medications and advances in technology, a great need for *Management of Benign Prostatic Hypertrophy* has arisen.

How best to approach patients is a common question posed by urologists. What is to be made of these newer therapies, and what are their roles vis-à-vis our more established treatments? *Management of Benign Prostatic Hypertrophy* is designed to address those needs for the practicing urologist who is often caught in the middle of these newer therapies and confused by the significant hype. Despite this clear need for interpretation of new data, a text that is not grounded in the principles and hallmarks of our specialty will offer little to budding urologists; rather, this text serves as a single source for quick reference on most aspects of this broad spectrum of BPH treatments.

Management of Benign Prostatic Hypertrophy is divided into three main categories: (1) pathophysiology and natural history of BPH, (2) epidemiology: definitions and prevalence of the disease, and (3) the urodynamic evaluation of lower urinary tract symptoms. The first category is also buttressed by a more current understanding and treatment of postobstructive diuresis, a significant medical complication and frequent source of urologic consultation. A second component of the text addresses medical therapies for BPH, namely α-adrenergic antagonists, 5α-reductase inhibitors, and their combination in the treatment of BPH. The most extensive portion of the text is an up-to-date, concise evaluation of each of the minimally invasive therapies as well as the time-tested surgical treatments.

I think you will find *Management of Benign Prostatic Hypertrophy* concise, readable, and up-to-date.

Kevin T. McVary, MD

v

Value-Added eBook/PDA

This book is accompanied by a value-added CD-ROM that
contains an eBook version of the volume you have just pur-
chased. This eBook can be viewed on your computer, and you can synchronize it to your
PDA for viewing on your handheld device. The eBook enables you to view this volume
on only one computer and PDA. Once the eBook is installed on your computer, you
cannot download, install, or e-mail it to another computer; it resides solely with the
computer to which it is installed. The license provided is for only one computer. The
eBook can only be read using Adobe(r) Reader(r) 6.0 software, which is available free
from Adobe Systems Incorporated at www.Adobe.com. You may also view the eBook
on your PDA using the Adobe(r) PDA Reader(r) software that is also available free
from Adobe.com.

You must follow a simple procedure when you install the eBook/PDA that will require
you to connect to the Humana Press website in order to receive your license. Please read
and follow the instructions below:

1. Download and install Adobe(r) Reader(r) 6.0 software
   You can obtain a free copy of the Adobe(r) Reader(r) 6.0 software at
   www.adobe.com
   *Note: If you already have the Adobe(r) Reader(r) 6.0 software installed,
   you do not need to reinstall it.
2. Launch Adobe(r) Reader(r) 6.0 software
3. Install eBook:
      Insert your eBook CD into your CD-ROM drive
      PC:
      Click on the "Start" button, then click on "Run"
      At the prompt, type "d:\ebookinstall.pdf" and click "OK"
      *Note: If your CD-ROM drive letter is something other than d: change
      the above command accordingly.
      MAC: Double click on the "eBook CD" that you will see mounted on
      your desktop.
      Double click "ebookinstall.pdf"
4. Adobe(r) Reader(r) 6.0 software will open and you will receive the message
   "This document is protected by Adobe DRM"
   Click "OK"
      *Note: If you have not already activated the Adobe(r) Reader(r)
      6.0 software, you will be prompted to do so. Simply follow the
      directions to activate and continue installation.
      Your web browser will open and you will be taken to the Humana
      Press eBook registration page. Follow the instructions on that page to
      complete installation. You will need the serial number located on the
      sticker sealing the envelope containing the CD-ROM.

If you require assistance during the installation, or you would like more information
regarding your eBook and PDA installation, please refer to the eBookManual.pdf
located on your cd. If you need further assistance, contact Humana Press eBook
Support by e-mail at ebooksupport@humanapr.com or by phone at 973-256-1699.

*Adobe and Reader are either registered trademarks or trademarks of Adobe Systems Incorporated in the United States and/or other countries.

Contents

Preface v

CD-ROM Instructions vi

List of Contributors ix

1 Prostate Anatomy and Causative Theories, Pathophysiology,
   and Natural History of Benign Prostatic Hyperplasia 1
   Jeffrey A. Stern, John M. Fitzpatrick, and Kevin T. McVary

2 The Definition of Benign Prostatic Hyperplasia:
   Epidemiology and Prevalence 21
   Glenn S. Gerber

3 Pathophysiology, Diagnosis, and Treatment
   of the Postobstructive Diuresis 35
   Chris M. Gonzalez

4 Urodynamics and the Evaluation
   of Male Lower Urinary Tract Symptoms 47
   J. Quentin Clemens

5 α-Adrenergic Antagonists in the Treatment
   of Benign Prostatic Hypertrophy-Associated
   Lower Urinary Tract Symptoms 61
   Ross A. Rames and David C. Horger

6 5α-Reductase Inhibitors 79
   Robert E. Brannigan and John T. Grayhack

7 Transurethral Needle Ablation of the Prostate 97
   Timothy F. Donahue and Joseph A. Costa

8 Transurethral Microwave Thermotherapy 109
   Jonathan N. Rubenstein and Kevin T. McVary

9 Transurethral Incision of the Prostate 125
   Robert F. Donnell

10 Interstitial Laser Coagulation and High-Intensity Focused Ultrasound
   for the Treatment of Benign Prostatic Hyperplasia 141
   Christopher M. Dixon

11 Transurethral Resection of the Prostate 163
   Harris E. Foster, Jr. and Micah Jacobs

12 Transurethral Vaporization of the Prostate 195
   Joe O. Littlejohn, Young M. Kang, and Steven A. Kaplan

13 Treatment of Benign Prostatic Hyperplasia with Ethanol Injections,
      Water-Induced Thermotherapy,
      and Prostatic Urethral Luminal Stents 211
    Jay Y. Gillenwater

14 Suprapubic Transvesical Prostatectomy
      and Simple Perineal Prostatectomy for the Treatment
      of Benign Prostatic Hyperplasia...221
    James M. Kozlowski, Norm D. Smith, and John T. Grayhack

    Index 263

Contributors

ROBERT E. BRANNIGAN, MD • *Department of Urology, Northwestern University Feinberg School of Medicine, Chicago, IL*

J. QUENTIN CLEMENS, MD, MSCI • *Section of Voiding Dysfunction and Female Urology, Department of Urology, Northwestern University Feinberg School of Medicine, Chicago, IL*

JOSEPH A. COSTA, DO • *Department of Urology, National Naval Medical Center; Department of Surgery, Uniformed Services University of Health Sciences, Bethesda, MD*

CHRISTOPHER M. DIXON, MD • *Division of Urology, New York University School of Medicine, New York, NY*

TIMOTHY F. DONAHUE, MD • *Department of Urology, National Naval Medical Center; Center for Prostate Disease Research, Department of Surgery, Uniformed Services University of Health Sciences, Bethesda, MD*

ROBERT F. DONNELL, MD, FACS • *Prostate Center, Clinical Trials (Urology), The Medical College of Wisconsin, Milwaukee, WI*

JOHN M. FITZPATRICK, MD • *Department of Surgery, Mater Misericordiae Hospital; University College of Dublin, Dublin, Ireland*

HARRIS E. FOSTER, JR., MD • *Section of Urology, Yale University School of Medicine, New Haven, CT*

GLENN S. GERBER, MD • *Section of Urology, Department of Surgery, University of Chicago Pritzker School of Medicine, Chicago, IL*

JAY Y. GILLENWATER, MD • *Department of Urology, University of Virginia Health Sciences Center, Charlottesville, VA*

CHRIS M. GONZALEZ, MD • *Department of Urology, Northwestern University Feinberg School of Medicine, Chicago, IL*

JOHN T. GRAYHACK, MD • *Section of Urologic Oncology, The Robert H. Lurie Comprehensive Cancer Center, Northwestern University Feinberg School of Medicine, Chicago, IL*

DAVID C. HORGER, MD • *Department of Urology, Medical University of South Carolina, Charleston, SC*

MICAH JACOBS, BA • *Yale University School of Medicine, New Haven, CT*

YOUNG M. KANG, MD • *Department of Urology, College of Physicians and Surgeons, Columbia University, New York Presbyterian Hospital, New York, NY*

STEVEN A. KAPLAN, MD • *Department of Urology, College of Physicians and Surgeons, Columbia University, New York Presbyterian Hospital, New York, NY*

JAMES M. KOZLOWSKI, MD, FACS • *Section of Urologic Oncology, The Robert H. Lurie Comprehensive Cancer Center, Northwestern University Feinberg School of Medicine, Chicago, IL*

JOE O. LITTLEJOHN, MD • *Department of Urology, College of Physicians and Surgeons, Columbia University, New York Presbyterian Hospital, New York, NY*

KEVIN T. MCVARY, MD, FACS • *Department of Urology, Northwestern University Feinberg School of Medicine, Chicago, IL*

ROSS A. RAMES, MD • *Department of Urology, Medical University of South Carolina, Charleston, SC*

JONATHAN N. RUBENSTEIN, MD • *Department of Urology, Northwestern University Feinberg School of Medicine, Chicago, IL*

NORM D. SMITH, MD • *Section of Urologic Oncology, The Robert H. Lurie Comprehensive Cancer Center, Northwestern University Feinberg School of Medicine, Chicago, IL*

JEFFREY A. STERN, MD, MPH • *Department of Urology, Northwestern University Feinberg School of Medicine, Chicago, IL*

1

Prostate Anatomy and Causative Theories, Pathophysiology, and Natural History of Benign Prostatic Hyperplasia

Jeffrey A. Stern, MD, John M. Fitzpatrick, MD, and Kevin T. McVary, MD

CONTENTS

INTRODUCTION
ANATOMY
NORMAL GROWTH AND DEVELOPMENT
   OF HUMAN PROSTATE
BENIGN PROSTATIC HYPERPLASIA
SUMMARY
REFERENCES

INTRODUCTION

The prostate is the major accessory sex gland of the male. It provides exocrine function, but it has no established endocrine or secretory function. Its secretion provides fluid that comprises 15% of the ejaculate. These secretions produce a volume-expanding vehicle for sperm, yet no reproductive function has been identified. The gland has been the subject of much study because it is the site of infection as well as benign and malignant neoplasm. The prostate's intimate anatomic relationship with the bladder neck and urethra increases the importance of these pathologic changes and is the focus of this chapter.

From: *Management of Benign Prostatic Hypertrophy*
Edited by: K. T. McVary © Humana Press Inc., Totowa, NJ

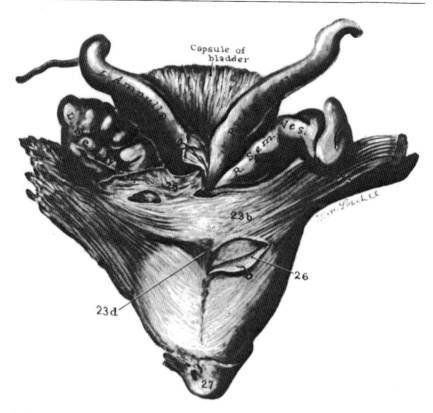

Fig. 1. This dorsal view of the prostate reveals its relationship with the seminal vesicles, the ampulla, and the bladder. The median sulcus separates the prostate into halves (23 d). The anterior layer of Denonvielliers fascia (26) comprises the dorsal capsule of the prostate. The urogenital diaphragm (27) merges with the distal end of the prostate. (From *3* and *12* with permission.)

ANATOMY

The prostate is a compound tubuloalveolar gland. It is adjacent to the bladder neck proximally and merges with the membranous urethra to rest on the urogenital diaphragm distally. The intact adult gland resembles a blunted cone, weighing approx 18 to 20 g. The gland measures about 4.4 cm transversely across its base, and it is 3.4 cm in length and 2.6 cm in anteroposterior diameter *(1)*. The urethra enters the prostate near the middle of its base and exits the gland on its anterior surface just before the apical portion. The ejaculatory ducts enter the base on its posterior aspect and run in an oblique fashion, terminating adjacent to the verumontanum. The capsule of the prostate gland is incomplete at the apex and does not represent a true capsule *(2)*. Fibrous septa emanate

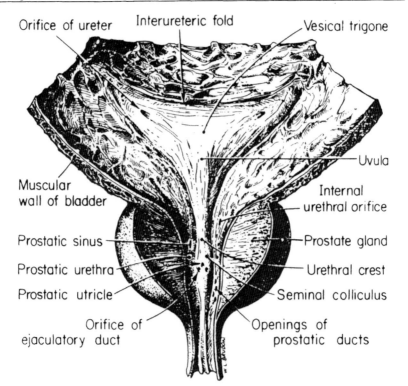

Orifice of ureter   Interureteric fold   Vesical trigone

Uvula

Muscular
wall of bladder   Internal
                                                     urethral orifice

Prostatic sinus   Prostate gland

Prostatic urethra   Urethral crest

Prostatic utricle   Seminal colliculus

Orifice of   Openings of
ejaculatory duct   prostatic ducts

Fig. 2. This frontal view of the prostate reveals its ductal system in continuity with the bladder and the urethra. The prostatic utricle rests atop the verumontanum. The majority of the prostatic ducts drain distal to the verumontanum. The bladder neck (internal sphincter) is comprised of the area extending from the trigone to the termination of the prostatic urethra. (From *3,* with permission.)

from the capsule, pierce the underlying parenchyma, and divide it into glandular units called lobules *(3).* Most of these units empty their contents into the prostatic urethra near the verumontanum *(4).* The anatomic details are illustrated in Figs. 1 and 2.

The endopelvic fascia represents the fusion of extraperitoneal connective tissue that forms a subserous covering for the pelvic viscera and envelops its neurovascular supply. A sheetlike proliferation of this fascia contributes to the formation of the puboprostatic ligaments. They anchor the anterior and lateral aspect of the prostate to the posterior aspect of the pubis *(5).*

The lateral pelvic fascia, also described as the parietal layer of the endopelvic or prostatic fascia, serves as the fascial envelope to the levator ani muscle and maintains continuity with the capsule of the prostate along its anterior and anterolateral aspects. Anatomic dissections by Walsh and Donker revealed that the major neurovascular bundles to the prostate were contained posterolaterally within the lateral leaves of this fascia (5).

Neurovascular Supply

The prostatovesicular artery, the major arterial supply to the prostate and seminal vesicles, is a branch of the inferior vesical artery. It originates from the anterior division of the hypogastric artery and courses medially on the levator muscle to the bladder base. The artery has tiny branches that go to the bladder base, prostate, and tip of the seminal vesicles. These urethral and capsular branches are the prostate's main arterial supply (1). The urethral branches course along the posterolateral aspect of the vesicoprostatic junction and usually enter the bladder neck and periurethral aspect of the prostate gland at the 5 and 7 o'clock positions (Fig. 3). The anterior division of the hypogastric artery also supplies the inferior aspect of the prostate, the seminal vesicles, and the vas deferens with accessory vessels from the middle hemorrhoidal and internal pudendal arteries (1,3).

Wide, thin-walled veins on the lateral and anterior aspect of the prostate gland merge with veins of the vesical plexus and the deep dorsal vein of the penis to form the plexus of Santorini within the puboprostatic space. This confluence of veins empties into the hypogastric vein.

In 1982, Walsh and Donker published landmark observations descr~2ing the anatomic relationship of the pelvic (autonomic)*ÿlexus and the prostate gland (6). The prostate, the other pelvic organs, and the corpora cavernosa receive their autonomic innervation from the pelvic plexus, a fenestrated 4-cm long, 2.5- to 3.0-cm high rectangular plate lying retroperitoneally adjacent to the rectum (7). Both the parasympathetic and sympathetic divisions of the autonomic nervous system contribute to the plexus. Parasympathetic visceral efferent preganglionic nerve fibers from the second through fourth levels of the sacral cord enter the plexus by way of the pelvic splanchnic nerve (nervi erigentes). This nerve is a composite of five or six branches rather than a discrete entity. The sympathetic component emanates from the thoracolumbar center (T11 to L2) and courses through the hypogastric nerve.

Normal Internal Architecture

The proposed organization of the fetal, newborn, and adult prostate into discrete lobes has been regarded with skepticism (8–12). With a

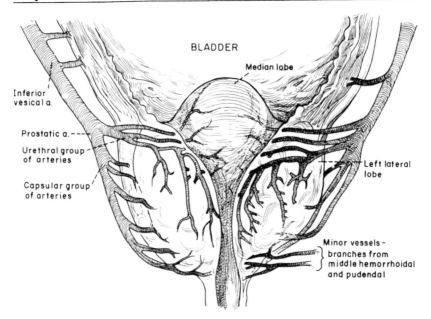

Fig. 3. The arterial blood supply to the prostate. The prostatovesicular artery is a terminal branch of the inferior vesical branch, arborizing into urethral and capsular tributaries. The urethral branches typically enter the bladder neck at the 5- and 7-o clock positions. The anterior division of the hypogastric artery supplies the inferior vesicle, the middle rectal, and the pudendal branches to the prostate gland. (From *12*, with permission.)

focus on the development of benign prostatic hypoplasia (BPH), Franks conceptualized a prostate with an inner (urethral) and outer glandular configuration *(13,14)*. McNeal *(15)* argued, as did Lowsley *(8)*, that the urethral (inner) glands should be considered separately from the prostate and its intrinsic architecture. However, the major physiologic and biochemical similarities of these glands and those of the prostatic parenchyma weigh against this concept.

McNeal has proposed and promoted acceptance of the theory of anatomic subdivisions with probable pathophysiologic significance in the adult prostate *(4,15)*. In his studies, McNeal emphasized the use of coronal and oblique coronal sections of prostates obtained between puberty and the third decade of life to study normal anatomy. Tisell and Salander, who used meticulous dissection techniques, observed subdivisions of the prostate gland that had several similarities to those reported by McNeal, but they interpreted these as evidence for the existence of prostatic lobes *(16)*.

McNeal observed that the urethra separates the prostate into ventral (fibromuscular) and dorsal (glandular) portions. Approximately midway between the apex and base, the posterior wall of the urethra undergoes an acute 35° ventral angulation that segregates the urethra into proximal and distal segments. The verumontanum and ejaculatory duct orifices exist exclusively within the distal segment. McNeal separated the glandular prostate into four distinct regions: peripheral zone, central zone, transition zone, and periurethral gland region (Fig. 4).

The peripheral zone constitutes approx 75% of the glandular prostate. Its ductal system enters the urethra along the posterolateral recesses of the urethra and extends from the verumontanum distally to the prostatic apex. The wedge-shaped central zone, the base of which is positioned superiorly at the bladder neck, occupies approx 20% of the glandular prostate. Its ductal network closely follows the ejaculatory ducts to the urethra and empties adjacent to orifices of the ejaculatory ducts on the apex of the verumontanum. The transition zone, accounting for 4–5% of the adult glandular prostate, is not well defined in the prepubertal prostate (17). It consists of two modest lobules of paraurethral tissue anterior to the peripheral zone. Its ducts empty in the posterior lateral recess of the urethra just proximal to peripheral zone ducts. The transition zone is lateral to McNeal's preprostatic sphincter, a smooth muscle cylinder enveloping the proximal urethra from the bladder neck to the base of the verumontanum. The last anatomically discrete area within the glandular prostate is the periurethral gland region, which represents less than 1% of the total volume of the glandular prostate. Its ductal network represents a more proximal extension of the networks of the peripheral and transition zone areas. These regions have differing acinar, stromal, and cellular configurations. McNeal postulated that the anatomic and histologic similarities of the peripheral and transition zones and periurethral gland region were attributable to a common urogenital sinus embryonic origin.

The anterior fibromuscular stroma forms an apron that extends distally, covers the entire anterolateral aspect of the glandular prostate, and is responsible for the anterior convexity of the prostate gland. It represents approximately one-third of the tissue within the prostate capsule (4). This unusually distinct area, composed predominantly of smooth-muscle fibers, maintains continuity proximally with the detrusor muscle fibers of the bladder neck.

Prostatic stroma consists predominantly of smooth muscle cells and fibroblasts arranged in close proximity to the distinct basal lamina of the epithelium. The fibroblasts, however, tend to be organized parallel to the long axis of these tubulosaccular glands and form a more predict-

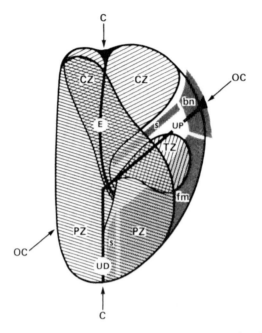

Fig. 4. This sagittal diagram of the prostate demonstrates its distinct zones: central zone (CZ), peripheral zone (PZ), and transitional zone (TZ). Its urethral segments, distal (UD), proximal (UP), and ejaculatory ducts (E) are illustrated along with nonglandular tissues [bladder neck (bn), anterior fibromuscular stroma (fm), preprostatic sphincter (s), distal striated sphincter (s)]. C and OC delineate the coronal and oblique coronal planes, respectively. (From *17*, with permission.)

able relationship with the basement membrane *(18).* The smooth muscle surrounds individual glands and is thought to play a pivotal role in the release of glandular secretions. Contraction of the circular smooth muscle of the bladder neck and preprostatic sphincter assists in the elimination of secretions within the prostatic urethra; this smooth muscle probably forms the major working element of the internal urethral sphincter. The anterior and anterolateral aspects of the prostate contain smooth and skeletal muscle, joining the fibers of the external sphincter and augmenting urinary control *(19).*

NORMAL GROWTH AND DEVELOPMENT
OF HUMAN PROSTATE

The human prostate increases in size and develops histologic evidence of stimulated growth during three periods of life: before and at birth, during puberty, and with achievement of advancing age *(20)*. The evidence for prostatic stimulation during gestation and at birth is based on histologic studies. During development, the prostatic tubules progress from solid cellular buds at the ends of ducts to bud acinar combinations and then to acinar tubular clusters arranged in lobules. The tubules gradually regress after the first month of life *(21)*. The secretions stain with variable intensity with periodic acid Schiff stain but stain only weakly for prostate-specific antigen *(11)*.

At puberty, the prostate demonstrates marked histologic evidence of stimulation, progressing from enlargement of the end buds of the prostatic ducts to development of somewhat distended alveoli and tall columnar epithelium. Although stromal cells are the predominant prostate tissue, the relative smooth muscle contribution decreases in the first and second decade of life and increases to neonatal levels in the third *(22)*. During the third decade, there is a gradual, irregular increase in the infolding of the alveolar epithelium. After the fourth decade, fewer of these infoldings are seen, and the tendency to cystic dilatation becomes evident.

BENIGN PROSTATIC HYPERPLASIA

Urinary obstruction resulting from benign prostatic disease was described in the earliest days of medicine. Initially formalized by Riolan in the 17th century, the relationship between BPH and urinary obstruction was further elucidated by Morgani in the mid-18th century; he provided one of the earliest descriptions of BPH and its sequelae *(23)*. More specific recognition of the pathologic process has been credited to Virchow in the last quarter of the 19th century. Despite a greater understanding of benign prostate growth, however, identification of its cause remains elusive.

Incidence

Autopsy studies have repeatedly demonstrated an association between BPH and aging based on histologic criteria, prostate weight, and prostate volume. Randall found histologic evidence that the incidence of BPH exceeded 50% in men over 50 yr of age and rose to 75% as men entered their 80s *(24)*. The age-related prevalence of histologic BPH found at autopsy is similar in several countries despite population diversity (Fig. 5; *25*). Mass producing BPH, however, occurs in approximately half of men with presumed histologic BPH and is clinically manifested in only half of those *(25)*. Its reported clinical incidence varies appreciably in different parts of the world *(26)*. Based on the combined

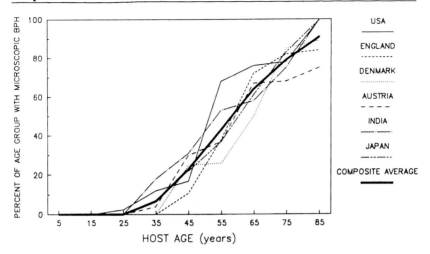

Fig. 5. This graph illustrates the strikingly similar age-specific prevalence of histologic BPH among different populations (From *25*, with permission.)

data from 10 autopsy studies, Berry et al. constructed curves for the prevalence of BPH with age (Fig. 6; *27*). Their analysis implies that BPH begins before the age of 30. Their calculated doubling time for BPH weight varies with age: 4.5 yr in the 31- to 50-yr age group, 10 yr in the 51- to 70-yr age group, and more than 100 yr in the greater than 70-yr age group. The autopsy finding of increased weight of glands requiring surgical intervention compared with the weight of those glands with hyperplasia only reinforces the potential role of prostate mass in BPH voiding dysfunction, as suggested in the Olmsted county male voiding pattern studies *(28)*.

   Although the literature on the racial and regional impact of BPH is difficult to interpret critically because of variable sampling and evaluation criteria, it clearly indicates an increasing but quantitatively variable incidence of pathologic and clinical BPH with aging *(29–31)*. The studies suggest that black and white populations in the United States have a similar incidence of BPH, although symptoms most likely develop earlier in blacks *(32)*. Blacks in the United States have a higher prevalence of adenomatous hyperplasia than blacks on the African continent. Moreover, data from the first half of the 20th century indicated a much lower prevalence of BPH in native Chinese and Japanese than in white populations *(31,33)*. These results were reaffirmed by a recent mass screening in Japan, which reported a 9.9 and 11.6% prevalence of

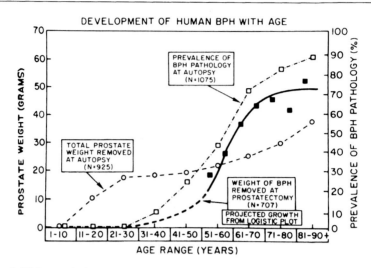

Fig. 6. This graph demonstrates the relationship between age-related changes in histologic BPH and prostate size. The increasing prevalence of BPH is far more apparent than the increase in prostate weight. (From *27*, with permission.)

BPH in men 70–79 and more than 80 yr of age, respectively *(31)*. Prospective ultrasound evaluation of monozygotic and dizygotic twins coupled with historic assessments of twins and of families with a high incidence of prostatectomy in men under age 64 support possible genetic factors in development of BPH *(34–36)*. Meikle et al., who studied twins, suggested that hereditary factors contributed substantially to symptomatology, but that nongenetic factors have more influence on zonal volumes of the prostate *(34,37)*. Overall, the data suggest that race and genetics have a limited role in the prevalence of histologic BPH, and that the environment, dietary intake, and genetic factors play a greater role in the rate and degree of development of mass-producing BPH.

Natural History of Anatomic BPH

The first pathologic evidence of BPH occurs in less than 10% of men in the 31- to 40-yr-old group (Table 1). Thus, either the initiating factor is present in most men of this age and only clinically evident in a few, or young men with recognizable BPH have a discrepancy between physiologic and chronologic aging. Evidence of histologic and anatomic BPH increases with age; by the ninth decade approx 90% of men have histologic evidence of BPH, and more than half have anatomic evidence of BPH *(38)*. The initial lesion of BPH typically occurs in the periurethral

Table 1
Prevalence of Pathologic BPH with Age in 1075 Human Prostates Collected at Autopsy

Age range (yr)	Autopsy studies					Combined data	
	Pradhan and Chandra (69)	Swyer (20)	Harbitz and Haugen (38)	Franks (14)	Moore (70)	Prevalence of human benign prostatic hyperplasia	
	No. with benign prostatic hyperplasia/total no. (%)	No. with benign prostatic hyperplasia/total no. (%)	No. with benign prostatic hyperplasia/total no. (%)	No. with benign prostatic hyperplasia/total no. (%)	No. with benign prostatic hyperplasia/total no. (%)	No. with benign prostatic hyperplasia/total no. (%)	% Mean ± standard error of mean
1–10	0/11 (0)	0/16 (0)				0/27 (0)	0 ± 0
11–20	0/21 (0)	0/13 (0)		0/1 (0)		0/35 (0)	0 ± 0
21–30	0/37 (0)	0/21 (0)		0/4 (0)	0/24 (0)	0/86 (0)	0 ± 0
31–40	7/38 (18)	0/31 (0)		0/8 (0)	1/28 (4)	8/105 (8)	8 ± 8.5
41–50	6/19 (31)	2/28 (7)	4/6 (67)	3/18 (17)	7/23 (30)	22/94 (23)	23 ± 30.4
51–60	9/17 (53)	11/33 (33)	21/38 (5)	16/38 (42)	24/65 (37)	81/191 (42)	42 ± 9.7
61–70	7/12 (58)	23/33 (69)	49/66 (74)	40/54 (74)	52/77 (67)	171/242 (71)	71 ± 7.2
71–80	3/4 (75)	14/17 (82)	64/67 (96)	57/70 (81)	43/63 (68)	181/221 (82)	82 ± 11.1
81–>90	2/2 (100)		27/29 (93)	16/19 (84)	18/24 (75)	65/74 (88)	88 ± 10.9
Totals	34/16	50/192	165/206	132/212	145/304	528/1075	

area proximal to the verumontanum. Although descriptions of the ductal and glandular structure of this area vary, it is generally agreed that BPH arises from an inner set of prostatic ducts and glands that reside within the urethral wall or adjacent to it. The paraurethral portion of this tissue comprises approx 5% of the normal gland and is designated the transition zone. However, once the process is initiated, all elements of the normal prostate, both stromal and glandular, participate to a variable degree in its progression. Glands in the hyperplastic nodules have the capacity to bud and form new ducts and acini; in contrast to normal tissue, these new glandular elements grow toward each other. Pure stromal nodules rarely reach large size. The variable local response to a postulated inductive agent is evident from the nodular nature of the BPH. Both the average weight of the prostate and the incidence of prostatectomy by decade suggest that once BPH develops, it is progressive in most men. The rate of growth calculated by Berry et al. indicates a prolongation of the doubling time with age (27). The important issue of whether established BPH stabilizes or regresses spontaneously cannot be evaluated from the current literature.

Cause

Identifying the cause of BPH remains a continuing challenge. The universal regional development of histologic BPH in aging men, with testes that produce an androgen-diminished environment, is an unexplained paradox independent of race and environment (25,39). The subsequent development of mass-producing BPH is selective and is potentially related to a variety of factors, some of which are associated with environment and lifestyle (25). When proposing causative factors for this common benign growth, one must consider the unusual pathologic features of BPH, including nodular growth and stromal predominance, and also its characteristic periurethral localization. Newly identified systemic or local prostatic growth-promoting agents traditionally receive prompt consideration. Currently, the following four hypotheses regarding the cause of BPH are most prominent:

1. The dihydrotestosterone (DHT) or altered hormone environment hypothesis
2. The embryonic reawakening hypothesis (15)
3. The stem cell hypothesis (25)
4. The nonandrogenic testis secretory factor hypothesis (40).

Two of these, the embryonic reawakening hypothesis and the stem cell hypothesis, focus on intrinsic cellular phenomena. The embryonic reawakening theory proposes that the interaction between glandular tissue of prostatic origin and stroma related to the bladder produces a reawakening of embryonic inductive interactions, resulting in tissue with growth characteristics and leading to the development of BPH[xv]. Subsequent growth of BPH is postulated to be multifactorial, with altered hormonal environment as well as stromal epithelial interaction having varying degrees of prominence in this phenomenon (41,42). The stem cell hypothesis proposes that an increase in the number of prostate stem cells and in their amplifying and transient cells is the basic phenomenon that leads to the development of BPH. However, neither the embryonic reawakening nor the stem cell hypothesis proposes an identifiable inducing mechanism to initiate or sustain the phenomena proposed.

The other two hypotheses, the DHT hypothesis, which is perhaps more appropriately termed the altered hormonal environment hypothesis, and the nonandrogenic testis secretory factor (NATF) hypothesis center on alterations in testis secretory function or changes in hormone metabolism that occur with age and may initiate and/or sustain phenomena leading to the development of BPH. Several studies have demonstrated that androgen levels diminish in the human male with aging. This decrease in systemic androgen is accompanied by stable or possibly slightly altered systemic estrogen and increased steroid hormone-binding serum levels (39,43,44). The latter further decreases the biologically available systemic testosterone. Although DHT and androgen receptor concentrations in BPH tissue are high, they do not differ from peripheral or normal prostate levels. The evidence suggests that androgens are necessary but not sufficient to induce development of BPH. Estrogens have demonstrated physiologic effects on male accessory sex gland growth, including the prostate, in animals; this primarily involved the stromal tissue (45,46). BPH can be induced in dogs by coadministration of androstandiol and estrogen (42,47). The recent discovery of a second estrogen receptor, estrogen receptor-β (ER-β), has stimulated additional speculation about potential mechanisms for and the role of estrogen in BPH growth. Of interest, genistein and other phytoestrogens have a much higher affinity for ER-β than for ER-α (48). However, despite the wealth of information from animal experimentation, human tissue, and serum hormone analysis, the role of estrogen in the development and progression of BPH remains controversial. Attempts to correlate serum hormone levels with benign prostate disease in radical prostatectomy specimens, with prostate size and anatomical configuration in twins, and with clinical manifestations of BPH have also failed to provide insight into the cause of BPH (34,49,50). Excluding the possible significant effects of estrogen imprinting on the neonatal prostate, these data suggest that estrogen may share a potential role in BPH mass development with a variety of other variously derived agents (51,52). Overall, studies of changes in known steroid hormone secretory products of the testis have not provided a likely explanation for the critical role of the testis in the development and growth of BPH.

The NATF hypothesis proposes that the testes secrete a nonandrogenic prostate growth stimulating factor that plays a critical role in the development of histologic BPH and most likely plays a contributory role in the subsequent development of mass-producing BPH (53,54).

Biologic evidence supporting the presence of a nonandrogenic male accessory sex gland growth-stimulating substance was derived from the assessment of age-related changes in the concentration of selected prostate and seminal vesicle secretory products and seminal vesicle weight (55,56). The testes were identified as a source of this hypothesized prostate growth-stimulating agent based on evidence that neither endogenous or exogenous testosterone nor estradiol could replace a normally functioning testis in producing BPH in dogs (57,58). This identification was also based on evidence for a systemic prostate growth-stimulating substance that was not a steroid in the testis intact but not the castrated rat.

The results of animal studies indicate that the prostate is exposed to NATF by a systemic delivery route. Moreover, the presence of NATF in the testosterone-rich testicular epididymal plasma fosters potential exposure of periurethral prostatic tissue to these independent and synergistic prostate growth-stimulating compounds. It has been postulated that this exposure induces the almost universal periurethrally localized development of histologic BPH. Subsequent selective stimulation of prostatic mass is thought to be induced by multiple factors, with a significant but less well-defined role for exposure to systemic and/or local NATF.

Pathophysiology

The development and progression of mechanical obstruction from the prostatic mass has been the traditional focus regarding the sequelae resulting from BPH. The perception that the mass and configuration of the hyperplasia dictated the degree of outflow blockage undoubtedly resulted from early experience treating patients with acute and chronic urinary retention. Renal failure, urinary tract infection, and calculi were common indications for various approaches to relieve bladder neck obstruction. The reversal of these serious secondary phenomena and restoration of improved voiding patterns reinforced the mass concept. Failures in both of these therapeutic goals were overshadowed by the frequent correction of the problems that existed. In the last 20 years, intrinsic prostatic tension from contracting prostate stromal smooth muscle and/or extrinsic tension on the BPH prostate mass by a contracting prostate capsule have been proposed as having potentially important roles in primary or persistent bladder outlet obstruction (59–62). The proposed role of stromal smooth muscle-mediated increased intrinsic prostate tension has been reinforced substantially by in vitro physiologic and, to a lesser degree, by clinical observations with both α-adrenergic agonists and antagonists (60). The proposed role of peripheral capsular tension on bladder outlet obstruction is supported by the results of transurethral incision (63,64). Although α-agonist mechanisms may adversely impact voiding in a variety of ways that may complement the effects of BPH[Ix], these secondary phenomena are unlikely to play a direct role in the primary BPH-mediated effects on voiding.

BPH-mediated bladder outlet obstruction results in a series of changes in bladder tissue mass, composition, and function. It also affects blood supply and nerve status and function. The degree and persistence of the obstruction is thought to play a pivotal role in the subsequent anatomic and functional bladder effects. Obstruction can be the primary source of physiologic change, with results varying from hyperfunction and hyperirritability to nonfunction or atony. Evaluation of this spectrum of functional states can be difficult and confusing. Consequently, evidence of bladder changes associated with outflow obstruction is derived largely from observations in animals. In general, partial bladder obstruction initially results in reversible detrusor hypertrophy and increased bladder weight (65,66). The increased muscle mass is associated with increased intravesical pressure (67). Studies in obstructed pigs demonstrate a decrease in functional bladder capacity, increased residual urine, detrusor instability associated with incontinence, and a prolonged period of hypoperfusion with associated tissue hypoxia (66). The human and the pig generally develop a thickened, trabeculated bladder in response to outflow obstruction. However, chronic retention of urine can lead to a thin-walled, flaccid bladder in both the obstructed pig and in the human. Moreover, obstruction is associated with increased collagen deposition and decreased compliance in man (65). Rabbits with bladder outlet obstruction show changes in detrusor muscle myosin phenotype, suggesting a trend to a dedifferentiated phenotype (65).

The anatomic and physiologic alterations that occur in response to obstruction probably play a major role in the specific bladder and renal changes that occur in individual patients. Currently, loss of bladder compliance is most likely the principal factor in producing upper urinary tract functional and anatomic damage. The cause of the obstruction-related involuntary bladder contractions remains elusive, but in vitro pig studies suggest a myogenic, not a neurogenic, basis *(58,66)*. Cellules, sacules, and diverticula are recognized related anatomic bladder changes that develop and progress unpredictably and may have clinical significance. Based on their extensive experience with the pathophysiology of obstruction-induced bladder changes, Levin et al. suggested that bladder outlet obstruction should be relieved as soon as possible after diagnosis to maximize the opportunity for bladder recovery *(66)*.

SUMMARY

The prostate has a unique anatomy and physiology that determines its high clinical relevance. This gland is separated into four distinct regions: the peripheral zone, the central zone, the transition zone, and the periurethral gland region. These zonal variations impact the internal architecture as well as the various functions of the gland and determine the clinical impact in disease progression. The prostate undergoes histologic evidence of growth from before birth and continues with advancing age. The environment, dietary intake, and genetic factors appear to play a large role in the development of mass-producing BPH. There is no consensus about the exact cause of the histologic and pathophysiologic process we call BPH. Regardless, despite our deficiencies in these aspects, this disease will remain an important topic for physicians and urologists alike.

REFERENCES

1. Lich R Jr, Howerton LW, Amin M. Anatomy and surgical approach to the urogenital tract in the male. In: Harrison JH, Gittes RF, Perlmutter AD, et al., eds., Campbell's Urology, vol. 1, ed. 4, Philadelphia: WB Saunders Co, 1978, p. 3.
2. Ayala RG, Ro JU, Babaian R, et al. The prostate capsule: does it exist? Its importance in the staging and treatment of prostate cancer. Am J Surg Pathol 1989;13:21–27.
3. Woodburne RT. Pelvis. In: Woodburne RT, ed., Essentials of Human Anatomy, New York: Oxford University Press, 1978, p. 479.
4. McNeal JE. Normal histology of the prostate. Am J Surg Pathol 1988; 12:619–633.
5. Walsh PC, Lepor H, Eggleston JC. Radical prostatectomy with preservation of sexual function: anatomical and pathological considerations. Prostate 1983b; 4:473–485.
6. Walsh PC, Donker PJ. Impotence following radical prostatectomy: insight into etiology and prevention. J Urol 1982;128:492–497.
7. Lepor H, Gregerman M, Crosby R, et al. Precise localization of the autonomic nerves from the pelvic plexus to the corpora cavernosa: a detailed anatomical study of the adult male pelvis. J Urol 1985;133:207–212.

8. Lowsley OS. The development of the human prostate gland with reference to the development of other structures at the neck of the urinary bladder. Am J Anat 1912;13:299–349.
9. Lowsley OS. The gross anatomy of the human prostate gland and contiguous structures. Surg Gynecol Obstet 1915;20:183–192.
10. Aumuller G. Prostate Gland and Seminal Vesicles. New York: Springer-Verlag, 1979.
11. Xia TG, Blackburn WR, Gardner WA Jr. Fetal prostate growth and development. Pediatr Pathol 1990;10:527–537.
12. Grayhack JT, Kozlowski JM. Benign prostatic hyperplasia. In: Gillenwater J, Grayhack J, Howards S, eds., Adult and Pediatric Urology, vol. 2, ed. 2, St. Louis, MO: Mosby, 1991, pp. 1211–1276.
13. Franks LM. Atrophy and hyperplasia in the prostate proper. J Pathol Bacteriol 1954a;68:617–621.
14. Franks LM. Benign prostatic hyperplasia: gross and microscopic anatomy. In: Grayhack JT, Wilson JD, Scherbenske MJ, eds., Benign Prostatic Hyperplasia: NIAMDD Workshop Proceedings, Feb 20-21, 1975. US Department of Health, Education, and Welfare publication no. (NIH) 76-1113, 1976, p. 63.
15. McNeal JE. Developmental and comparative anatomy of the prostate. In: Grayhack JT, Wilson JD, Scherbenske MJ, eds., Benign Prostatic Hyperplasia, NIAMDD Workshop Proceedings, Feb 20–21, 1975. US Department of Health, Education, and Welfare publication no. (NIH) 76-1113, 1976, pp. 1–10.
16. Tisell LE, Salander H. The lobes of the human prostate. Scand J Urol Nephrol 1975;9:185–191.
17. McNeal J. Pathology of benign prostatic hyperplasia: insight into etiology. Urol Clin N Am 1990;17:477–486.
18. Mostofi FK, Price EB. Tumors of the male genital system. In: Atlas Tumor Pathology, series 2, fascicle 8. Washington, DC, Armed Forces Institute of Pathology, 1973, pp. 196–219.
19. Manley CB Jr. The striated muscle of the prostate. J Urol 1966;95:234–240.
20. Swyer GI. Post-natal growth changes in the human prostate. J Anat 1944;78:130.
21. Zondek LH, Zondek T. Congenital malformation of the male accessory sex glands in the fetus and neonate. In: Spring-Mills E, Hafez ESE, eds., Male Accessory Sex Glands, New York: Elsevier North-Holland Biomedical Press, 1980, p. 17.
22. Shapiro E, Hartanto V, Perlman EJ, et al. Morphometric analysis of pediatric and nonhyperplastic prostate glands: evidence that BPH is not a unique stromal process. Prostate 1997;33:177–182.
23. Morgagni GB. The Seats and Causes of Disease Investigated by Anatomy, book 3, London: Johnson & Paine, 1760, p. 460.
24. Randall A. Surgical Pathology of Prostatic Obstruction, Baltimore, MD: Williams & Wilkins Co, 1931.
25. Isaacs JT, Coffey DS. Etiology and disease process of benign prostatic hyperplasia. Prostate 1989;suppl 2:33–50.
26. Ekman P. BPH epidemiology and risk factors. Prostate 1989;suppl 2:23–31.
27. Berry SJ, Coffey DS, Walsh PC, et al. The development of human benign prostatic hyperplasia with age. J Urol 1984;132:474–479.
28. Girman CJ. Population-based studies of the epidemiology of benign prostatic hyperplasia. Br J Urol 1998;suppl 1:34–44.
29. Lytton B, Emery JM, Harvard BW. The incidence of benign prostatic obstruction. J Urol 1968;99:639–645.

30. Meigs JB, Mohr B, Barry MJ, Collins MM, McKinlay JB. Risk factors for clinical benign prostatic hyperplasia in a community-based population of healthy aging men. J Clin Epidemiol 2001;54(9):935–944.
31. Ohnishi K, Boyle P, Barry MJ, et al. Epidemiology and natural history of benign prostatic hyperplasia. 4th International Consultation on BPH, Paris, July 2–5, 1997. Editors: Denis L, Griffiths K, Khoury S, et al., p. 16.
32. Derbes VDP, Leche SM, Hooker CC. The incidence of benign prostatic hypertrophy among the whites and negroes of New Orleans. J Urol 1937;38:383–388.
33. Rotkin ID. Origins, distribution and risk of benign prostatic hypertrophy. In: Hinman F Jr, ed., Benign Prostatic Hypertrophy, New York: Springer-Verlag, 1983 pp. 10–21.
34. Meikle AW, Stephenson A, Lewis CM, et al. Age, genetic, and nongenetic factors influencing variation in serum sex steroids and zonal volumes of the prostate and benign prostatic hyperplasia in twins. Prostate 1997;33:105–111.
35. Partin AW, Sanda MG, Page WF, et al. Concordance rates for benign prostatic disease among twins suggest hereditary influence. Urology 1994;44:646–650.
36. Sanda MG, Beaty TH, Stutzman RE, et al. Genetic susceptibility of benign prostatic hyperplasia. J Urol 1994;152:115–119.
37. Meikle AW, Bansal A, Murray DK, et al. Heritability of the symptoms of benign prostatic hyperplasia and the roles of age and zonal prostate volumes in twins. Urology 1999;53:701–706.
38. Harbitz TB, Haugen OA. Histology of the prostate in elderly men: a study in an autopsy series. Acta Pathol Microbiol Immunol Scand 1972;80:756–768.
39. Gray A, Feldman HA, McKinlay JB, et al. Age, disease, and changing sex hormone levels in middle-aged men: results of the Massachusetts male aging study. J Clin Endocrinol Metab 1991;73:1016–1025.
40. Grayhack JT, Sensibar JA, Ilio KY, et al. Synergistic action of steroids and spermatocele fluid on in vitro proliferation of prostate stroma. J Urol 1998a; 159:2202–2209.
41. Lee C, Kozlowski JM, Grayhack JT. Intrinsic and extrinsic factors controlling benign prostatic growth. Prostate 1997;31:131–138.
42. Partin AW. Etiology of benign prostatic hyperplasia in prostatic diseases. In: Lepor H, ed., Philadelphia, PA: W. B. Saunders, 2000, pp. 95–105.
43. Nankin HR, Calkin JH. Decreased bioavailable testosterone in aging normal and impotent men. J Clin Endocrinol Metab 1986;63:1418–1420.
44. Griffith K. Molecular control of prostate growth. In: Kirby R, McConnell J, Fitzpatrick J, Roehrborn C, Boyle P, eds., Textbook of Benign Prostatic Hyperplasia, Oxford, UK: Isis Med Medico, 1996, pp. 22–55.
45. Mann T, Lutwak-Mann C. Male reproductive function and semen. New York: Springer-Verlag, 1981.
46. Janulis L, Nemeth JA, Yang T, Lang S, Lee C. Prostatic luminal cell differentiation and prostatic steroid-binding protein (PBP) gene expression are differentially affected by neonatal castration. Prostate 2000;43:195–204.
47. Walsh PC, Wilson JD. The induction of prostatic hypertrophy in the dog with androstanediol. J Clin Invest 1976;57:1093–1099.
48. Chang WY, Prins GS. Estrogen receptor-β: Implications for the prostate gland. Prostate 1999;40:115–124.
49. Partin AW, Oesterling JE, Epstein JI, et al. Influence of age and endocrine factors on the volume of benign prostatic hyperplasia. J Urol 1991;145:405–409.
50. Gann PH, Hennekens CH, Longcope C, et al. A prospective study of plasma hormone levels, non hormonal factors and development of benign prostatic hyperplasia. Prostate 1995;26:40–49.

51. Prins GS, Birch L. Neonatal estrogen exposure up-regulates estrogen receptor expression in the developing and adult rat prostate lobes. Endocrinol 1997; 138:1801–1809.
52. Naslund MJ, Coffey DS. The differential effects of neonatal androgen, estrogen and progesterone on adult rat prostate growth. J Urol 1986;136:1136–1140.
53. Grayhack JT, Kozlowski JM, Lee C. The pathogenesis of benign prostatic hyperplasia: A proposed hypothesis and critical evaluation. J Urol 1998b; 160(suppl):2375–2380.
54. Ilio K, Kasjanski RZ, Sensibar JA, et al. Identification of a non-androgenic prostate stimulating factor from the testis. J Urol 2000;163(suppl):204A.
55. Grayhack JT. Changes with aging in human seminal vesicle fluid fructose concentration and seminal vesicle weight. J Urol 1961;86:142–148.
56. Grayhack JT, Kropp KA. Changes with aging in prostatic fluid: citric acid, acid phosphatase and lactic dehydrogenase concentration in man. J Urol 1965;93:258–262.
57. Grayhack JT, Lee C, Brand W. The effect of testicular irradiation in established BPH in the dog: evidence of a non-steroidal testicular factor for BPH maintenance. J Urol 1985;134:1276–1281.
58. Juniewicz PE, Berry SJ, Coffey DS, et al. The requirement of testes in establishing the sensitivity of the canine prostate to develop benign prostatic hyperplasia. J Urol 1994;152:996–1001.
59. Caine M, Pfau A, Perlberg S. The use of alpha-adrenergic blockers in benign prostatic obstruction. Br J Urol 1976;48:255–263.
60. Lepor H. Adrenergic blockers for the treatment of benign prostatic hyperplasia. In: Prostatic Diseases. Lepor H, ed., Philadelphia: WB Saunders, 2000, pp. 297–307.
61. Hutch JA, Rambo ON Jr. A study of the anatomy of the prostate, prostatic urethra and the urinary sphincter system. J Urol 1970;104:443–452.
62. Ohnishi K. A study of the physical properties of the prostate (the second part). The relationships between dysuria and the strength of the surgical capsule in benign prostatic hypertrophy. J Jpn Urol Assoc 1986;77:1388–1399.
63. McConnell JD, Barry MS, Bruskewitz RC, et al. Benign Prostatic Hyperplasia: Diagnosis and Treatment. Clinical practice guideline No. 8, US Dept. Health and Human Services. Public Health Service Agency for Health Care Policy and Research, Rockville, MD, 1994.
64. Mebust WK. Transurethral resection of the prostate and transurethral incision of the prostate. In: Prostate Diseases. Lepor H, Lawson RK, eds., Philadelphia: WB Saunders, 1993, pp. 150–163.
65. McConnell JD. Bladder responses to obstruction. In: Kirby R, McConnell J, Fitzpatrick J, Roehrborn C, Boyle P, eds., Textbook of Benign Prostatic Hyperplasia, Oxford, UK: ISIS Medical Media, 1996, pp. 105–108.
66. Levin RM, Brading AF, Mills IW, et al. Experimental models of bladder outlet obstruction in prostatic disease. In: Prostatic Diseases. Lepor H, ed., Philadelphia, PA: WB Saunders, 2000, pp. 169–196.
67. Claridge M, Shuttleworth KE. The dynamics of obstructed micturition. Invest Urol 1964;25:188–199.
68. Schoenberg HW, Gutrich JM, Cote R. Urodynamic studies in benign prostatic hypertrophy. Urology 1979;14:634–637.
69. Pradhan BK, Chandra K. Morphogenesis of nodular hyperlasia—prostate. J Urol 1975;113(2):210–213.
70. Moore RA. Benign hypertrophy of the prostate: a morphology study. J Urol 1943;50:680.

2 The Definition of Benign Prostatic Hyperplasia
Epidemiology and Prevalence

Glenn S. Gerber, MD

CONTENTS

INTRODUCTION
BPH DEFINITIONS
PREVALENCE
EPIDEMIOLOGY OF BPH
ECONOMICS OF BPH
SUMMARY
REFERENCES

INTRODUCTION

Benign prostatic hyperplasia (BPH) is the most common neoplasm in men and is a significant cause of urinary symptoms in the aging male *(1)*. Although much is unknown about the pathophysiology of BPH, the condition results in a diminished quality of life for many patients. The symptoms of BPH can be broadly divided into obstructive and irritative components. The former symptoms include a weakened urinary stream, hesitancy, and the need to push or strain to initiate micturition. Irritative symptoms can be much more bothersome for many men and include frequency, nocturia, and urgency *(2)*. When assessing the importance and magnitude of BPH, one must consider several factors. First, the typical symptoms of BPH are nonspecific *(3)*. There are many other potential causes of urinary symptoms in aging men, including diabetes mellitus, Parkinson's disease, and stroke, which can lead to the

From: *Management of Benign Prostatic Hypertrophy*
Edited by: K. T. McVary © Humana Press Inc., Totowa, NJ

same urinary problems seen in men with prostatic enlargement. Second, unlike most other common, chronic medical disorders such as diabetes, hypertension, or hypercholesterolemia, there is no standardized medical test or measurement that can be used to quantify the problem or assess the response to treatment for men with BPH. Rather than lowering blood pressure or maintaining blood glucose levels in the desired range, the primary goal in the management of BPH for most patients is a subjective improvement in urinary symptoms and quality of life. Although objective measurements such as urinary flow rate and postvoid residual urine volume can be used to evaluate BPH, the reproducibility and correlation of these measures with urinary symptoms is often limited (4,5). Finally, much is unknown about the natural history of BPH, and this may dramatically impact our understanding of the magnitude and prevalence of the problem (6).

BPH DEFINITIONS

One of the most basic, yet most important, difficulties in the evaluation and management of men with BPH concerns definitions. In a strict sense, BPH is a histologic diagnosis that is established by the presence of hyperplastic glands on pathologic inspection of prostatic tissue (1). In common usage, however, the term BPH is used to indicate that a patient has an enlarged prostate or that the patient has urinary symptoms that are believed to be the result of bladder outlet obstruction by the prostate. Peak urinary flow rate (Qmax) has also been used by many investigators to help define the presence of BPH (3,4). A decrease in Qmax is a nonspecific finding and may be attributable to detrusor dysfunction rather than bladder outlet obstruction (4,5). Nevertheless, BPH has commonly been defined as Qmax less than 15 mL/s on a voided volume of at least 125–150 mL and has been diagnosed based on this finding.

Issues regarding the definition of BPH may be confusing for both patients and primary care physicians, and it is important to keep this in mind when counseling men regarding BPH. In addition, there is a poor correlation between histologic changes within the gland, the size of the prostate, and the severity of urinary symptoms (3). These confounding relationships may be attributed in part to physiologic changes in the aging bladder, alterations in the volume and pattern of urine production, and/or other unspecified factors (7). To help clarify the terminology associated with the diagnosis of BPH and to focus attention on the lack of specificity of urinary symptoms, the alternative definition of lower urinary tract symptoms (LUTS) has been recommended and should be used when referring to such patients (8).

Although beyond the scope of this chapter, it is generally accepted that the most important cause of LUTS in aging males is bladder outlet obstruction resulting from prostatic enlargement *(3)*. However, as discussed above, urinary symptoms commonly attributed to BPH are nonspecific and may result from a variety of other causes. An important but largely unanswered issue concerns the relationship between LUTS and bladder outlet obstruction. The gold standard in defining such obstruction is urodynamic study, in which the detrusor pressure is measured during voiding *(9)*. The single most important measure of obstruction is detrusor pressure at Qmax *(10)*. Using urodynamic evaluation, it has been demonstrated that as many as one-third of men with urinary symptoms attributed to BPH do not have obstruction *(9,11)*. Further evidence supporting the disparity between LUTS and prostatic obstruction comes from studies of age-matched women, who have been shown to have urinary symptoms similar to those of men with BPH *(12)*. Overall, the nonspecific nature of LUTS and the lack of concordance between symptoms and obstruction make it very difficult to arrive at a generally accepted definition of what constitutes BPH.

One of the most important developments in defining the extent and magnitude of BPH has been the introduction of validated symptom scores *(13)*. Health measurement scales such as the American Urological Association (AUA) symptom score must have demonstrated reliability and validity to be clinically useful *(14)*. Several factors must be considered when determining the utility of such measures. First, internal-consistency reliability must be considered. This refers to the relatedness of the different items in the scale and is evaluated by administering the questionnaire to a group of subjects *(2)*. Second, the test-retest reliability of the questionnaire must be established. This can be accomplished by demonstrating that there is minimal change in the results when the test is given to the same patients after a short interval *(2)*. Third, a questionnaire such as the AUA symptom score should have the same degree of accuracy as any other diagnostic test used to assess a disease process *(2)*. To be valid, the symptom score results should accurately quantify the severity of BPH in the same manner that serum lipid levels reflect the disease status in patients with hypercholesterolemia. Finally, health measurement scales must be responsive to be useful in discriminating among patients who get better, get worse, or remain the same with or without treatment over time *(2,15)*.

Based on the criteria described above, the AUA symptom score has been shown to be reliable and valid in the assessment of patients with BPH *(7,13)*. The seven questions that comprise the symptom score address seven separate but related urinary symptoms that are typically associated with prostatic enlargement in the aging male. The results of these questions are scored from 0 to 5 based on the frequency of occurrence of each symptom. The scores for the seven questions may then be added to give a total score of 0–35. Based on this score, patients can be categorized as having mild (0–7 points), moderate (8–19 points), or severe (20–35 points) LUTS. In addition, an impact question designed to assess the overall quality of life associated with urinary symptoms has been added to the AUA symptom score (16). The initial seven questions plus the quality of life question comprise the International Prostate Symptom Score (I-PSS) (16). This questionnaire has been translated into many languages and has been used worldwide to measure the incidence and prevalence of BPH in many countries (17,18).

Because the I-PSS has been the benchmark evaluation used to establish the prevalence of BPH across the world, it is important to understand the extent and reliability of testing that has been used to determine its validity. Statistical measurements of internal consistency reliability and 1-wk test–retest correlation have been shown to be 0.86 and 0.92, respectively (13). Both of these measures highly support the reliability of the I-PSS in these areas. Because there is no gold standard comparison for assessing the presence and severity of LUTS, it is also important that the I-PSS be tested in other ways to determine its validity (2). The I-PSS has been shown to correlate well with older questionnaires used to assess voiding symptoms in men with BPH (19). Higher scores in the I-PSS have also been demonstrated to correlate well with health measurement scales designed to evaluate general health and well-being (2,20). Additionally, the symptom score has been shown to be a reliable predictor of whether men would choose to undergo prostatectomy for BPH and in determining the response to surgical and medical therapy (2,13,21,22). Overall, the I-PSS has been shown to be reliable and valid through a variety of testing modalities. Therefore, its use in measuring the prevalence of BPH and helping to understand the quality of life changes, epidemiology, and health care costs associated with prostatic enlargement is extremely valuable.

PREVALENCE

BPH is one of the most common conditions for which patients seek medical attention. In recent years, a variety of factors have led to further increases in the number of men evaluated and/or treated for LUTS. These include increased attention to prostate diseases in the lay press, the escalating use of the Internet as a source of information for patients, advertising by pharmaceutical companies in mainstream publications, and the growing elderly population in the United States and other developed countries. In addition to those patients diagnosed with BPH, surveys of men over 40 yr of age have demonstrated a significant incidence of urinary symptoms among unevaluated groups (17,18,23).

Using a histologic definition, the prevalence of BPH is greater than 50% by age 60 and almost 90% by age 85 (1). It is estimated that about half of these men will have detectable prostatic enlargement and that half of those will seek medical attention because of LUTS (1). The Agency for Health Care Policy and Research Diagnostic and Treatment Guidelines for BPH in 1994 estimated that approx 25% of white males in the United States in 1990 had an AUA symptom score of 8 or greater (moderate-to-severe symptoms) and Qmax less than 15 mL/s (1). Additional information concerning the prevalence and demographics of BPH has come from the Rochester Epidemiology Project, which has studied the population of Olmstead County, Minnesota (24). Based on symptom questionnaires administered to unselected men living in this community, it was found that moderate-to-severe urinary symptoms were present in 13% of men between 40 and 49 yr and in 28% of those older than 70 yr (24). Longitudinal studies in this group have demonstrated that the 10-yr cumulative risk acute urinary retention developing in a man with moderate symptoms is almost 14% (2,24). In addition, a consistent decline in Qmax was noted when this parameter was measured longitudinally in this community-based cohort (25). Although most American studies of BPH prevalence have focused on white men, there does not appear to be an increased risk of BPH in African Americans (26).

Investigators in other countries have studied the prevalence of BPH using symptom questionnaires and have found similar results (17,18,23,27). Chicharro-Molero et al. evaluated 1106 men in a Spanish community using the I-PSS (17). In addition, prostate size was measured by transrectal ultrasonography (TRUS), and Qmax was measured. Overall, the prevalence of moderate or severe symptoms was approx 25% and, as expected, tended to increase with age. Using the impact question (quality of life measure) from the I-PSS, it was concluded that 12.5% of men had a poor quality of life. Interestingly, among younger men, moderate symptoms were perceived as resulting in poor quality of life, whereas the same symptoms in older men led to a subjective sense of a good quality of life. Qmax less than 15 mL/s was noted in more than 55% of men. Using a definition of BPH that included an I-PSS more than 7, prostate size more than 30 g, and Qmax less than 15 mL/s, the authors found that the prevalence of BPH in this population was 11.8%. Among patients less than 50 yr of age, however, the prevalence

Table 1
Prevalence of LUTS in 2096 Austrian Men

Age (yr)	Mean I-PSS	Moderate to severe LUTS	Previous TURP
20–29	2.1	6.3%	0%
30–39	2.6	8.4%	0%
40–49	3.0	11.1%	0%
50–59	5.8	27.1%	1.3%
60–69	5.7	28.3%	4.2%
70–79	6.4	36.0%	20.9%
80 or greater	6.1	35.7%	27.5%

Adapted from ref. *18*.

using this definition was less than 1%, and in men older than 70 yr, the prevalence using this definition was 30%. In another study, the I-PSS was administered to 2096 men 20 yr or older in Austria, who also underwent a digital rectal examination (DRE) and provided a detailed urologic history *(18)*. When stratified by decade, patients with advancing age showed an increase in the I-PSS and the incidence of previous surgical treatment for BPH (Table 1).

The prevalence of BPH was also studied in a Dutch population of 502 men between the ages of 55 and 74 yr who had no history of prostate cancer or surgical treatment for BPH *(27)*. In addition to the I-PSS, prostate volume, Qmax, and postvoid residual urine volumes (PVR) were measured. Using the I-PSS, moderate or severe symptoms were noted in 24% and 6% of men, respectively. A good correlation was found between the total symptom score and the single disease-specific quality of life question included with the I-PSS. However, weak correlations were noted between the I-PSS results and prostate volume, Qmax, PVR, and age. Based on the poor correlation between the magnitude of urinary symptoms and the observed objective measures, the authors of this study concluded that symptom scores should not be independently used as a criterion for determining the prevalence of clinical BPH.

A subsequent Dutch study of nearly 4000 men between 50 and 75 yr of age further demonstrated the difficulty in defining the clinical prevalence of BPH *(28)*. In this trial, men completed the I-PSS and also underwent physical examination, measurement of prostate volume by TRUS, and determination of Qmax. To define the prevalence of BPH, a variety of definitions of BPH that had been suggested by earlier studies to be most valid were assessed *(29,30)*. Using an I-PSS of eight or greater to define the presence of clinical BPH, the overall incidence in this study among all men was 25% *(28)*. However, there were significant differences in the prevalence of BPH when alternative definitions were used. As defined by a symptom score of eight or greater and a prostate volume of more than 30 g, the incidence of BPH in this study was 14%. When also requiring a Qmax of less than 15 mL/s, 12% of men met the criteria used to define the presence of BPH. Because no clear consensus has been reached as to how BPH should be defined, it is apparent that there will be wide differences in the reported prevalence rates depending on the choice of criteria used.

EPIDEMIOLOGY OF BPH

A number of investigators have studied the epidemiology of BPH. Clearly, the most important demographic factor in the incidence and severity of BPH is aging. Not only does prostate size correlate closely with age, but worsening LUTS is also seen commonly as men get older. Rhodes et al. studied men using serial prostatic ultrasonography performed during a follow-up period of approx 7 yr *(31)*. In general, higher prostate growth rates were seen in men with larger baseline glands, and the average annual change was 1.6% across all age groups. Although urinary symptoms may worsen because of ongoing prostatic enlargement, it is also likely that some component of symptom progression is attributable to increased bladder dysfunction associated with aging and other factors.

In addition to aging, a variety of other factors have been investigated in men with BPH. In many cases, disparate results have been noted in different trials. Platz et al. studied the role of racial or ethnic origin in the prevalence of BPH among American male health professionals *(26)*. Included in the study were 1508 men who underwent surgery for BPH between 1986 and 1994 and 1837 men who had moderate-to-severe LUTS during approximately the same time period. In addition, more than 23,000 asymptomatic men were also included. The authors of this study found that African-American men were not at increased risk for BPH compared with white men. Although Asian men were less likely to have undergone surgery for BPH than white men, the relative risk for symptoms was similar in the two groups. White men of Scandinavian heritage had a slightly decreased likelihood of BPH symptoms than white men of southern European origin. Homma et al. studied approx 7500 men in Asia and Australia using the I-PSS and compared their results to those found in studies of men in Europe and North America *(32)*. They concluded that the prevalence of symptomatic men in Asia and Australia is similar or greater than the number among the comparison group. Studies have also been conducted concerning the role of family history in the development of BPH and urinary symptoms (33). Using the Olmstead County population in Minnesota, 2119 men completed symptom scores, had their flow rates measured, and were questioned regarding their family history of BPH and prostatic enlargement (33). The age-adjusted odds ratio of having moderate or severe urinary symptoms was elevated to 1.3 among those with a family history. The relative risk was also greater for men with relatives diagnosed with BPH at a younger age. Finally, men with a family history were also 1.3 times more likely to have a diminished Qmax.

The role of a variety of lifestyle factors in the development of BPH has also been investigated. Three studies have addressed the effect of cigarette smoking on prostate size and BPH (34–36). Meigs et al. followed 1709 men age 40 to 70 yr for a mean of 9 yr (34). Men were classified with clinical BPH if they reported frequent or difficult voiding and were told by a physician that they had an enlarged prostate, or if they had undergone surgery for BPH. Using this classification, cigarette smoking appeared to lower the risk of developing clinical BPH. Similarly, in a study of Japanese men who underwent transrectal ultrasonography with measurement of prostate size, it was found that men who smoked cigarettes had a lower risk of prostatic enlargement (35). Contrasting results regarding the effects of cigarette smoking were noted, however, in a study of Greek men (36). In this investigation, which included men who were surgically treated for BPH and normal controls, cigarette smoking had no major effect on the incidence of BPH.

The relationship between diet and BPH has been explored by several investigators (34,35,37). Lagiou et al. studied Greek men with and without prostate disease and found that increased consumption of both butter and margarine was positively associated with the risk of BPH (37). In addition, fruit intake appeared to lower the risk of BPH. In an American study, no association between total or fat calorie intake and the development of BPH was noted (34). Nukui has reported that higher serum levels of β-carotene were seen in men with BPH compared to those without prostate disease (35). In addition to dietary factors, it has been suggested that obesity may play a role in the development of BPH (38). Possible reasons for this include the increase in estrogen-androgen ratio that occurs in obesity and greater sympathetic nervous system activity (38). Giovannucci et al. studied the association between obesity and BPH in men age 40 to 75 yr who were participants in the Health Professionals Follow-Up Study (38). These investigators found that abdominal obesity may increase the frequency and severity of urinary obstructive symptoms and did increase the likelihood of men undergoing surgical treatment for BPH. In contrast to these results, Meigs et al.

reported that body mass index and waist-hip ratio were not helpful in predicting the presence of clinical BPH *(34)*.

Hyperinsulinemia has been suggested to be a risk factor for the development of BPH *(39)*. Hammarsten and Hogstedt studied 307 men with LUTS to investigate the effects of metabolic disease and fasting plasma insulin levels on the annual growth rate of the prostate *(39)*. Prostate volume was determined by serial transrectal ultrasound, and insulin levels were assessed from fasting blood samples. Serum cholesterol levels, blood pressure, history of hypertension, body height and weight, and body mass index were also assessed. In the entire group of patients, the median annual prostatic growth rate was 1.03 mL/yr. This growth rate was significantly faster in men with metabolic disease, noninsulin-dependent diabetes mellitus, treated hypertension, obesity, and dyslipidemia. In addition, the prostatic growth rate correlated positively with the diastolic blood pressure and the body mass index and correlated negatively with the high-density lipoprotein cholesterol level. High fasting plasma insulin levels also correlated with the annual prostate growth rate and were an independent predictor of prostate gland volume using multivariate analysis. The authors of this study concluded that hyperinsulinemia is a causative factor in the development of BPH and felt that their findings supported the concept of increased sympathetic activity in men with BPH.

Oh et al. investigated the association of BPH and male-pattern baldness *(40)*. Both are androgen-dependent and it is logical to presume that there may be an increased incidence of prostatic enlargement and/or BPH symptoms among bald men. The study involved 225 patients with BPH and 160 controls of similar age *(40)*. Baldness was graded on a scale of 1 to 7 (Norwood classification), and BPH was evaluated using the I-PSS. The investigators found that patients with BPH had a higher grade of male-pattern baldness compared with controls. Overall, the proportion of men with baldness of grade 4 or greater in the BPH group was significantly larger than that of the control group (54 vs 37%). Finally, limited study suggests that physical exercise may have a protective effect against the development of clinical BPH, and alcohol intake was not helpful in predicting the presence of BPH *(34,35)*.

ECONOMICS OF BPH

It is likely that the cost of treatment associated with BPH will continue to rise in upcoming years for a variety of reasons. The aging population in the United States and other Western countries will result in a greater number of men with BPH who will require treatment. It has been estimated that by the year 2020 there will be 65 million Americans 65 yr of age or older *(41)*. In addition, new pharmacologic and techno-logic developments are likely to improve the therapy of BPH and lower the incidence of side effects, thus leading more men to choose to be treated. Newer technology is generally more expensive, however, which will further increase costs. Finally, a greater awareness among layper-sons regarding prostate disease and treatment options is likely to increase the number of men seeking medical attention for BPH.

There is a great deal of information that is unknown regarding the cost-effectiveness associated with the evaluation and management of men with BPH *(42)*. Although the details are beyond the scope of this chapter, a variety of diagnostic methods are available to the physician when assessing men with LUTS. There remains much controversy sur-rounding the use of these tests, and no clear consensus has been reached in many cases. Similarly, the growing treatment options available for men with BPH have only added to the confusion regarding the best and/or most cost-effective options. Although medical therapy may be less expensive in the short term, surgical or device therapy may ulti-mately be less expensive when long-term costs are considered *(43)*. Much work needs to be done in these areas as we strive to define the best approach to evaluate and manage men with BPH.

SUMMARY

BPH is an important cause of diminished quality of life among aging men, and the prevalence of this condition in the United States is likely to grow as the population ages. A variety of definitions of BPH is avail-able based on the presence of urinary symptoms, prostatic enlargement, and/or the histologic finding of hyperplastic glands. In addition, urodynamic results demonstrating decreased urinary flow rates or blad-der outlet obstruction may also be used to help define the presence of BPH. Although nonspecific, the presence of LUTS such as frequency, hesitancy, or nocturia are most commonly used to define the prevalence of BPH. Overall, the introduction and validation of symptom question-naires such as the I-PSS has added greatly to our understanding of the extent and magnitude of BPH in a variety of populations.

A number of epidemiologic factors have been investigated among men with BPH. Although aging clearly has the most important effect on the development of prostatic enlargement and urinary symptoms, a variety of other factors may also play a role in the occurrence of BPH. It appears that racial or ethnic background may play a minor role in the incidence of BPH. However, African-American men do not appear to be at increased risk compared with whites and other groups. Although a family history of BPH appears to increase the overall likelihood that urinary symptoms and prostatic enlargement will occur, the ambiguity associated with the definition of BPH among relatives is a limiting factor. Among lifestyle factors, cigarette smoking seems to lower the risk of BPH, whereas obesity and a high-fat diet may increase the incidence of prostatic enlargement. Conflicting results have been reported, however, in different studies, and the precise role of many factors in the development of BPH remains largely unknown. As the importance of BPH grows, it is likely that further information will become available regarding the role of epidemiologic factors in BPH.

REFERENCES

1. McConnell JD, Barry MJ, Bruskewitz RC, et al. Benign Prostatic Hyperplasia: Diagnosis and Treatment. Clinical Practice Guideline, Number 8. Rockville, MD, Agency for Health Care Policy and Research, US Public Health Service, US Dept of Health and Human Services, 1994. AHCPR Publication No. 94-0582.
2. Barry MJ. Evaluation of symptoms and quality of life in men with benign prostatic hyperplasia. Urology 2001;58(suppl 6a):25.
3. Barry MJ, Cockett ATK, Holtgrewe HL, et al. Relationship of symptoms of prostatism to commonly used physiologic and anatomical measures of the severity of benign prostatic hyperplasia. J Urol 1993;150:351.
4. Andersen JT, Nordling J, Walter S. Prostatism: I. The correlation between symptoms, cystometric and urodynamic findings. Scand J Urol Nephrol 1979;13:229.
5. Brooks ME, Hanani D, Braf ZF. Relationship between subjective complaints and urinary flow. Urology 1983;22:449.
6. Jacobsen SJ, Girman CJ, Lieber MM. Natural history of benign prostatic hyperplasia. Urology 2001;58(suppl 6a):5.
7. Yalla SV, Sullivan MP, Lecamwasam HS, et al. Correlation of American Urological Association symptom index with obstructive and non-obstructive prostatism. J Urol 1995;153:674.
8. Abrams P. New words for old: lower urinary tract symptoms for "prostatism". BMJ 1994;308:929.
9. Schafer W, Rubben H, Noppeney R, Deutz FJ. Obstructed and unobstructed prostatic obstruction. A plea for urodynamic objectivation of bladder outflow obstruction in benign prostatic hyperplasia. World J Urol 1989;6:198.
10. Abrams P. Objective evaluation of bladder outlet obstruction. Br J Urol 1995;76(suppl):11.
11. Rollema HJ, van Mastrigt R. Improved indication and follow up in transurethral resection of the prostate using the computer program CLIM: a prospective study. J Urol 1992;148:113.
12. Lepor H, Machi G. Comparison of the AUA symptom index in unselected males and females between 55 and 79 years of age. Urology 1993;42:36.
13. Barry MJ, Fowler FJ Jr., O'Leary MP, et al. The American Urological Association symptom index for benign prostatic hyperplasia. J Urol 1992;148:1549.
14. Streiner D, Norman G. Health Measurement Scales: A Practical Guide to Their Development and Use, Oxford, Oxford University Press, 1989, pp. 4–10.

15. Wright JG, Young NL. A comparison of different indices of responsiveness. J Clin Epidemiol 1997;50:239.

16. Barry MJ, Adolfsson J, Batista J, et al. Committee 6: measuring the symptoms and health impact of benign prostatic hyperplasia and its treatments. In Denis L, Griffiths K, Khoury S, et al., eds., Proceedings of the Fourth International Consultation on Benign Prostatic Hyperplasia. Plymouth, UK: Health Publications, Ltd, 1998, pp. 265–321.

17. Chicharro-Molero JA, Burgos-Rodriguez R, Sanchez-Cruz JJ, et al. Prevalence of benign prostatic hyperplasia in Spanish men 40 years old or older. J Urol 1998;159:878.

18. Madersbacher S, Haidinger G, Temml C, Schmidbauer CP. Prevalence of lower urinary tract symptoms in Austria as assessed by an open survey of 2,096 men. Eur Urol 1998;34:136.

19. Barry MJ, Fowler FJ Jr, O'Leary MP, et al. Correlation of the American Urological Association symptom index with self-administered versions of the Madsen-Iversen, Boyarsky and Maine Medical Assessment Program symptom indexes: Measurement committee of the American Urological Association. J Urol 1992;148:1558.

20. Barry MJ, Fowler FJ, Jr, O'Leary MP, et al. Measuring disease-specific health status in men with benign prostatic hyperplasia. Med Care 1995;33:AS145.

21. Barry MJ, Fowler FJ, Mulley AG, et al. Patient reactions to a program designed to facilitate patient participation in decisions for benign prostatic hyperplasia. Med Care 1995;33:771.

22. Barry MJ, Williford WO, Chang Y, et al. Benign prostatic hyperplasia specific health status measures in clinical research: how much change in the American Urological Association symptom index and the benign prostatic hyperplasia impact index is perceptible to patients? J Urol 1995;154:1770.

23. Haidinger G, Madersbacher S, Waldhoer T, et al. The prevalence of lower urinary tract symptoms in Austrian males and associations with sociodemographic variables. Eur J Epidemiol 1999;15:717.

24. Chute CG, Panser LA, Girman CJ, et al. The prevalence of prostatism: a population-based survey of urinary symptoms. J Urol 1993;150:85.

25. Roberts RO, Jacobsen SJ, Jacobsen DJ, et al. Longitudinal changes in peak urinary flow rates in a community based cohort. J Urol 2000;163:107.

26. Platz EA, Kawachi I, Rimm EB, et al. Race, ethnicity and benign prostatic hyperplasia in the health professionals follow-up study. J Urol 2000;163:490.

27. Bosch JL, Hop WC, Kirkels WJ, Schroder FH. The International Prostate Symptom Score in a community-based sample of men between 55 and 74 years of age: prevalence and correlation of symptoms with age, prostate volume, flow rate and residual urine volume. Br J Urol 1995;75:622.

28. Blanker MH, Groeneveld FP, Prins A, et al. Strong effects of definition and nonresponse bias on prevalence rates of clinical benign prostatic hyperplasia: the Krimpen study of male urogenital tract problems and general health status. BJU Int 2000;85:665.

29. Garraway WM, Collins GN, Lee RJ. High prevalence of benign prostatic hypertrophy in the community. Lancet 1991;338:469.

30. Bosch JL, Hop WC, Kirkels WJ, Schroder FH. Natural history of benign prostatic hyperplasia: appropriate case definition and estimation of prevalence in the community. Urology 1995;46:34.

31. Rhodes T, Girman CJ, Jacobsen SJ, et al. Longitudinal prostate growth rates during 5 years in randomly selected community men 40-79 years old. J Urol 1999;161:1174.

32. Homma Y, Kawabe K, Tsukamoto T, et al. Epidemiologic survey of lower urinary tract symptoms in Asia and Australia using the international prostate symptom score. Int J Urol 1997;4:40.
33. Roberts RO, Rhodes T, Panser LA, et al. Association between family history of benign prostatic hyperplasia and urinary symptoms: results of a population-based study. Am J Epidemiol 1995;1:142.
34. Meigs JB, Mohr B, Barry MJ. Risk factors for clinical benign prostatic hyperplasia in a community-based population of healthy aging men. J Clin Epidemiol 2001;54:935.
35. Nukui M. Epidemiological study on diet, smoking and alcohol drinking in the relationship to prostatic weight. Nippon Hinyokika Gakkai Zasshi 1997;88:950.
36. Signorello LB, Tzonou A, Lagiou P, et al. The epidemiology of benign prostatic hyperplasia: a study in Greece. BJU Int 1999;84:286.
37. Lagiou P, Wuu J, Trichopoulou A, et al. Diet and benign prostatic hyperplasia: a study in Greece. Urology 1999;54:284.
38. Giovannucci E, Rimm EB, Chute CG, et al. Obesity and benign prostatic hyperplasia. Am J Epidemiol 1994;140:989.
39. Hammarsten J, Hogstedt B. Hyperinsulinaemia as a risk factor for developing benign prostatic hyperplasia. Eur Urol 2001;39:151.
40. Oh BR, Kim SJ, Moon JD, et al. Association of benign prostatic hyperplasia with male pattern baldness. Urology 1998;51:744.
41. Holtgrewe HL, et al. The economics of the management of lower urinary tract symptoms and benign prostatic hyperplasia. In: Denis L, Griffiths K, Khoury S, et al., eds., Proceedings of the 4th International Consultation on BPH, Plymouth, UK: Health Publication Ltd, 1998, pp. 63–81.
42. Stoevelaar HJ, McDonnell J. Changing therapeutic regimens in benign prostatic hyperplasia. Clinical and economic considerations. Pharmacoeconomics 2001;19:131.
43. McDonnell J, Busschbach JJ, Kok E, et al. Lower urinary tract symptoms suggestive of benign prostatic obstruction- Triumph: health-economical analysis. Eur Urol 2001;39(suppl 3):37.

3 Pathophysiology, Diagnosis, and Treatment of the Postobstructive Diuresis

Chris M. Gonzalez, MD

CONTENTS

CASE REPORT
BASIC PATHOPHYSIOLOGY
DIAGNOSIS
LABORATORY DATA
TREATMENT
CONCLUSION
REFERENCES

CASE REPORT

A 68-year-old man was seen in the emergency room with a 4-d complaint of dribbling urination and lower abdominal discomfort. His medical history included hypertension controlled on two medications and benign prostatic hyperplasia (BPH) treated with an α1-receptor antagonist. The patient's vital signs revealed a temperature of 99°F, blood pressure of 132/80, pulse of 65 beats per min, and respiratory rate of 10. On physical examination, the patient was alert and responsive to commands and had lower abdominal distension with moderate edema of the lower extremities. His serum electrolyte levels were normal, with serum blood urea nitrogen (BUN) level and creatinine levels of 42 and 3.5, respectively. A Foley catheter was placed in the patient's bladder and 2 L of urine were drained. Urinalysis revealed 3 white blood cells per high-powered field with eventual culture showing no bacterial growth. Renal ultrasound revealed bilateral hydroureteronephrosis with no evidence of parenchymal abnormalities or echogenic foci.

From: *Management of Benign Prostatic Hypertrophy*
Edited by: K. T. McVary © Humana Press Inc., Totowa, NJ

The patient was given free access to oral fluids and observed in the emergency room for the next 4 hr, with urine output of 1200 mL during that time. Repeat serum electrolyte testing was normal and showed a urine osmolality of 150 mosM/L, spot urine sodium excretion of 50 meq/L, and fractional excretion of sodium (FENa) > 1. The patient was admitted to the hospital for observation. Over the next 24 hr, he was given free access to oral intake, and his urine output remained high at 250 mL/hr. His mental status, physical examination, vital signs, and serum electrolyte levels remained normal throughout this time; however, he did have persistent azotemia, with a serum BUN/creatinine of 42/3.4, urine osmolality of 1.000, and FENa > 1.

He was started on intravenous D5 half-normal saline with milliliter-for-milliliter fluid replacement of the previous 2-hr urine output. He was still granted free access to oral fluids at this time. His vital signs remained stable over the next 12 hr, with normal serum electrolyte levels and a repeat serum BUN/creatinine of 21/2.3. At this time, the urine specific gravity was 1.010, urine osmolality was 350 mosM/L, and FENa was > 1. Intravenous fluid replacement was continued over the next several hours, and the urine output remained brisk at 200 mL/hr with no change in the patient's vital signs or mental status. Twelve hours later, the serum electrolyte levels were normal and serum BUN/creatinine was 12/1.1. The intravenous fluids were stopped, and the patient was discharged home. Over the next 72 hr, the patient's urine output slowed to 2500 mL/d with moderate oral intake. Repeat renal ultrasound revealed resolution of the hydronephrosis, and the patient underwent successful transurethral prostatic resection one month later.

This case report demonstrates a management scheme for the patient with postobstructive diuresis (POD) after relief of a bladder neck obstruction. Complete urinary tract obstruction impedes the ability of the kidneys to concentrate and regulate the urine properly. After relief of the obstructive process, there may be a marked diuresis of solutes and water that ranges from mild and self-limiting to severe and potentially life-threatening. Although most patients do not exhibit POD of water and solutes, it is important to have a high index of suspicion for this condition so that it can be recognized promptly and managed. This chapter will attempt to provide a basic, simplified guide toward understanding issues related to the pathophysiology, diagnosis, and treatment of POD.

BASIC PATHOPHYSIOOGY

A description of renal physiology is beyond the scope of this chapter, and the reader is referred elsewhere for a review of this subject. Complete obstruction of the urinary tract refers to a process that involves both kidneys or a solitary kidney. At the basis of this pathophysiologic milieu is an elevation of ureteral pressure that is ultimately transmitted to the level of Bowman's capsule. This increased intratubular pressure causes a decrease in hydrostatic pressure at the interface of Bowman's capsule and the glomerulus, causing vasoconstriction of the glomerular vessels and a reduced glomerular filtration rate (GFR). This decrease in GFR causes further vasoconstriction of the afferent renal arterioles and leads to an overall decrease in renal blood flow (1). This entire process begins within the first 24 hr of complete obstruction and will progress rapidly if unaltered.

Decreased blood flow to the obstructed kidney(s) leads to azotemia, ischemia, and eventual acute tubular necrosis (ATN), all of which impair the kidney's ability to maintain a normally hyperosmotic medullary interstitium. It is this hyperosmotic medullary gradient maintained through the tubular regulation and reabsorption of sodium, urea, and water that is responsible for the kidney's ability to concentrate urine. The two main tubular areas that are damaged from ischemia and ATN are the normally water-impermeable, thick ascending limb of Henle and the collecting duct. Damage to these tubular structures prevents the reabsorption of sodium and chloride in the thick ascending limb and prevents the reabsorption of urea in the collecting duct. The inability to reabsorb these particular solutes prevents the maintenance of the hyperosmolar medullary gradient and the subsequent ability of the kidneys to concentrate the urine before excretion (2). In addition to causing the tubular damage that leads to POD, the solutes and water that are retained as a result of the obstructed urinary tract accumulate within the tubules and interstitium of the kidney and lead to an overall volume expansion of the patient. Once the obstructed urinary tract is relieved, the restored blood flow to the kidney and specifically to the medullary interstitium causes a washout of the retained solutes and water from the tubules and interstitium of the kidney. This washout of the hyperosmolar medullary gradient in concert with excretion of the retained water and solutes in the POD leads to the indiscriminate diuresis seen in some patients (2–5).

Hormones also have a role in urinary tract obstruction and possibly in POD. Secretion of atrial natriuretic peptide in response to stretch of the right atrium has been reported in patients with an obstructed urinary tract (6). Elevated serum levels of atrial natriuretic peptide have also been found to increase the GFR through afferent arteriolar smooth muscle relaxation and to improve the filtration of plasma at the glomerular/tubular interface (3,6,7). Because of these natriuretic (sodium excretion) and diuretic affects, this peptide has been implicated as a cause of POD, along with fluid overload and tubular injury. This hypothesis, however, is controversial, and further data are needed (8). The role of the secretion and regulation of antidiuretic hormone during POD is still unclear.

Clinically, three types of POD have been described: physiologic, pathologic, and iatrogenic (5,9,10). The basis of a physiologic POD includes the loss of iso-osmotic urine (300 mosM/L) without excessive solute loss (sodium and urea) from the kidney. The excessive urine output in this process stems from the excretion of the retained sodium, potassium, urea, and water within the tubules and interstitium of the kidney during the obstructive process. Because these substances could not be reabsorbed or excreted during the obstructive process, they are removed by means of a relatively limited physiologic water diuresis after the obstruction has been relieved. This type of POD is generally self-limited and subsides within 24 hr after the excess free water and solutes have been excreted and renal function normalizes. Prolonged azotemia and congestive heart failure (CHF) can potentiate this physiologic subtype of POD, and these patients should be monitored closely.

Less common is a pathologic POD that involves the excessive loss of sodium from the tubules because of ATN incurred during the obstructive process. This excessive loss of sodium is not related to the excretion of retained sodium during the obstructive process but rather to the injured renal tubule's inability to reabsorb this solute. Sodium losses in this condition can be massive and are associated with equal losses of free water (9,11). Because this condition is usually associated with acute renal failure and rapid volume depletion as a result of enormous sodium and water losses, intensive monitoring and aggressive volume replacement should be instituted.

Finally, iatrogenic POD involves the excessive intravenous replacement of glucose to the patient. Large amounts of this solute can overload the proximal tubule's ability to reabsorb it and POD can be prolonged. Management involves the elimination of excessive glucose from the intravenous fluids.

DIAGNOSIS

POD refers to the potential polyuria that can occur after relief of an obstructed urinary tract involving either both kidneys or a solitary kidney. Generally, obstruction occurs at the level of the bladder neck in male patients, but rarely, obstruction can involve an extrinsic or intrinsic process that occludes both ureters or the ureter of a solitary kidney. Although there are many potential causes of complete urinary tract obstruction, there does not appear to be any relationship between the cause of the obstructive process and the incidence or severity of resultant POD. Therefore, the importance of taking a thorough medical history, performing a good physical examination, and appropriately interpreting laboratory data are mandatory to identify those with or at risk for POD.

The most important issue for a patient with an obstructive uropathy is immediate, definitive relief of the occluded kidneys. Maneuvers such as clamping the Foley catheter for a time after each half-liter of urine is drained has no physiologic basis and only delays the complete relief of total urinary obstruction. Once the patient's urinary tract has been completely relieved, close monitoring of the patient's overall fluid status and urine output is mandatory. The definition of POD is sustained urine output of more than 200 mL/ hr for 24 hr; however, it is wise to assume that this process is underway if urine output remains more than 200 mL/hr for the first 2 to 3 hr after relief of obstruction. Factors such as high glucose-containing intravenous fluid preparations, uncontrolled diabetes, or excessive hypertonic fluid replacement should be recognized and addressed before making a diagnosis of POD.

Historic elements that are important include renal insufficiency, CHF, hypertension, recent hypotension, dizziness, or mental status impairment. Any of these conditions can place the patient at high risk for possible POD, and close monitoring should be instituted (5). Vital signs and urine output should be monitored every 2 hr in these high-risk patients once the obstructive process has been relieved.

The patient's general appearance and mental status should be closely followed once urinary obstruction has been relieved because altered sensorium may indicate an underlying metabolic disturbance that will affect the patient's ability to take oral replacement for ongoing water and solute loss. A complete physical examination should be conducted with special attention to findings consistent with volume overload such as jugular venous distension, presence of rales on auscultation of the lungs, and lower extremity edema. Serum chemistries including BUN, creatinine, electrolyte, magnesium, phosphorous, calcium, and glucose levels should be obtained. Obtaining BUN and serum creatinine levels when the patient is first seen is important because a patient with azotemia is also considered to be at high risk for POD and should be managed accordingly. Urine sodium, potassium, chloride, and creatinine levels in addition to specific gravity should be obtained if urine output remains high and POD is suspected. Urine is sent for analysis and culture, and empiric antibiotic therapy should be instituted in the presence of pyuria or bacteruria.

LABORATORY DATA

The frequency of obtaining serum and urine chemistries is according to the judgment of the clinician and largely depends on the overall condition of the patient and the severity of the diuresis. At the minimum, the basic serum and urine chemistries should be ordered once the diagnosis of POD is suspected or if a patient has the previously mentioned high risk factors for the condition. From the results of serum and urine chemistries, the clinician can calculate many important characteristics of the diuresis, which will guide management (Table 1).

Urine osmolality is an important parameter used to guide the treatment of POD. The inability of the kidneys to concentrate urine is one of the first renal functions impaired in the azotemic patient because of the pathophysiologic mechanisms described earlier. A simple way to estimate urine osmolality while waiting for this value to be automated is through urine specific gravity. It is important to note that the more consecutive readings taken of the urine osmolality and specific gravity, the more accurate the data regarding POD. If the specific gravity is 1.010, this is consistent with a urine osmolality of 300 mosM/L and thus the urine is iso-osmotic with serum. This indicates that the kidneys are unable to or do not need to maximally concentrate the urine, and an iso-osmotic diuresis is in progress. This most commonly represents physiologic POD, which is a self-limiting process of excreting retained solutes and water. A specific gravity of 1.020 is consistent with a higher urine osmolality in the range of 700 to 800 mosM/L, indicating that the urine-concentrating ability of the kidneys is intact and recovery is complete or near complete. The presence of glycosuria (severe diabetes) and proteinuria can cause a false elevation of the urine osmolality, and these factors should be excluded before the urine is determined to be hyperosmolar. Finally, a low specific gravity of 1.000 correlates with a urine osmolality of 50–100 mosM/L, indicating hypo-osmolality of the urine. This inability of the kidneys to concentrate urine should prompt serial readings of the urine because the pathologic salt-wasting subtype of POD most commonly is shown by hypotonic urine.

Serum osmolarity is calculated as 2 × (serum sodium) + serum glucose/2.8 + BUN/18. This calculated value should be within 10 mosM/L of the automated measured serum value. Patients with azotemia or diabetes may have raised serum osmolarity as the result of elevated BUN (urea) or glucose levels, respectively. All efforts should be made to correct these parameters as soon as possible in the face of POD. A self-limited rise in the serum osmolarity level can sometimes be seen in the

Table 1
Calculation of Serum and Urine Parameters Used in the Evaluation of POD

	Calculation	Comments
Urine Osmolality	Automated	Urine-specific gravity correlates with the urine osmolality. Specific gravity of 1.000 correlates with a urine osmolality of 50–100 mosM (low osmolality).
Serum Osmolarity	2 × (serum sodium) + serum glucose / 2.8 + BUN / 18	Normal is 280 mosM/L
FeNa	$\dfrac{\text{(urine spot sodium)} \times \text{(serum sodium)}}{\text{(serum creatinine)} \times \text{(urine creatinine)}} \times 100$	FeNa < 1 suggests a salt-conserving condition. FeNa < 1 suggests a salt-wasting condition.
Creatinine Clearance	(140 − age) × (kg weight)/72 × serum creatinine	The value for women is that of men × 0.85.
Spot Urine Electrolytes	Sodium, potassium, chloride	Serial levels should be taken. Sodium > 40 meq suggests a salt-wasting condition.

earlier phases of POD because of retention of these respective solutes and sodium during the obstructive process.

Fractional excretion of sodium is also an important measurement to obtain in a patient with suspected severe POD, namely the salt-wasting variety. It is simply calculated as:

$$FeNa = [\text{Urine spot sodium} \times \text{serum creatinine}/ \\ \text{serum sodium} \times \text{urine creatinine}] \times 100.$$

If the FeNa value is less than 1, this indicates that sodium is being conserved and that the patient's intravascular volume is depleted (dehydration). If the FeNa is more than 1, this indicates that sodium is being inappropriately lost from the kidneys. Massive sodium loss is very serious and is consistent with the pathologic salt-wasting variety of POD, which requires intensive monitoring and intervention.

Creatinine clearance can be performed as a rough estimate of overall renal function and may be an adjunctive way to monitor recovery of renal function if desired. The optimal way to calculate this value is 24-h urine collection, although this can be somewhat impractical in the setting of POD. A simple way to calculate this value is as follows:

$$\text{Men: Creatinine clearance in mL/min} = (140 - \text{age}) \times (\text{kg weight}) / \\ 72 \times \text{serum creatinine}$$

$$\text{Women: Absolute value calculated in men} \times 0.85$$

Spot urine electrolyte levels also provide valuable information, but variations can be seen with isolated values. Much like urine osmolality and the fractional excretion of sodium, the more consecutive spot urine electrolyte readings taken over a set period of time, the more indicative these values are of the underlying condition. Generally a spot urine sodium level more than 40 meq/L during prolonged POD indicates sodium wasting that is most likely associated with tubular injury and the inability to appropriately absorb this solute. A spot urine potassium level more than 20 meq/L and chloride level more than 20 meq/L also indicates the inability to reabsorb these solutes and the corresponding presence of tubular injury. If large amounts of solutes continue to be excreted, serum levels of the corresponding solutes should be checked every 4 to 8 h and replaced as needed.

Radiologic imaging after relief of obstructive uropathy associated with azotemia generally includes a renal and bladder ultrasound. In the presence of azotemia, bilateral hydronephrosis is generally seen, and this finding warrants a repeat ultrasound within the next several days to ensure resolution of the obstruction. If azotemia does not improve after 48 to 72 h, further imaging should be obtained to ensure complete relief of the urinary tract. Noncontrast computed tomography scan of the abdomen and pelvis may be a useful adjunct to the renal ultrasound to investigate hydronephrosis and obstruction of the urinary tract. Intravenous contrast should not be given in this situation because it may exacerbate the existing azotemia and acute tubular necrosis. All medications given to the patient with azotemia should be adjusted accordingly.

TREATMENT

Treatment of POD should be directed toward complete relief of urinary tract obstruction, replacement of electrolytes, correction of intravascular volume, and appropriate patient monitoring. If the patient has signs of urosepsis, draw appropriate blood and urine cultures before administering broad-spectrum intravenous antibiotics. Because many patients with POD have azotemia, dose adjustment of antibiotics should be made, and some agents (i.e., gentamicin) should be avoided.

Awake, conscious patients should have free access to fluids, and intravenous fluid replacement is unnecessary (4,6,8). These patients can be monitored by measuring weight daily, taking vital signs every 6 to 8 hr, and measuring serum electrolyte levels every 12 to 24 hr. Once azotemia resolves and serum BUN and creatinine levels return to baseline, the urine output will quickly normalize and patients can be followed on an outpatient basis. The vast majority of patients with POD fall into this category of physiologic diuresis, and there is no need to make serial serum or urine studies in these patients. However, if POD continues 48 h after relief of obstruction and azotemia persists, intravenous fluid replacement should be considered in addition to more frequent monitoring of urine and serum electrolyte levels, and the pathologic form of POD should be considered (8). Imaging should be repeated to rule out persistent obstruction of the urinary tract.

Patients with overt volume overload, CHF, hypertension, and altered mental status represent more of a treatment challenge for the urologist. These patients will need intensive hemodynamic monitoring and will require hourly measurement of urine output values, serial measurement of urine and serum electrolyte levels, and judicious intravenous fluid replacement. For patients with pathologic salt-wasting POD or persistent physiologic POD, there are two objectives of treatment: identification and correction of abnormal serum electrolytes and restoration of the GFR and subsequent renal blood flow through appropriate volume expansion. Data have shown that intravenous fluids containing sodium may provide a more expeditious recovery of GFR as a result of maintaining intravascular volume. Therefore, patients without overt volume overload or CHF should be given intravenous fluid replacement with a physiologic solution (D5 half-normal saline) milliliter-for-milliliter of the previous hour's urine output *(4,6)*. The patient should be monitored closely by means of vital sign measurements, physical examination, fractional excretion of sodium determination, and serum/urine electrolyte determinations to document progress and make adjustments in the intravenous replacement fluid content or volume. In patients with normal mental status, free access to oral fluids is granted.

Some patients may demonstrate signs and symptoms of CHF or volume overload at the time of diagnosis or during resuscitation for POD. The most prudent course of management for these patients is to avoid intravenous fluid replacement and allow natural diuresis of the extra fluid. A central venous catheter or pulmonary artery catheter may be needed to manage these potentially complicated patients. Serum electrolyte values should be monitored every 4 to 6 h and corrected as needed.

The endpoint of intravenous fluid replacement for any patient with POD involves assessing the overall renal function. Once the renal function returns to normal, there is no longer a need for intravenous fluid replacement, and the patient can remain on free access to fluids if mentally alert. If the patient is not mentally alert, a daily maintenance rate of physiologic intravenous solution is provided. As mentioned earlier, if POD continues and azotemia persists, repeat renal ultrasound along with cystoscopy, retrograde pyelograms, and possible stent placement for unrecognized obstruction of the ureter(s) should be pursued. At last resort, if POD continues and the patient continues to have azotemia and fluid overload, hemodialysis may be used to relieve fluid overload, uremia, or persistent electrolyte derangements. If patients demonstrate hypotension and hemodynamic instability, venovenous hemofiltration may be used to complete the dialysis.

CONCLUSION

Most patients who undergo relief of complete urinary tract obstruction will retain or quickly recover normal renal function and accordingly avoid POD. Patients at high risk for POD should be identified and appropriately monitored. Most patients with POD will be alert and able to restore intravascular volume and eventual renal function with oral intake alone. In the more complicated patient, serial urine and serum parameters should be used to guide appropriate intravenous fluid replacement with the endpoint of maintaining intravascular volume and restoring baseline renal function.

REFERENCES

1. Vaughan ED Jr, Sorenson EJ, Gillenwater JY. The renal hemodynamic response to chronic unilateral complete ureteral occlusion. Invest Urol 1970;8:78.
2. Gonzalez JM, Suki WN. Polyuria and nocturia. In: Massry SG, Glassock RJ, ed., Textbook of Nephrology, 3rd ed., Baltimore: Williams & Wilkins, 1995, pp. 547–552.
3. Gulmi FA, Mooppan UMM, Chou S, Kim H. Atrial natriuretic peptide in patients with obstructive uropathy. J Urol 1989;142:268–272.
4. Gulmi FA, Felson D, Vaughan ED Jr. Management of post-obstructive diuresis. AUA Update Series, lesson 23. 1998;27:178–183.
5. Loo MH, Vaughan ED Jr. Obstructive nephropathy and postobstructive diuresis. Urology Update series, lesson 9. 1985.
6. Gulmi FA, Matthews GJ, Marion D, et al. Volume expansion enhances the recovery of renal function and prolongs the diuresis and natriuresis after release of bilateral ureteral obstruction: a possible role for atrial natriuretic peptide. J Urol 1995;153:1276–1283.
7. Cogan MG. Atrial natriuretic peptide. Kidney Int 1990;37:1148–1160.
8. Gulmi FA, Felsen D, Vaughan ED Jr. Pathophysiology of urinary tract obstruction. In: Walsh PC, Retik AB, Stamey TA, Vaughan ED Jr, eds., Campbell's Urology, 7th ed., vol. 1, Philadelphia: WB Saunders Co, 1998, pp. 342–385.
9. Earley LE. Extreme polyuria in obstructive uropathy: report of a case of "water losing nephritis" in an infant with a discussion of polyuria. N Engl J Med 1956;255:600.
10. Muldowney FP, Duffy GJ, Kelly DG, et al. Sodium diuresis after relief of obstructive uropathy. N Engl J Med 1966;1294–1298.
11. Howards S. Postobstructive diuresis: a misunderstood phenomenon. J Urol 1973;110:537.

4   Urodynamics
and the Evaluation of Male
Lower Urinary Tract Symptoms

J. Quentin Clemens, MD, MSCI

CONTENTS

INTRODUCTION
UROFLOWMETRY
PRESSURE-FLOW STUDIES
VIDEOURODYNAMICS
CYSTOMETRY
SYMPTOMS AND URODYNAMIC FINDINGS
PREDICTIVE VALUE OF URODYNAMICS
INDICATIONS FOR URODYNAMIC STUDIES
    IN MEN WITH LUTS
CONCLUSION
REFERENCES

INTRODUCTION

The purpose of urodynamic testing is to reproduce the patient's symptoms in a controlled laboratory setting. A variety of measurements (bladder and urethral pressures, urine flow rate, fluoroscopic imaging) are made, and based on these observations and the clinical acumen of the examining physician, a diagnosis can be found that explains the patient's complaints. In men with lower urinary tract symptoms (LUTS), the primary urodynamic question is whether or not there is bladder outlet obstruction. A variety of urodynamic techniques may be used to address this question.

From: *Management of Benign Prostatic Hypertrophy*
Edited by: K. T. McVary © Humana Press Inc., Totowa, NJ

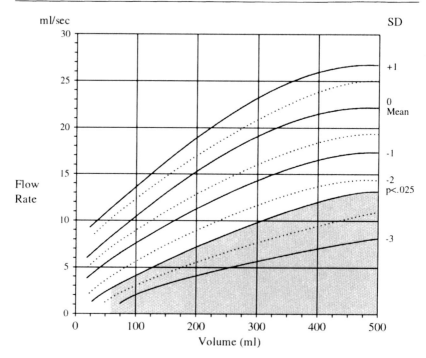

Fig. 1. Siroky nomogram for evaluation of uroflow results. The peak flow rate (vertical axis) and total bladder volume (voided volume plus residual volume, horizontal axis) are plotted as a single point on the nomogram. The shaded zone indicates values that occur in < 2.5% of the normal male population.

UROFLOWMETRY

Uroflowmetry is an attractive test for both clinician and patient because it is simple to perform and noninvasive. The most clinically useful measurement is the maximum urinary flow rate (Qmax), which is measured in milliliters per second. Other information that may be obtained includes the flow pattern (continuous or intermittent), average flow rate, shape of the flow curve, flow time, and time to maximum flow. Postvoid residual bladder volume may also be assessed with ultrasonography after the void. Uroflowmetry may be done with the patient in the standing or supine position to best mimic normal voiding patterns at home.

In general, Qmax of < 10 mL/s is considered abnormal; Qmax of > 15 mL/s is normal; and Qmax of 10–15 mL/s is equivocal (*1,2*). It is advisable to perform multiple measurements because intraindividual variation for this test is high (*3*). Interestingly, the variability appears to be increased in men with LUTS as a result of benign prostatic hyperplasia (BPH) when compared with asymptomatic controls *(4)*. At very low voided volumes (< 150 mL), uroflow results are quite inaccurate, and results from such voiding episodes should be viewed with a high degree of skepticism *(5)*. Furthermore, it must be remembered that normal flow-rate parameters vary with voided volume and with age. The progressive decrease in Qmax observed with age does not appear to be caused by an increased incidence of bladder outlet obstruction *(6,7)*. A variety of nomograms with volume- and/or age-adjusted normative flow rate calculations have been published. The Siroky nomogram is one of the most commonly used (Fig. 1) *(8)*.

The urinary flow rate is a product of both detrusor contractility and urethral resistance. A low flow rate may be caused by anatomic obstruction (BPH, urethral stricture), dynamic obstruction (incomplete external sphincter relaxation), poor detrusor contraction, or a combination of these factors. Similarly, a normal or supranormal flow rate may occur in the face of significant outlet obstruction by strong detrusor contraction. It is, therefore, not surprising that uroflowmetry results alone do not differentiate obstructed from unobstructed patients *(9–11)*. Nevertheless, the technique may have some merit as a screening test for obstruction, because in general, those with a low flow rate (<10 mL/s) are more likely to have obstruction *(7,12)*. In addition, uroflow results are a convenient way to assess response to therapy.

PRESSURE-FLOW STUDIES

Pressure-flow studies consist of the simultaneous measurement of bladder pressure, abdominal pressure, and uroflow. The patient has a full bladder, and a free (uncatheterized) urine flow rate is obtained. A small (7–8 Fr) dual-lumen catheter is placed in each urethra; one lumen is used to measure bladder pressure and the other is used to infuse room temperature water or saline. A rectal catheter is placed to measure abdominal pressure. Detrusor pressure is obtained by subtracting the abdominal pressure from the total bladder pressure. All pressure transducers are zeroed to atmospheric pressure at the level of the pubic symphysis before they are connected to the catheters. Electromyography (EMG) of the external urethral sphincter is usually also recorded by means of patch or needle electrodes on the perineum. The bladder is filled through the urethral catheter at a medium rate (10–50 mL/min). The patient is asked to void when his bladder feels full. A high detrusor pressure–low flow pattern indicates bladder outlet obstruction, whereas a low pressure–low flow pattern indicates impaired detrusor contractility. The EMG recording indicates the degree of external sphincter activ-

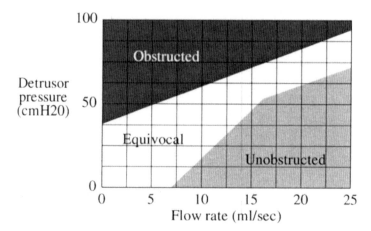

Fig. 2. Abram-Griffith nomogram for evaluation of pressure-flow data in men. The detrusor pressure at maximum flow (vertical axis) and peak flow rate (horizontal axis) are plotted as a single point. More sophisticated analyses may be performed to attempt to classify patients whose results are in the equivocal area.

ity and is most useful in identifying a lack of sphincter relaxation during voiding (dynamic obstruction).

There are a variety of ways in which the results of pressure-flow studies may be interpreted. In general, a detrusor pressure of more than 40 cm H_2O with a uroflow less than 12 mL is considered obstructed; a detrusor pressure of less than 30 cm H_2O with a uroflow less than 12 mL indicates impaired detrusor contractility; and detrusor pressures between 30 and 40 cm H_2O with a uroflow less than 12 mL is indeterminate (13). Another common way to analyze these studies is to plot the detrusor pressure at maximum flow vs the maximum flow rate. The Abrams-Griffiths nomogram is then used to divide results into obstructed, unobstructed, and equivocal categories (Fig. 2; 1).

Pressure-flow studies are advantageous because they can be used to differentiate detrusor hypocontractility from bladder outlet obstruction. They are considered the gold standard for the diagnosis of bladder outlet obstruction and are widely used for both clinical and research purposes. However, they are invasive, time-consuming, labor-intensive, and prone to measurement error. Two or three consecutive studies must be performed because the results of a single test are highly variable (14). There tends to be a decrease in obstructive parameters with successive tests so that as many as 28% of patients will be redefined into a less obstructive Abrams-Griffiths category if the first study is compared with subsequent studies (15,16). Furthermore, interpretation of the tests is not always straightforward, resulting in high intrainterpreter and inter-interpreter variability *(17)*.

VIDEOURODYNAMICS

Videourodynamic studies involve the measurement of urodynamic parameters along with the simultaneous fluoroscopic imaging of the bladder and urethra. For these studies, contrast material is infused into the bladder instead of saline or water. The term videourodynamics may be used to describe a number of different techniques. In some instances, fluoroscopy is simply added to the pressure-flow study as described previously. In other cases, a triple-lumen bladder catheter is used, with the third, proximal lumen used to measure intraluminal urethral pressure. During filling, the proximal urethral pressure transducer (which is marked with a radiopaque marker) is positioned at the area of maximum resting urethral pressure (the external sphincter), and the distal transducer remains in the bladder to record intravesical pressure. This technique gives a more direct measurement of external sphincter activity than EMG electrodes. Some urodynamicists also omit the rectal catheter and simply measure total vesical pressure and urethral pressure.

By adding fluoroscopic imaging to the measurements of pressures and flow rates, videourodynamic testing can be used to identify the location of bladder outlet obstruction (bladder neck, prostate, external urethral sphincter, bulbar urethra). Furthermore, other abnormalities such as vesicoureteral reflux or urinary incontinence are easily demonstrated.

One specific technique that uses fluoroscopic imaging to precisely localize obstruction is micturitional urethral pressure profilometry (MUPP) *(18)*. This technique uses a triple-lumen urethral catheter as detailed above. During voiding, the catheter is slowly withdrawn so that the urethral transducer records pressures from the bladder outlet to the supramembranous urethra. In the absence of obstruction, the pressure difference across these two areas is zero; whereas, when obstruction is present, the pressure difference is greater than 20 cm H_2O *(19,20)*. By moving the catheter proximally and distally, the exact point of obstruction can be identified. The obstruction can be confirmed fluoroscopically by observing a narrowing of the urinary stream. This technique correlates well with results of pressure-flow studies and is less prone to technical difficulty *(19)*.

Despite the apparent advantages of videourodynamic studies, there has been no systematic evaluation of the utility of these studies in the evaluation of men with LUTS.

CYSTOMETRY

Cystometry is routinely performed as part of a pressure-flow or videourodynamics study. Pertinent abnormalities on cystometry include detrusor instability and diminished bladder compliance. Detrusor instability (DI) can be documented in approx 50% of men with LUTS and 40% of men with documented obstruction (21–25). In patients who have DI before surgery, up to half may continue to have DI after prostatectomy, a suboptimal result (21,22,26). Unfortunately, there are currently no clinical or urodynamic criteria to determine which patients with bladder outlet obstruction and DI will do well after relief of the obstruction, and which patients will continue to have DI.

Diminished bladder compliance has been demonstrated in 25–35% of men with bladder outlet obstruction (23,27). Older patients and those with severe obstruction demonstrate more significant compliance abnormalities than patients who are younger and have less obstruction (27). This loss of compliance appears to be a generic response of the detrusor to obstruction (28–30). This finding is quite important because severe compliance abnormalities are clearly associated with the development of hydronephrosis and postrenal azotemia (28,31). Surgical intervention should be strongly considered for patients with significantly diminished compliance and bladder outlet obstruction. Such patients should have close urodynamic follow-up to assess for improvements in compliance following relief of the obstruction.

SYMPTOMS AND URODYNAMIC FINDINGS

Bladder outlet obstruction from BPH may result in medical conditions (urinary retention, renal insufficiency, bladder stones, recurrent urinary tract infections) that warrant surgical therapy. However, most men with prostatism do not have such conditions but instead have bothersome voiding symptoms. Traditionally, it has been held that these symptoms are the direct result of mechanical outlet obstruction by the prostatic adenoma. However, it is now clear that they are bladder symptoms that are not specific to obstruction, and in fact, are just as common in women as in men (32–34). Numerous studies have failed to show any type of reproducible urodynamic finding that correlates with specific symptomatic complaints (35–38). Therefore, validated symptom scores for BPH are helpful to quantitate symptoms and assess response to therapy but cannot be used to diagnose bladder outlet obstruction. Similarly, urodynamic evidence of obstruction may be found in asymptomatic patients, and documented relief of obstruction following surgery does not always correlate with symptomatic improvement *(39–42)*. Urodynamic studies and symptom assessments appear to measure separate aspects of lower urinary tract function that are probably related to some degree, but the nature of that relationship has not yet been defined.

PREDICTIVE VALUE OF URODYNAMICS

Most patients with LUTS initially undergo medical treatment with α-adrenergic receptor antagonists or 5α-reductase inhibitors. Although the morbidity of these therapies is minimal, the costs are not inconsequential, and not all patients benefit from these treatments. A number of investigators have examined pretreatment urodynamic findings to correlate them with eventual symptomatic outcome. Lepor and associates found that those with peak urinary flow rates more than 15 mL/s had similar symptomatic improvement after treatment with α-blockers as those with peak flow rates less than 15 mL/s *(43)*. Other studies indicate that those who are not obstructed by pressure-flow criteria appear to derive equivalent benefit from medical therapy when compared with patients who have obstruction *(24,44–47)*. Furthermore, in those with symptomatic improvement following α-blocker therapy, no significant urodynamic changes could be demonstrated *(44)*. Two conclusions may be drawn from these data. First, there appears to be no cost-benefit advantage to performing routine urodynamic testing before initiating medical therapy for BPH. Second, the symptomatic improvement seen from medical therapy is likely to be the result, at least in part, of effects other than the relief of bladder outlet obstruction.

The morbidity of surgical therapy for BPH may be considerable, and therefore, much attention has been directed at identifying urodynamic parameters that may improve outcomes and minimize unnecessary surgery. It is clear that 20–50% of men with LUTS do not have bladder outlet obstruction *(24,45,48,49)*. Because the decision to perform surgery is often based on symptoms alone, one would expect that an equivalent proportion of patients undergoing surgery would also be unobstructed. Indeed, studies that report such data show that to be true *(24,42,50,51)*. Improvements in obstructive urodynamic parameters are seen uniformly following surgery, and as expected, these improvements are more pronounced in patients who are obstructed preoperatively *(46,52)*. If relief of obstruction equates with symptomatic success, one would expect limited symptomatic relief in those who are unobstructed preoperatively, but the literature on this point is inconclusive.

A variety of studies have stratified symptomatic outcome based upon preoperative uroflowmetry results. Jensen and co-workers performed a prospective study of 139 men undergoing prostatectomy and found that those with a preoperative Qmax of greater than 15 mL/s had an increased likelihood of symptomatic treatment failure at 6 mo *(53)*. Others have found decreased global satisfaction or increased symptom scores for those with preoperative flow rates more than 10 mL/s when compared with those whose preoperative flow rate was less than or equal to 10 mL/s *(54,55)*. However, the majority of studies have failed to demonstrate a clear relationship between preoperative flow rate and symptomatic outcome following surgery *(26–58)*.

Pressure-flow studies have been extensively evaluated as potential predictors of treatment response following surgery (TURP or open prostatectomy). Some evidence exists that urodynamic data may yield relevant prognostic information. Abrams et al. reported a 72% success rate (symptomatic and flow rate improvement), which increased to 88% if pressure-flow criteria were used to select patients for surgery *(41)*. However, this study has been criticized for the unusually high failure rate (28%) in the initial group *(59)*. Rollema et al. reported a better symptomatic outcome in 19 preoperatively obstructed patients when compared with 10 unobstructed patients *(50)*. Interestingly, 3 of the 10 unobstructed patients reported significant postoperative improvement despite no demonstrable urodynamic changes. Jensen et al. demonstrated a 93% subjective satisfaction rate in the obstructed patients compared with a rate of 78% in unobstructed patients *(42)*. Kuo and Tsai reported a good outcome in 94% of men with high-pressure obstruction and in only 12% of those who were not obstructed *(60)*. Data from these studies indicate that a policy of reserving surgical therapy for patients with demonstrated obstruction on preoperative pressure-flow studies may improve treatment outcomes, although most of these studies indicate a significant benefit to unobstructed patients as well.

Other studies have shown no clear benefit to the routine performance of pressure-flow studies before surgery. Kaplan et al. performed a retrospective review of 121 patients after TURP, with a mean follow-up of more than 4 yr *(24)*. There was no correlation with level of satisfaction with therapy and the presence or absence of bladder outlet obstruction on preoperative urodynamic tests *(24)*. Neal et al. conducted a prospective study of 217 men who underwent pressure-flow studies before TURP *(26)*. Those with low or normal preoperative voiding pressures as a group had lower satisfaction with surgical results at 11 mo follow-up, but outcomes could not be predicted accurately in individual patients using urodynamic measurements *(26)*. In another prospective study of 56 patients, Roehrborn et al. reported no association between degree of preoperative obstruction and 6-mo symptomatic response following TURP *(58)*.

Limited data exist regarding the prognostic value of performing urodynamic studies before initiating alternative, minimally invasive treatments for BPH. Initial experience indicates that uroflowmetry results do not predict treatment response before transurethral needle ablation (TUNA) or transurethral microwave thermotherapy (TUMT) *(58,61,62)*. TUMT treatment has been reported to have higher efficacy in men with higher grades of obstruction by some authors, whereas others could not demonstrate a correlation with pressure-flow studies and outcome *(46,63,64)*. The few reports of the predictive value of urodynamics before TUNA indicate that degree of obstruction does not affect treatment results *(58,65)*.

INDICATIONS FOR URODYNAMIC STUDIES IN MEN WITH LUTS

To date, no urodynamic criteria have been found that predict treatment response to medical therapy for men with LUTS. Therefore, urodynamic testing has a limited role before the initiation of medical therapy. The role of routine urodynamic testing before surgery is controversial. Urodynamic testing does appear to lower the surgical failure rate to some degree. Furthermore, although a significant number of unobstructed patients benefit from surgery, in such cases it is unclear what is being treated. Alternative therapies such as anticholinergic agents or biofeedback-assisted pelvic floor muscle exercises may be equally beneficial and less morbid. However, the cost of performing routine urodynamic testing before surgery in all patients would be significant. Also, relief of symptoms can be seen in up to 90% of men selected without urodynamic data *(56,66)*. The decision to obtain urodynamic studies must be individualized, but the eventual decision is largely based on the treatment philosophy of the physician.

In some situations, the benefits of urodynamic testing appear to be clear cut (Table 1). Men with persistent symptoms following surgical treatment to relieve bladder outlet obstruction should be studied. Such patients may have persistent obstruction, detrusor hypocontractility, detrusor instability, or diminished bladder compliance *(67,68)*. The treatment for each of these conditions is different; therefore, tailored therapy based on a specific urodynamic diagnosis is likely to be more successful than empiric treatment. Similarly, those with known or suspected neurologic disease may exhibit a wide range of urodynamic abnormalities. Proceeding with TURP or open prostatectomy in these patients should be done only after other potential sources of voiding dysfunction have been identified and treated. Men with previous pelvic

Table 1
Indications for Urodynamic Studies in Men with LUTS

Absolute Indications
    Failure of previous surgery
    Known or suspected neurologic disease
    Prior pelvic radiation
    Prior radical pelvic surgery
Relative Indications
    Severe symptoms and normal uroflow
    Young age
    Isolated symptoms of urgency and urge incontinence

radiation or major pelvic surgery should also undergo urodynamic testing because these treatments may result in impaired bladder storage function, which could result in suboptimal results following surgery. In men with atypical clinical presentations (isolated symptoms of urgency and urge incontinence, severe symptoms and normal uroflow, young age), BPH-induced bladder outlet obstruction is less likely to be the cause of the symptoms, and it would therefore seem prudent to make the diagnosis clearly before proceeding with surgical therapy.

CONCLUSION

A variety of urodynamic techniques exist to help assess for the presence of bladder outlet obstruction. Physicians who order and interpret these tests must be aware of the specific strengths and weaknesses of each technique. The predictive value of urodynamic testing in the routine evaluation of men with LUTS has not yet been well defined. However, if used intelligently, urodynamic testing can be very helpful in the assessment of these patients.

REFERENCES

1. Abrams PH, Griffiths DJ. The assessment of prostatic obstruction from urodynamic measurements and from residual urine. Br J Urol 1979;51:129–134.
2. Andersen JT. Prostatism. Clinical, radiological and urodynamic aspects. Neurourol Urodyn 1982;1:241–293.
3. Feneley MR, Dunsmuir WD, Pearce J, Kirby RS. Reproducibility of uroflow measurement: experience during a double-blind, placebo-controlled study of doxazosin in benign prostatic hyperplasia. Urology 1996;47(5):658–663.
4. Golomb J, Lindner A, Siegel Y, Korczak D. Variability and circadian changes in home uroflowmetry in patients with benign prostatic hyperplasia compared to normal controls. J Urol 1992;147:1044–1047.
5. Drach GW, Layton TN, Binard WJ. Male peak urinary flow rate: relationships to volume voided and age. J Urol 1979;122:210–214.

6. Girman CJ, Panser LA, Chute CG, et al. Natural history of prostatism: urinary flow rates in a community-based study. J Urol 1993;150:887–892.
7. Madersbacher S, Klingler CH, Schatzl G, et al. Age related urodynamic changes in patients with benign prostatic hyperplasia. J Urol 1996;156:1662–1667.
8. Siroky MB, Olsson CA, Krane RJ. The flow rate nomogram I: Development and II: Clinical correlation. J Urol 1979;122:665–668. 1980;123:208–210.
9. Chancellor MB, Blaivas JG, Kaplan SA, Axelrod S. Bladder outlet obstruction versus impaired detrusor contractility: the role of outflow. J Urol 1991;145: 810–812.
10. Rollema HJ, van Mastrigt R. Detrusor contractility before and after prostatectomy. Neurourol Urodyn 1987;6:220–221.
11. Poulsen AL, Schou J, Puggaard L, Torp-Pedersen S, Nordling J. Prostatic enlargement, symptomatology and pressure/flow evaluation: interrelations in patients with symptomatic BPH. Scand J Urol Nephrol 1994;157:67–73.
12. Reynard JM, Yang Q, Donovan JL, et al. The ICS-'BPH' Study: uroflowmetry, lower urinary tract symptoms and bladder outlet obstruction. Br J Urol 1998;82:619–623.
13. Blaivas JG. Obstructive uropathy in the male. Urol Clin N Am 1996;23(3):373.
14. Sonke GS, Kortmann BBM, Verbeek ALM, et al. Variability of pressure flow studies in men with lower urinary tract symptoms. Neurourol Urodyn 2000; 19:637–656.
15. Tammela TLJ, Schafer W, Barrett DM, et al., for the Finasteride Urodynamics Study Group. Repeated pressure-flow studies in the evaluation of bladder outlet obstruction due to benign prostatic enlargement. Neurourol Urodyn 1999;18: 17–24.
16. Madsen FA, Rhodes PR, Bruskewitz RC. Reproducibility of pressure-flow variables in patients with symptomatic benign prostatic hyperplasia. Urology 1995;46:816–820.
17. Kortmann BBM, Sonke GS, Wijkstra H, et al. Intra- and inter-investigator variation in the analysis of pressure-flow studies in men with lower urinary tract symptoms. Neurourol Urodyn 2000;19:221–232.
18. Yalla SV, Sharma GV, Barsamian EM. Micturitional static urethral pressure profile: a method of recording urethral pressure profile during voiding and the implications. J Urol 1980;124:649–656.
19. DuBeau CE, Sullivan MRP, Cravalho E, Resnick NM, Yalla SV. Correlation between micturitional urethral pressure profile and pressure-flow criteria in bladder outlet obstruction. J Urol 1995;154:498–503.
20. McGuire EJ. Urodynamic studies in prostatic obstruction. In: Fitzpatrick JM, Krane RJ, eds., The Prostate, New York: Churchill Livingstone, 1989, pp. 103–109.
21. Jensen KME, Jorgensen JB, Mogensen P. Urodynamics in prostatism. III. Prognostic value of medium-fill water cystometry. Scand J Urol Nephrol 1988; S114:78–83.
22. Dorflinger T, Frimodt-Moller PC, Bruskewitz RC, et al. The significance of uninhibited detrusor contractions in prostatism. J Urol 1985;133:819–821.
23. Sullivan MP, Yalla SV. Detrusor contractility and compliance characteristics in adult male patients with obstructive and non-obstructive voiding dysfunction. J Urol 1996;155:1995–2000.
24. Kaplan SA, Bowers DL, Te AE, Olsson CA. Differential diagnosis of prostatism: a 12-year retrospective analysis of symptoms, urodynamics and satisfaction with therapy. J Urol 1996;155:1305–1308.

25. Knutson T, Edlund C, Fall M, Dahlstrand C. BPH with coexisting overactive bladder dysfunction- an everyday urological dilemma. Neurourol Urodyn 2001;20(3);237–247.

26. Neal DE, Ramsden PD, Sharples L, et al. Outcome of elective prostatectomy. BMJ 1989;299:762–767.

27. Madersbacher S, Pycha A, Klingler CH, et al. Interrelationships of bladder compliance with age, detrusor instability, and obstruction in elderly men with lower urinary tract symptoms. Neurourol Urodynam 1999;18:3–15.

28. George NJ, O'Reilly PH, Barnard RJ, Blacklock NJ. High pressure chronic retention. BMJ 1983;286(6380):1780–1783.

29. Styles RA, Ramsden PD, Neal DE. Chronic retention of urine. The relationship between upper tract dilatation and bladder pressure. Br J Urol 1986;58(6): 647–651.

30. McGuire EJ, Woodside JR, Borden TA, Weiss RM. Prognostic value of urodynamic testing in myelodysplastic patients. J Urol 1981;126:205–209.

31. Wang SC, McGuire EJ, Bloom DA. A bladder pressure management system for myelodysplasia- clinical outcome. J Urol 1988;140:1499–1502.

32. Chai TC, Belville WD, McGuire EJ, Nyquist L. Specificity of the American Urological Association voiding symptom index: comparison of unselected and selected samples of both sexes. J Urol 1993;150:1710–1713.

33. Lepor H, Machi G. Comparison of AUA symptom index in unselected males and females between fifty-five and seventy-nine years of age. Urology 1993; 42:36–40.

34. Jolleys JV, Jolleys JC, Wilson J, et al. Does sexual equality extend to urinary symptoms? Neurourol Urodyn 1993;12:391–392.

35. Yalla SV, Sullivan MP, Lecamwasam HS, et al. Correlation of American Urological Association symptom index with obstructive and nonobstructive prostatism. J Urol 1995;(3 Pt 1):679–680.

36. de la Rosette JJMCH, Witjes WPJ, Schafer W, et al., for the ICS-BPH Study Group. Relationships between lower urinary tract symptoms and bladder outlet obstruction: results from the ICS-BPH Study. Neurourol Urodyn 1998;17: 99–108.

37. Sirls LT, Kirkemo AK, Jay J. Lack of correlation of the American Urological Association Symptom 7 index with urodynamic bladder outlet obstruction. Neurourol Urodyn 1996;15:447–456.

38. Ko DS, Fenster HN, Chambers K, Sullivan LD, Jens M, Goldenberg SL. The correlation of a multichannel urodynamic pressure-flow studies and American Urological Association symptom index in the evaluation of benign prostatic hyperplasia. J Urol 1995;154 (2 Pt 1):396–398.

39. Botker-Rasmussen I, Bagi P, Jorgensen JB. Is bladder outlet obstruction normal in elderly men without lower urinary tract symptoms? Neurourol Urodyn 1999;18:545–552.

40. Walker RMH, Romano G, Davies AH, et al. Pressure flow study in data in a group of asymptomatic male control patients 45 years old or older. J Urol 2001;165;683–687.

41. Abrams PH, Farrar DJ, Turner WRT, et al. The results of prostatectomy: a symptomatic and urodynamic analysis of 152 patients. J Urol 1979;121:640–642.

42. Jensen KME, Jorgensen JB, Mogensen P. Urodynamics in prostatism. II. Prognostic value of pressure-flow study combined with stop-flow test. Scand J Urol Nephrol 1988;S114:72–77.

43. Lepor H, Nieder A, Feser J, O'Connell C, Dixon C. Effect of terazosin on prostatism in men with normal and abnormal peak urinary flow rates. Urology 1997;49:476–480.

44. Rossi C, Kortmann BBM, Sonke GS, et al. (alpha)-Blockade improves symptoms suggestive of bladder outlet obstruction but fails to relieve it. J Urol 2001;165:38–41.

45. Gerber GS, Kim JH, Contreras BA, Steinberg GD, Rukstalis DB. An observational urodynamic evaluation of men with lower urinary tract symptoms treated with doxazosin. Urology 1996;47:840–844.

46. Witjes WP, Robertson A, Rosier PF, et al. Urodynamic and clinical effects of noninvasive and minimally invasive treatments in elderly men with lower urinary tract symptoms stratified according to the grade of obstruction. Urology 1997;50:55–61.

47. Arnold EP. Tamsulosin in men with confirmed bladder outlet obstruction: a clinical and urodynamic analysis from a single centre in New Zealand. BJU Int 2001;87(1):24–30.

48. Eckhardt MD, Venrooij GE, Boon TA. Interactions between prostate volume, filling cystometric estimated parameters, and data from pressure-flow studies in 565 men with lower urinary tract symptoms suggestive of benign prostatic hyperplasia. Neurourol Urodyn 2001;20(5):579–590.

49. Fusco F, Groutz A, Blaivas JG, Chaikin DC, Weiss JP. Videourodynamic studies in men with lower urinary tract symptoms: a comparison of community based versus referral urological practices. J Urol 2001;166:910–913.

50. Rollema HJ, Van Mastrigt R. Improved indication and followup in transurethral resection of the prostate using the computer program CLIM: a prospective study. J Urol 1992;148:111–116.

51. Schafer W, Noppeney R, Ruben H, Lutzeyer W. The value of free flow rate and pressure/flow-studies in the routine investigation of BPH patients. Neurourol Urodyn 1988;7:219–221.

52. Bosch J, Ruud LH. Urodynamic effects of various treatment modalities for benign prostatic hyperplasia. J Urol 1997;158:2034–2044.

53. Jensen KME, Jorgensen JB, Mogensen P. Urodynamics in prostatism. I. Prognostic value of uroflowmetry. Scand J Urol Nephrol 1988;S114:63–71.

54. Jensen KM, Bruskewitz FC, Iversen P, Madsen PO. Spontaneous uroflowmetry in prostatism. Urology 1984;24:403–409.

55. Meyhoff HH, Nordling J, Hald T. Clinical evaluation of transurethral versus transvesical prostatectomy. A randomized study. Scand J Urol Nephrol 1984; 18:201–209.

56. Wasson JH, Reda DJ, Bruskewitz RC, et al., for the Veterans Affairs Cooperative Study Group on Transurethral Resection of the Prostate. A comparison of transurethral surgery with watchful waiting for moderate symptoms of benign prostatic hyperplasia. N Engl J Med 1995;332:75–79.

57. Pannek J, Berges RR, Haupt G, Senge T. Value of Danish prostate symptom score compared to the AUA symptom score and pressure/flow studies in the preoperative evaluation of men with symptomatic benign prostatic hyperplasia. Neurourol Urodyn 1998;17(1):9–18.

58. Roehrborn CG, Burkhard FC, Bruskewitz RC, et al. The effects of transurethral needle ablation and resection of the prostate on pressure flow urodynamic parameters: analysis of the United States randomized study. J Urol 1999;162: 92–97.

59. McConnell JD. Why pressure-flow studies should be optional and not manda-
    tory studies for evaluating men with benign prostatic hyperplasia. Urology
    1994;44:156.

60. Kuo HC, Tsai TC. The predictive value of urine flow rate and voiding pressure
    in the operative outcome of benign prostatic hypertrophy. Taiwan I Hsueh Hui
    Tsa Chih 1988;87:323–330.

61. Hallin A, Berlin T. Transurethral microwave thermotherapy of benign prostatic
    hyperplasia: do any pretreatment conditions predict the result? Eur Urol
    1996;30(4):429–436.

62. Eliasson TU, Abramsson LB, Pettersson GT, Damber JE. Responders and non-
    responders to treatment of benign prostatic hyperplasia with transurethral
    microwave thermotherapy. Scand J Urol Nephrol 1995;29(2):183–191.

63. Bursa B, Wammack R, Djavan B, et al. Outcome predictors of high-energy
    transurethral microwave thermotherapy. Tech Urol 2000;6(4):262–266.

64. Floratos DL, Kiemeney LALM, Rossi C, et al. Long-term follow-up of random-
    ized tranurethral microwave thermotherapy versus transurethral prostatic resec-
    tion study. J Urol 2001;165:1533–1538.

65. Campo B, Bergamaschi F, Corrada P, Ordesi G. Transurethral needle ablation
    (TUNA) of the prostate: a clinical and urodynamic evaluation. Urology 1997;
    49:847–850.

66. McConnell JD, Barry MJ, Bruskewitz RC, et al. Benign prostatic hyperplasia:
    diagnosis and treatment. Clin Pract Guidel No 8 AHCPR Publ No 94-0582.
    Rockville, MD: Agency Health Care Policy and Research, US Dept Health
    Human Services, 1994.

67. Nitti VW, Kim Y, Combs AJ. Voiding dysfunction following transurethral
    resection of the prostate: symptoms and urodynamic findings. J Urol 1997;
    157:600–603.

68. Seaman EK, Jacobs BZ, Blaivas JG, Kaplan SA. Persistence or recurrence of
    symptoms after transurethral resection of the prostate: a urodynamic assess-
    ment. J Urol 1994;152:935–937.

5

α-Adrenergic Antagonists in the Treatment of Benign Prostatic Hypertrophy-Associated Lower Urinary Tract Symptoms

Ross A. Rames, MD and David C. Horger, MD

CONTENTS

INTRODUCTION
MECHANISM OF ACTION
RECEPTOR CLASSIFICATION
INITIAL EVALUATION AND SELECTION OF THERAPY
SELECTION OF AN α-ANTAGONIST AGENT
α-ANTAGONISTS IN NON-BPH PATIENTS
CONCLUSIONS
REFERENCES

INTRODUCTION

The development of benign prostatic hypertrophy (BPH) is common among aging men. Accompanying the development of BPH may be impairment of the bladder's ability to store and empty urine. Symptoms may include frequent urination, urgent voiding, an intermittent and diminished urinary stream, straining to void, nocturia, and a sense of incomplete bladder emptying. Collectively, these symptoms may be referred to as lower urinary tract symptoms, or LUTS. In advanced stages, elevated postvoid residual urine, urinary tract infections, hydronephrosis, impairment of renal function, and urinary retention may develop.

From: *Management of Benign Prostatic Hypertrophy*
Edited by: K. T. McVary © Humana Press Inc., Totowa, NJ

Transurethral resection of the prostate (TURP) is the gold standard of BPH treatment in terms of symptom relief. It remains one of the most effective methods of treating this disease. Newer technologies now offer comparable symptom relief without the need for anesthetic administration and subsequent hospitalization. Most patients, however, prefer to avoid invasive treatments if possible *(1)*. It is from this desire that the popularity of medically managing BPH-associated LUTS emerged.

Currently two classes of medications are commonly used to treat BPH-associated LUTS: αl-adrenergic antagonists and 5α-reductase inhibitors. The 5α-reductase inhibitors act to decrease the size of the adenomatous component of the prostate and are covered elsewhere in this text. This chapter will address the use of α-adrenergic antagonists, or α-blockers, in the treatment of BPH-associated LUTS.

The use of α-blockers to treat BPH originated in the 1970s. Although the early trials of α-blockers demonstrated clinical efficacy, cardiovascular and central nervous system side effects limited their usefulness. The development of agents more specific to the α-receptor sites in the prostate resulted in fewer troublesome side effects and the same beneficial effects. With safe and effective medical treatment available, primary care physicians assumed a more active role in the treatment of BPH, along with urologists, and a dramatic decline in the surgical treatment of male LUTS ensued. The α-receptor antagonists are now considered the first line of therapy for most patients with BPH-associated LUTS *(2)*.

MECHANISM OF ACTION

Many organs in the human body contain α-adrenergic receptors. Those in the urinary tract that are of primary concern are located in the prostate and urethra, with less density of receptors in the bladder *(3)*. Binding of the neurotransmitter norepinephrine to α-receptors in the urinary tract leads ultimately to smooth muscle contraction. The resultant increase in smooth muscle tone may create a restriction of urinary outflow and aggravate voiding symptoms. It has been estimated that approx 40% of bladder outlet obstruction may be caused by smooth muscle contraction. Alpha stimulation has been demonstrated urodynamically to increase resistance to urinary flow *(4)*. As outflow is restricted, changes in detrusor muscle occur and spinal reflexes that may contribute to LUTS also develop *(5)*.

Adenomatous tissue found in BPH tends to have a higher stroma to epithelial ratio when compared to normal prostate. Because smooth muscle is primarily located in the stromal component of prostate, patients with BPH may be hypersensitive to α-adrenergic stimulation *(6)*.

The α-antagonists evoke their pharmacologic effect by blocking the postsynaptic α-receptor sites. In the urinary tract, this ultimately results in decreased smooth muscle tone in the prostate and urethra, with reduction in the restriction of urinary flow and subsequent relief of voiding symptoms. This mechanism may not fully explain the ability of α-blockers to significantly reduce LUTS and improve quality of life. Urodynamic studies on the therapy showed that α-blockers lowered detrusor pressure at maximum flow only 4 cm H2O (7). Symptom relief may be the result of other responses mediated by α1D-receptors (8). The usefulness of α-blockers in the treatment and prevention of acute urinary retention has also been demonstrated (9,10).

Most of the side effects of α-blockers are caused by α-receptors located in vascular smooth muscle, in the brain, and in the spinal cord. Blockade of these receptors can result in commonly reported adverse side effects, including orthostatic hypotension, asthenia, and dizziness.

RECEPTOR CLASSIFICATION

The α- and β-adrenergic receptors differ in location, structure, and function. The β-receptors are located on the smooth muscle of blood vessels, airways, and the uterus, as well as on cells of the pancreas, heart, juxtaglomerular apparatus of the kidney, and the liver. The α-receptors are found on the smooth muscle of blood vessels and the urinary tract and in the central nervous system.

The α-receptors are subdivided into α1 and α2 subgroups. The α2-receptors are presynaptic and, when bound with norepinephrine, act by feedback inhibition to reduce further release of norepinephrine from the stimulated neuron (Fig. 1). The α1-receptors are located on the cell membranes of the target organs, and the binding site located deep within the membrane; they are a subtype of G-protein-coupled receptors (11).

Binding of norepinephrine to the receptor site prompts binding of G-protein, with subsequent disassociation of the α-subunit of the G-protein. This is then activated by means of phosphorylation, and the activated G-protein subunit subsequently binds with and activates phospholipase C. Phospholipase C hydrolyzes membrane phospholipids, yielding second messengers. One of these, inositol triphosphate, causes release of calcium from the sarcoplasmic reticulum and subsequent smooth muscle contraction.

The α-blockers exert their therapeutic effect by inhibiting the binding of norepinephrine to the postsynaptic α1 site (12). Subsequent reduction of intracellular calcium release reduces smooth muscle contraction and decreases the tone of the end organ. Nonspecific α-blockers

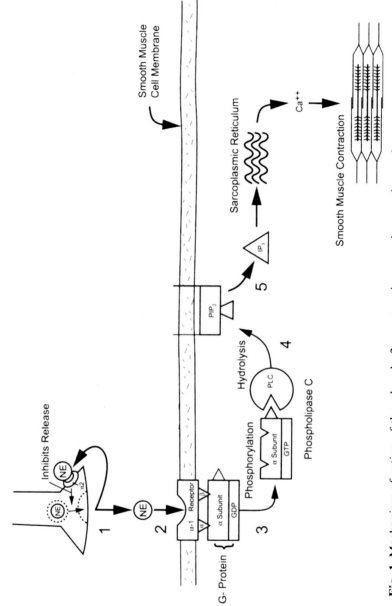

Fig. 1. Mechanism of action of the α1 and α2 receptors in prostatic smooth muscle.

such as phenoxybenzamine block both the α1- and α2-receptors. The α1-specific blockers such as alfuzosin, doxazosin, prazosin, tamsulosin, and terazosin block the α1 sites preferentially.

The α1-receptors have been further classified into subtypes by radioligand binding studies. These include α1A-, α1B-, and α1D-receptors *(13)*. The α1A-receptors constitute approx 70% of the prostatic α1-receptors *(14)*. Subtypes of α1A-receptors include α1A1-receptors (wild type), α1A2-receptors, α1A3-receptors, and α1A4-receptors. These four subtypes demonstrate identical ligand (drug-binding) and second messenger-coupling properties *(13)*.

The α1D-receptor subtypes are found primarily in the bladder and in sacral cord. The α1A-and α1B-receptors are found in human vascular smooth muscle. Their primary effect is exerted in the resistance vessels. As aging occurs, α1B-receptors become predominant.

INITIAL EVALUATION AND SELECTION OF THERAPY

The Agency for Healthcare Policy and Research clinical guidelines for the diagnosis and treatment of BPH provide an approach to the evaluation and therapy for this disease *(15)*. On initial evaluation, taking a medical history and performing a physical examination, including a digital rectal exam, are recommended. Laboratory evaluation includes a urinalysis, creatinine measurement, and optional prostate-specific antigen test.

Surgical intervention should be considered primary therapy for those patients with refractory retention, recurrent urinary tract infection, recurrent or persistent gross hematuria, bladder stones, or renal insufficiency secondary to bladder outlet obstruction. For the remaining patients, quantitative symptom assessment with instruments such as the International Prostate Symptom Score (I-PSS) provide a standardized measurement of symptoms *(16)*. The I-PSS includes a quality of life scale to determine the degree of bother experienced by the patient. The symptom score may be used to monitor response to therapy as well.

Patients with mild symptoms may be offered watchful waiting, medical management, or more invasive therapy. Those with moderate-to-severe symptoms should be considered for more thorough evaluation, including measurement of urinary flow rate and residual urine and pressure/flow studies. If those studies are consistent with bladder outlet obstruction, surgical and medical therapy may be offered along with watchful waiting. Patients with symptoms not caused by BPH should be treated according to the established diagnosis.

Cystoscopy and prostate ultrasonography are optional by the Agency for Healthcare Policy and Research BPH guidelines if they are important in planning the operative approach. Certainly cystoscopy is useful in evaluating patients with hematuria and those with risk factors for transitional cell carcinoma.

Voiding diaries are invaluable in evaluating symptoms and correlate well with symptom scores and quality of life assessments (17). Measurement of volume and voiding frequency will determine bladder functional capacity and may elucidate urine volume abnormalities such as polyuria and nocturnal diuresis. Poorly controlled diabetes mellitus, diabetes insipidus, peripheral edema, or diuretic therapy may produce urine volume abnormalities with complaints similar to those caused by BPH. These symptoms will not likely respond to therapy directed at BPH and should be addressed by treatment of the underlying cause. Voiding diaries may identify problems that may be corrected with lifestyle changes, such as the reduction of caffeine, alcohol, and excess fluid consumption.

In summary, medical therapy of BPH-associated male LUTS is appropriate in patients with mild, moderate, and severe symptoms. Patients desiring medical management do not require invasive testing before initiating therapy. The α-antagonists are an appropriate choice for most patients who desire medical management of LUTS. Those patients with higher prostate-specific antigen levels and larger prostates are those most likely to respond favorably to 5α-reductase inhibitors (18).

SELECTION OF AN α-ANTAGONIST AGENT

Several effective agents are available for those patients with BPH-associated voiding symptoms for whom treatment with α-antagonists is deemed appropriate. These are summarized in Table 1 and will be reviewed in detail.

Phenoxybenzamine

Phenoxybenzamine is presented for historical perspective; it no longer indicated in clinical treatment of BPH. A long-acting, nonselective α-blocker with affinity for both α1- and α2-receptors, its current indication is for treatment of hypertension and sweating associated with pheochromocytoma. Demonstrable pharmacologic effects may persist for 3–4 d after intravenous administration (19).

Early studies of phenoxybenzamine demonstrated therapeutic effect in patients with BPH-associated voiding symptoms. In two large reviews, 80–90% of treated patients reported symptomatic improvement (20,21). Maximum urinary flow rate improvements were noted as well. Significant adverse effects occurred in approx 30% of treated

Table 1
Summary of α-Antagonists in Current Clinical Use for the Treatment of Male LUTS

	Doxazosin	Terazosin	Alfusozin	Tamsulosin
Dosage	1 mg QD, titrate up to 8 mg QD	1 mg QHS, titrate up to 10 mg QHS	2.5 mg TID, or SR 10 mg QD	0.4–0.8 mg QD
Half-life (h)	22	9–12	10	9–15
Drug responses vs placebo (shown in parentheses)				
Change in max flow rate (mL/sec)	2.3–3.3 (0.1–0.7)	2.6–3.0 (1.0–1.4)	1.8–2.6 (0.3–1.1)	1.5–1.8 (0.5–0.9)
Change in max flow rate	23–31% (7–21%)	30–35% (10–16%)	15–29% (3–14%)	15.0–18.6% (5–9%)
Reduction in AUA symptom score	21–37% (12–31%)	42–45% (11–30%)	31–42% (18–32%)	28–48% (19–28%)
Common Adverse Effects				
Hypotension/postural hypotension	1.7%	0.6–3.9%	0.4–0.6%	0.2–0.4%
Headache	9.9%	4.9%	2.4–3.0%	19.3–21.1%
Dizziness	15.6%	9.1%	5.7–9.0%	14.9–17.1%
Asthenia	8%	7.4%	2.7–4.2%	7.8–8.5%
Syncope	0.5%	0.6%	0.2–0.6%	0.2–0.4%
Somnolence	3%	3.6%	1.6%	3.0–4.3%
Erectile/ejaculatory dysfunction	1.1%	1.6%	1.5–2.1%	8.4–18.1%
Nausea	1.5%	1.7%	2.4%	2.6–3.9%
URI symptoms	1.1%	1.9%	5.7–6.1%	13.1–17.9%

Data from references 19,40,41,54.

patients and included dizziness, weakness/lethargy, and palpitations. Side effects were severe enough in 10% of those treated to cause withdrawal from study (20,21).

Ultimately, the long-term use of phenoxybenzamine for LUTS was limited by frequent bothersome side effects, including postural hypotension, tachycardia, ejaculatory dysfunction, nasal congestion, miosis, drowsiness, and fatigue.

Prazosin

Prazosin was already in use for the treatment of hypertension when it became the next α-blocker used for the treatment of BPH. Currently, in the United States it is indicated for the treatment of hypertension and is not in common use for LUTS. It is a short-acting, α1-specific antagonist. Rapid metabolism necessitates dosing two to three times per day. Approximately 1% of patients experience syncopal episodes within 30 to 90 min of the initial dose. Careful titration with initial doses no higher than 1 mg help to minimize this side effect (19).

An early double-blind, placebo-controlled crossover study with 20 patients demonstrated improvement in maximum flow rates and reduction of postvoid residuals with prazosin. Obstructive symptoms improved as well (22). Subsequently, a study involving 80 patients with BPH who were treated with 2 mg twice daily revealed improvement in maximum flow rates in 59% of treated patients vs 6% in the placebo group. Postvoid residuals and frequency decreased significantly. A high (32%) dropout rate was noted (23).

In 1992, 93 patients enrolled in a double-blind, placebo-controlled trial for 3 months compared treatment with 2 mg of prazosin twice daily to treatment with placebo (24). In the 75 patients completing the study, maximum flow rates increased by 2.4 mL/s from baseline in the treatment group. Significant side effects were associated with prazosin, including dizziness in 16.7 vs 10% of patients receiving placebo and headache in 12.6 vs 5% of placebo patients. Symptom relief was less than that found in earlier short-term studies.

Doxazosin

Doxazosin is a long-acting α1-specific antagonist. Peak plasma level after oral ingestion is attained at 2–3 h. After hepatic metabolism, most metabolites are excreted in the feces, with a small amount excreted in the urine. The medication's half-life is approx 22 h. Doxazosin is typically administered at bedtime, with dose titration from 1 mg up to 8 mg over the course of 1–2 wk to minimize hypotensive and syncopal events

(19). Doxazosin is available as an easily divided scored tablet, a feature that facilitates dose titration.

An early trial with a dose of 4 mg per day vs placebo demonstrated improvement in maximum and average urinary flow rates, although not to statistically significant levels. Adverse events were approximately equal in both the treatment and placebo groups *(25)*. Subsequent studies of the 4-mg dose vs placebo over 3 mo of therapy demonstrated no statistically significant improvement in maximum flow rates. There was significant improvement in symptoms of hesitancy, nocturia, urgency, and impaired stream *(26)*.

When higher doses of doxazosin were evaluated (most patients were taking 8 mg daily), there was statistically significant improvement in maximum urinary flow rates and symptom scores *(27)*. Maximum effect was reached after approx 6 wk in this study of 100 patients. Adverse effects were more common in the treatment group and included dizziness, fatigue, headache, somnolence, hypotension, diarrhea, and nausea. The treatment group also demonstrated a decrease in blood pressure. In subsequent large, long-term studies, only those patients receiving the 4-mg and 8-mg dosage had significant reduction in symptom scores, with the 8-mg dose demonstrating greatest efficacy *(28)*.

Terazosin

Terazosin is a long-acting α1-specific antagonist with Food and Drug Administration indications for the treatment of both hypertension and BPH-associated voiding symptoms. After oral administration, it reaches peak plasma levels in approx 1 h and has a serum half-life of 12 h. It undergoes hepatic metabolism, with 60% excretion in the stool and 40% in the urine *(19)*. To minimize risk of first-dose syncope and orthostatic hypotension, dosing is initiated at 1 mg and titrated up to 10 mg over 1–2 wk.

Boyarsky symptom score reduction was demonstrated in a double-blind, placebo-controlled study of 285 patients, and the greatest improvement was noted in the 10-mg dose group *(29)*. Of those receiving 10 mg, 69% had more than 30% improvement in symptom scores, whereas 40% of those receiving placebo experienced that level of symptom relief. Maximum urinary flow rate increased by more than 30% in 52% of those on 10 mg, with an average improvement of 3 mL/s. A greater than 30% improvement in maximum urinary flow rates was achieved in 26% of the placebo group.

Symptom improvement appears to be sustained over long-term treatment *(30)*. As with most trials, significant increases in the incidence of side effects were noted during treatment with terazosin. Dizziness occurred in 6.7%, asthenia in 3.8%, and somnolence in 2%. Other trials demonstrated similar significant side effects including dizziness, asthenia, peripheral edema, chest pain, nausea, and postural hypotension *(31)*.

Varying effects on blood pressure have been reported in patients taking terazosin. Lepor's large trial demonstrated minimal changes in blood pressure in normotensive participants *(30)*. Those with hypertension demonstrated mean reduction in systolic and diastolic blood pressures between 10 and 15 mg. Other reviews found significant decreases in blood pressure in both hypertensive and normotensive subjects *(31,32)*.

Tamsulosin

Tamsulosin is an α1A-specific subtype antagonist designed to maximize prostate activity and minimize systemic side effects. Pharmacologic studies demonstrate 10–12 times greater affinity for prostate receptors vs vascular and extraprostatic receptors *(33,34)*.

Tamsulosin is administered once daily, usually 0.4 mg one-half hour after breakfast. This method of administration is intended to reduce rapid peaking of plasma concentration and subsequently reduce undesirable side effects. The observed half-life of tamsulosin is 14.9 ± 3.9 h, with metabolism occurring primarily in the liver via cytochrome P450 enzymes *(19)*.

Early experience acquired in Europe has been presented. Meta-analysis presented by the European Tamsulosin Study Group reviewed 382 patients treated with tamsulosin in an open-label study *(35)*. Maximum flow rates demonstrated a small improvement, with increases of 1.6 mL/s compared with the placebo group's improvement of 0.6 mL/s. Boyarsky symptom scores improved, with a reduction of 3.3. in the treatment group vs 2.2 in placebo group. Other long-term, open-label studies have demonstrated clinically significant improvement in BPH symptoms in 70% of patients, a result maintained over 12 mo *(36)*.

Phase III clinical trials in the United States involving double-blind, randomized, placebo-controlled studies with 735 patients found doses of 0.4 mg and 0.8 mg to be superior to placebo in relieving symptoms in patients with moderate-to-severe BPH-associated voiding symptoms *(37)*. American Urological Association (AUA) symptom score reduction of greater than or equal to 25% was found in 56% of patients on 0.8 mg, in 55% on 0.4 mg, and in 40% of those on placebo. Symptom relief was found to be rapid in onset with statistically significant improvement in maximum flow rates 4–8 h after a single dose of 0.4 mg. Significant reduction in symptom scores was noted after 1 wk.

Adverse events included upper respiratory tract infections/colds, rhinitis, abnormal ejaculation, and dizziness. The incidence of asthenia was described as minimal. Investigators saw no clinically significant orthostatic hypotension or first-dose associated syncopal episodes but did note the incidence of dizziness and abnormal ejaculation. More patients receiving the 0.8-mg dosage elected to discontinue treatment, with 13% withdrawing from the study. A similar incidence of withdrawal from the study occurred in the placebo and 0.4-mg group, at 9% and 7%, respectively.

A total of 418 patients elected to continue into the extension phase of the study (38). This study demonstrated that symptom relief was durable, with AUA symptom score reduction greater than or equal to 25% found in 78% of those taking 0.8 mg, in 81% taking 0.4 mg, and in 59% of those taking placebo. Maximal flow rate increases of more than or equal to 30% occurred in 38% of those on 0.8 mg, in 40% on 0.4 mg, and in 22% of those on placebo. The 0.8-mg–dose group experienced more side effects than the placebo or 0.4-mg–dose groups. Side effects were similar in the 0.4-mg and placebo groups. The most common reported side effect was cold and upper respiratory infection. Cardiovascular side effects were similar throughout the treatment and placebo groups, ranging from 10 to 14%. Abnormal ejaculation was more common in the treatment arm, affecting 26% in the 0.8-mg group, 10% of those in the 0.4-mg group, and 0% in the placebo group. Adverse events were found to be similar at the end of 13 and 53 wk.

Extensive meta-analysis studies have confirmed the efficacy at commonly prescribed doses (39).

Tamsulosin offers α1A specificity and has therapeutic effects similar to other α-blockers but less significant effects on blood pressure and pulse and minimal cardiovascular adverse events. Rapid onset of clinical effect on voiding symptoms, along with no dose titration, allow rapid assessment of patient's response to therapy. When compared with terazosin and doxazosin, tamsulosin appears to have a lower incidence of dizziness and headaches but increased rates of ejaculatory dysfunction.

Alfuzosin

Alfuzosin has been evaluated and used extensively in Latin America, Asia, and Europe and is not currently in general clinical use in the United States. It has biochemical properties that differentiate it from the other α-antagonists. Although it doesn't demonstrate significant selectivity for receptor subtypes, tissue studies demonstrate high selectivity for prostate over vascular tissues. Animal studies also have demonstrated significantly lower hypotensive effects when administered intravenously in supraclinical dosages. Its chemical properties also impair penetration of the blood-brain barrier, which may reduce central nervous system side effects (40).

When initially introduced, alfuzosin required three-times-daily administration. A sustained release form was subsequently created allowing twice-daily dosing. Most recently, a prolonged-release system was created that allows a single 10-mg dose to be delivered consistently over 24 h. No dosage titration is required. Alfuzosin 10 mg once daily formulation should be administered with a meal to enhance bioavailability.

Early studies performed with 7.5–10 mg administered in three divided doses demonstrated statistically significant improvement in symptom scores, with no significant improvement in maximum flow rates (41). The side effect profile was similar to that of placebo. Alfuzosin has a rapid onset of action. Urodynamic studies have demonstrated significant decreases in maximum detrusor pressure during voiding (42). Postvoid residuals have been demonstrated to be significantly reduced when compared with placebo (43).

In studies comparing alfuzosin with prazosin, similar symptom relief was noted for both drugs, but alfuzosin had fewer side effects (44). A large French study involving 13,389 patients showed no serious adverse events, although some vasodilatory side effects were noted (45).

Double-blind, randomized studies of alfuzosin 10 mg once daily have demonstrated significant reductions of the I-PSS scores compared with placebo, significant improvement in disease-specific quality of life, and significant improvements in peak urinary flow rates (46). A multicenter, randomized, double-blind, placebo-controlled study performed in the United States demonstrated similar results (47). The 15-mg once-daily formulation did not appear to provide additional clinical benefit. The most commonly reported α-antagonist side effect was dizziness, occurring in 5% of those patients taking 10 mg vs 2.1% of those on placebo. The incidence of hypotension was less than 1% in the treatment arms. Ejaculatory dysfunction in one patient each of the 10- and 15-mg treatment groups resolved despite continuing therapy and was thought not to be related to the study medication. No significant cardiac or blood pressure events were noted compared with placebo.

Combination therapy using alfuzosin and finasteride has not been demonstrated to be more effective than alfuzosin alone (48).

α-ANTAGONISTS IN NON-BPH PATIENTS

The α-antagonists have been found to be of potential benefit for children with neuropathic and nonneuropathic voiding dysfunction (49).

Of 17 children with voiding dysfunction treated with doxazosin, 82% demonstrated symptomatic improvement, 59% had reduced postvoid residuals, and 18% demonstrated improvement in peak urinary flow. In two of three patients, new-onset hydronephrosis resolved while they were being treated with doxazosin. A reduction in leak point pressure was also noted on urodynamic studies in some patients. Patients with spinal cord injury and decreased bladder compliance have demonstrated urodynamic improvement when treated with terazosin (50).

Neurologically intact patients with overactive bladders were found to have a four-fold increase in α-receptor density in the detrusor muscle when compared with those with normal bladders. This may provide a possible explanation for the clinical usefulness of α-antagonists in this patient population (51).

Studies in women with LUTS have not shown definite benefit from α-blocker therapy. Further discouraging their use, the development of incontinence has been noted. A double-blind, randomized study comparing terazosin to placebo in women with significant LUTS failed to demonstrate any significant improvement in AUA symptom scores in the treatment group (52). Two patients in the treatment arm developed stress urinary incontinence necessitating cessation of the medication.

In a review of women treated with prazosin, terazosin, or doxazosin for hypertension, 40.8% were found to have complaints of urinary incontinence vs 16.3% in age- and parity-matched controls. After discontinuing the α-blockers, incontinence symptoms abated in 13 of 18 patients (53).

CONCLUSIONS

Although the improvement in symptom scores and urinary flow rates on treatment with α-blockers is not equivalent to the gold standard of TURP, significant clinical improvement is consistently demonstrated. This efficacy along with an acceptable side effect profile and the patient's desire to seek less invasive treatment has lead to a reduction in surgical management of BPH-associated LUTS. Medical management using α-blockers for these symptoms is now considered first-line therapy and is used safely by primary care physicians as well as urologists.

Comparing studies of α-blockers is difficult because of the different instruments used to measure symptom scores, varied exclusion criteria for studies, and varied, sometimes suboptimal, dosages of medication. Relatively large placebo effects are often noted. In general, the therapeutic effects are similar among α-antagonists, with symptom scores improving approx 30 to 50% compared with placebo improvements ranging from 10 to 30%. Whereas most trials have demonstrated clinically significant improvements in urinary symptoms, several trials failed to demonstrate this finding. Maximum urinary flow rates usually improved with α-antagonists, ranging from 20 to 50% vs 0 to 30% in placebo groups. This difference did not reach statistical significance in some trials.

REFERENCES

1. Kaplan SA, Golobuff ET, Olsson CA. Effect of demographic factors, urinary peak flow rates, and Boyarsky symptom scores on patient treatment choice in benign prostatic hypertrophy. Urology 1995;45:398–405.
2. Bruskewitz R. Management of symptomatic BPH in the US: who is treated and how? Eur. Urol. 1999;36(suppl 3):7–13.
3. Lepor H, Tang R, Kobayashi S. Localization of the alpha-1A adrenoreceptor in the human prostate. J Urol 1995;154:2096–2099.
4. Furuya S, Kumamoto Y, Yokoyama E. Alpha-adrenergic activity and urethral pressure in the prostate zone in benign prostate hypertrophy. J Urol 1982; 128:836–839.
5. Lepor H. The pathophysiology of lower urinary tract symptoms in the aging male population. Br J Urol 1998;81(suppl 1):29–33.
6. Bartsch G, Muller HR, Oberholzer M, Rohr HP. Light microscopic stereological analysis of the normal human prostate and of BPH. J Urol 1979;122:487–491.
7. Rossi C, Kortmann B, Sonke G, et al. Alpha-blockade improves symptoms suggestive of bladder outlet obstruction but fail to relieve it. J Urol 2001;165:38–41.
8. Schwinn D, Michelotti G. Alpha-1 adrenoreceptors in the lower urinary tract and vascular bed: potential role for the alpha-1D subtype in filling symptoms and effects of aging on vascular expression. Br J Urol 2000;85(suppl 2):6–11.
9. McNeill SA. Does acute urinary retention respond to alpha-blockers alone? Eur Urol 2001;39(suppl 6):7–12.
10. Hartung R. Do alpha-blockers prevent the occurrence of acute urinary retention? Eur Urol. 2001;39(suppl 6):13–18.
11. Schwinn DA, Price RR. Molecular pharmacology of human alpha 1-adrenergic receptors: unique features of the alpha 1a-subtype. Eur Urol 1999;36(suppl 1):7–10.
12. Schwinn DA. The role of alpha-1 adrenergic receptor subtypes in lower urinary tract symptoms. Br J Urol Int 2001;88(suppl 2):27–34.
13. Schwinn DA. Novel role for alpha-1 adrenergic receptor subtypes in lower urinary tract symptoms. Br J Urol Int 2000;86(suppl 2):11–20.
14. Price DT, Schwinn DA, Lomasney JW, et al. Identification, quantification, and localization of mRNA for three distinct alpha-1 adrenergic receptor subtypes in human prostate. J Urol 1993;150(2 Pt 1):546–551.
15. Benign Prostatic Hyperplasia: Diagnosis and Treatment. Clinical Practice Guideline No. 8. Agency for Health Care Policy and Research Pub. No. 94-0582: February 1994; ahcpr.gov/clinic/medtep/bphguide.htm.
16. El Din KE, Koch WF, de Wildt MJ, et al. Reliability of the International Prostate Symptom Score in the assessment of patients with lower urinary tract symptoms and/or benign prostatic hyperplasia. J Urol 1996;155:1959.
17. Van Venrooij GE, Eckhardt MD, Gisolf KW, Boon TA. Data from frequency-volume charts versus symptoms scores and quality of life score in men with lower urinary tract symptoms due to benign prostatic hyperplasia. Eur Urol 2001;39(1):42–47.

18. Roehrborn CG, Boyle P, Bergner D, et al. Serum prostate-specific antigen and prostate volume predict long-term changes in symptoms and flow rate: results of a four-year, randomized trial comparing finasteride versus placebo. PLESS study group. Urology 1999;54:662–669.
19. Phenoxybenzamine: 1345, Prazosin: 2278, Doxazosin: 2668, Terazosin: 3613, Tamsulosin: 1044. Physicians Desk Reference, Medical Economics Company, Inc., 2002. Package inserts, Montvale, NJ.
20. Caine M, Perlberg S, Shapiro A. Phenoxybenzamine for benign prostatic obstruction. Review of 200 cases. Urology 1981;17:542–546.
21. Abrams PH, Shah PJ, Stone R, Choa RG. Bladder outflow obstruction treated with phenoxybenzamine. Br J Urol 1982;54(5):527–530.
22. Hedlund H, Andersson KE, Ek A. Effects of prazosin in patients with benign prostatic obstruction. J Urol 1983;130:275–278.
23. Kirby RS, Coppinger SW, Corcoran MO, et al. Prazosin in the treatment of prostatic obstruction. A placebo-controlled study. Br J Urol 1987;60(2):136–142.
24. Chapple CR, Stott M, Abrams PH, Christmas TJ, Milroy EJ. A 12-week placebo-controlled double-blind study of prazosin in the treatment of prostatic obstruction due to benign prostatic hyperplasia. Br J Urol 1992;70(3):285–294.
25. Christensen MM, Holme J, Rasmussen PC, et al. Doxazosin treatment in patients with prostatic obstruction. Scand J Urol Nephrol 1993;27(1):39–44.
26. Chapple CR, Carter P, Christmas TJ, et al. A three month double-blind study of doxazosin as treatment for benign prostatic bladder outlet obstruction.: Br J Urol 1994;74(1):50–56.
27. Gillenwater JY, Mobley DL. A sixteen week, double blind, placebo-controlled, dose-titration study using doxazosin tablets for the treatment of benign prostatic hyperplasia (BPH) in normotensive males. J Urol 1993;149(suppl A):324.
28. Gillenwater JY, Conn RL, Chrysant SG, et al. Doxazosin for the treatment of benign prostatic hyperplasia in patients with mild to moderate essential hypertension: a double-blind, placebo-controlled, dose-response multicenter study. J Urol 1995;154(1):110–115.
29. Lepor H, Auerbach S, Puras-Baez A, et al. A randomized, placebo-controlled multicenter study of the efficacy and safety of terazosin in the treatment of benign prostatic hyperplasia. J Urol 1992;148(5):1467–1474.
30. Lepor H. Long-term efficacy and safety of terazosin in patients with benign prostatic hyperplasia. Terazosin Research Group. Urology 45(3):406–413.
31. Lowe FC. Safety assessment of terazosin in the treatment of patients with symptomatic benign prostatic hyperplasia: a combined analysis. Urology 1994; 44(1):46–51.
32. Wilde MI, Fitton A, Sorkin EM. Terazosin. A review of its pharmacodynamic and pharmacokinetic properties, and therapeutic potential in benign prostatic hyperplasia. Drugs Aging 1993;3(3):258–277.
33. Yamada S, Tanaka C, Kimura R, Kawabe K. Alpha-1 adrenoreceptors in human prostate: characterization and binding characteristics of alpha-1 antagonists. Life Sci 1994;54(24):1845–1854.
34. Yamada S, Tanaka C, Oukura T. High-affinity specific tamsulosin binding to alpha-1 adrenoreceptors in human prostates with benign prostatic hypertrophy. Urol Res 1994;22(5):273–278.
35. Chapple CR, Wyndaele JJ, Nordling J, et al. Tamsulosin, the first prostate-selective alpha 1A-adrenoceptor antagonist. A meta-analysis of two randomized, placebo-controlled, multicentre studies in patients with benign prostatic obstruction (symptomatic BPH). European Tamsulosin Study Group. Eur Urol 1996;29(2):155–167.

36. Schulman CC, Cortvriend J, Jonas U, et al. Tamsulosin, the first prostate-selective alpha 1A-adrenoceptor antagonist. Analysis of a multinational, multicentre, open-label study assessing the long-term efficacy and safety in patients with benign prostatic obstruction (symptomatic BPH). European Tamsulosin Study Group. Eur Urol 1996;29(2):145–154.

37. Lepor H. Phase III multicenter placebo-controlled study of tamsulosin in benign prostatic hyperplasia. Tamsulosin Investigator Group. Urology 1998; 51(6):892–900.

38. Lepor H. Long-term evaluation of tamsulosin in benign prostatic hyperplasia: placebo-controlled, double-blind extension of phase III trial. Tamsulosin Investigator Group. Urology 1998;51(6):901–906.

39. Wilt TJ, MacDonald R, Nelson D. Tamsulosin for treating lower urinary tract symptoms compatible with benign prostatic obstruction: a systematic review of efficacy and adverse effects. J Urol 2002;167:177–183.

40. Roehrborn CG. Alfuzosin: overview of pharmacokinetics, safety, and efficacy of a clinically uroselective alpha-blocker. Urology 2001;58(6 suppl 1):55–63.

41. Jardin A, Bensadoun H, Delauche-Cavallier MC, Attali P. Alfuzosin for treatment of benign prostatic hypertrophy. The BPH-ALF Group. Lancet 1991;337:1457–1461.

42. Martorana G, Giberti C, Di Silverio F, et al. Effects of short-term treatment with the alpha 1-blocker alfuzosin on urodynamic pressure/flow parameters in patients with benign prostatic hyperplasia. Eur Urol 1997;32(1):47–53.

43. McNeill SA, Hargreave TB, Geffriaud-Ricouard C, Santoni J, Roehrborn CG. Postvoid residual urine in patients with lower urinary tract symptoms suggestive of benign prostatic hyperplasia: pooled analysis of eleven controlled studies with alfuzosin. Urology 2001;57(3):459–465.

44. Buzelin JM, Hebert M, Blondin P. Alpha-blocking treatment with alfuzosin in symptomatic benign prostatic hyperplasia: comparative study with prazosin. The PRAZALF Group. Br J Urol 1993;72(6):922–927.

45. Lukacs B, Blondin P, MacCarthy C, et al. Safety profile of 3 months' therapy with alfuzosin in 13,389 patients suffering from benign prostatic hypertrophy. Eur Urol 1996;29(1):29–35.

46. van Kerrebroeck P, Jardin A, Laval KU, van Cangh P. Efficacy and safety of a new prolonged release formulation of alfuzosin 10 mg once daily versus alfuzosin 2.5 mg thrice daily and placebo in patients with symptomatic benign prostatic hyperplasia. ALFORTI Study Group. Eur Urol 2000; 37(3):306–313.

47. Roehborn C. Efficacy ans safety of once-daily alfuzonsin in the treatment of lower urinary tract symptoms and clinical benign prostatic hyperplasia: a randomized, placebo-controlled trial. Urology 2001;58(6):953–959.

48. Debryne FM, Jardin A, Collon D, et al. Sustained release alfuzosin, finasteride and the combination of both in the treatment of benign prostate hyperplasia. European ALFIN study group. Eur Urol 1998;34:169–175.

49. Austin PF, Homsy YL, Masel JL, et al. Alpha-adrenergic blockade in children with neuropathic and non-neuropathic voiding dysfunction. J Urol 1999; 162(3 Pt 2):1064–1067.

50. Swierzewski SJ, Gormley EA, Belville WD, et al. The effect of terazosin on bladder function in the spinal cord injured patient. J Urol 1994;151(4):951–954.

51. Restorick JM, Mundy AR. The density of cholinergic and alpha and beta adrenergic receptors in the normal and hyper-reflexic human detrusor. Br J Urol 1989;63:32–35.

52. Lepor H, Theune C. Randomized double-blind study comparing the efficacy of terazosin versus placebo in women with prostatism-like symptoms. J Urol 1995;154(1):116–118.
53. Marshall HJ, Beevers DG. Alpha-adrenoceptor blocking drugs and female urinary incontinence: prevalence and reversibility. Br J Clin Pharmacol 1996; 42(4):507–509.

6   5α-Reductase Inhibitors

Robert E. Brannigan, MD
and John T. Grayhack, MD

CONTENTS

INTRODUCTION
ANDROGEN AND PROSTATE GROWTH
DEVELOPMENT OF 5α-REDUCTASE INHIBITORS
FINASTERIDE MOLECULAR KINETICS
USE OF FINASTERIDE IN THE TREATMENT OF BPH
FINASTERIDE PHASE III CLINICAL TRIALS
PROSCAR LONG-TERM EFFICACY AND SAFETY STUDY
ADDITIONAL CLINICAL TRIALS
HISTOLOGIC EFFECTS OF FINASTERIDE THERAPY
LONG-TERM URODYNAMIC CHANGES
    WITH FINASTERIDE THERAPY
FINASTERIDE TREATMENT AND PSA CONCENTRATION
FUTURE DIRECTIONS IN FINASTERIDE THERAPY
REFERENCES

INTRODUCTION

Although transurethral resection of the prostate (TURP) has been the gold standard for management of symptomatic benign prostate hyperplasia (BPH) for more than 50 years, surgery is not appropriate for all patients. Issues such as risk of anesthesia, postoperative recovery time, potential complications associated with TURP, and a desire to avoid surgery lead many patients to pursue medical therapy. Surgical therapy will continue to be the treatment of choice in men with severe obstructive symptoms, but for men with mild-to-moderate symptoms and for those who are not candidates for TURP, medical therapy is a mainstay treatment option.

From: *Management of Benign Prostatic Hypertrophy*
Edited by: K. T. McVary © Humana Press Inc., Totowa, NJ

The two main classes of medications currently available for the treatment of symptomatic BPH target different prostatic-growth promoting characteristics. The α1-receptor blockers, discussed in a separate chapter, seek to alter smooth muscle tone. Alternatively, the 5α-reductase inhibitors discussed here seek to control and reverse androgen-induced prostate growth.

ANDROGEN AND PROSTATE GROWTH

The prostate gland is dependent on androgens that are produced exogenously by the testicles to facilitate normal development and to maintain normal structure and function (1). Briefly, the testes are stimulated to produce and secrete testosterone and other steroids by an exogenous protein, luteinizing hormone, which is made in the pituitary gland. Testosterone (T) is converted to its reduced form, dihydrotestosterone (DHT), by the enzyme 5α-reductase in the prostate. Both T and DHT bind to and activate the androgen receptor, causing a cascade of events that results in stimulation and maintenance of prostatic epithelial and stromal growth and secretion. DHT has a greater affinity for the androgen receptor than T and is normally the major prostate growth stimulant. Currently, attempts to interrupt or alter the stimulatory effects of exogenous factors that control prostate growth target aspects of the pituitary-testis-prostate axis. One approach is to alter the production and secretion of testosterone by altering pituitary function or removing the testis. Another method is inhibition of the prostate stimulatory effects of local conversion of T to the more biologically active DHT. A final method is prevention of activation of the anabolic metabolic cascade by interference with DHT/T androgen-receptor binding.

Androgen deprivation by any of these mechanisms leads to dramatic changes in both prostate anatomy and function. Flutamide, an oral nonsteroidal androgen-receptor antagonist, competitively inhibits testosterone and DHT binding to androgen receptor sites. This results in significant histologic changes in prostate tissue, including squamous metaplasia, fibrosis, basal cell hypertrophy, and lymphocytic infiltration (2). Functional prostatic changes represented by decreases in prostate secretions have also been noted in the ejaculate of patients treated with flutamide androgen blockade (3). It is known that surgical castration by means of orchiectomy also results in profound changes in prostate anatomy and physiology. In the 1940s, Huggins and Stevens demonstrated that significant prostatic atrophy occurred in patients with BPH within 3 mo after orchiectomy (4). Subsequent work has shown that castration results in increased DNA synthesis within the prostate,

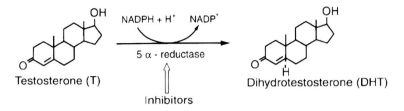

Fig. 1. Mechanism of conversion of testosterone (T) to dihydrotestosterone (DHT).

with an approx 90% decrease in the epithelial glandular component and an approx 20% involution of the stromal glandular component *(5,6)*. Medical and surgical castration lead to inducible gene expression, which is an active process that results in apoptosis in androgen-dependent prostate cells *(7,8)*. Impairment in prostate growth and function are changes associated with androgen depletion. Androgen levels can be restored in medically treated patients with cessation of therapy and in postorchidectomy patients who are given androgen-replacement therapy *(9)*.

T, the primary androgen secreted by the testis, has a direct stimulatory effect on androgen-dependent activities in skeletal muscle, in the brain, and in testicular seminiferous tubules. However, DHT is the primary androgen present in the prostate gland *(10)*. T is converted to DHT by 5α-reductase (Fig. 1). Two isozymes for 5α-reductase exist: type I and type II. Type I 5α-reductase is present in the liver and in the skin (sebaceous glands), and in small amounts in the prostate. Type II 5α-reductase is present in the prostate, liver, chest skin, beard, and scalp (hair follicles). Within the prostate gland, 90% of androgens are in the form of DHT. In 1970, Siiteri et al. postulated that DHT secretion might be associated with the development of BPH *(11)*. Although T and DHT both bind to the same androgen receptor, DHT binds with greater affinity and forms a more stable complex than T. Additionally, the DHT-receptor complex stimulates a greater increase in androgen-receptor concentration. The binding of the DHT-receptor complex to nuclear DNA initiates a cascade of androgen-dependent gene transcription and protein synthesis (Fig. 2).

The critical role of 5α-reductase in normal male development was documented in two important independent publications in 1974. These papers reported observations in two geographically separate groups in Texas and in the village of Salinas in the Dominican Republic *(12,13)*. The investigators described the development of male primary and secondary sexual characteristics within individuals with congenital

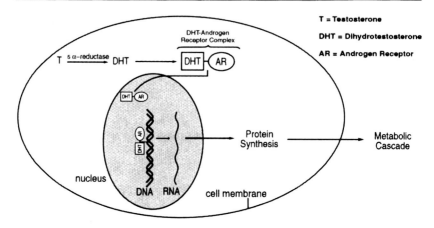

Fig. 2. Conversion of testosterone to dihydrotestosterone within the prostate.

deficiencies in 5α-reductase production. Men affected by this auto-somal-recessive disorder have impaired embryonic differentiation of the external genitalia and prostate glands. Phenotypically, these individuals, born as pseudohermaphrodites with a 46,XY karyotype, have normal testes (presenting as inguinal or labial masses), a scrotum resembling a labia, and normal epididymides and vas deferens. Although their underdeveloped phallus resembles a clitoris, they have severe hypospadias and a urogenital sinus with a blind-ending vaginal pouch. They routinely have a prostate gland that is poorly formed.

Walsh et al. examined a group of patients from Texas, and Imperato-McGinley studied a group of patients from a single village in the Dominican Republic, Salinas, where inbreeding was common *(12,13)*. Both studies are experiments of nature observed by two insightful groups, and the anatomic features as well as the natural history of the condition are detailed in these papers. Both groups of patients had congenital deficiency in 5α-reductase activity. The children from the Dominican Republic were typically raised as girls from birth until puberty, when they underwent virilizing changes. These changes included scrotal rugation and hyperpigmentation, penile growth and function, increase in skeletal muscle mass, deepening voice, testicular descent, and development of the ability to ejaculate. Testicular biopsies revealed complete spermatogenesis and normal Leydig cells. These individuals demonstrated male psychosocial orientation. Despite these masculinizing changes, several other hallmark features of puberty were missing in these individuals. Specifically, they developed a scanty beard, if any at all. Also, the 5α-reductase-deficient group experienced neither male-pattern baldness nor acne. More importantly, it was observed that their prostate glands, which were poorly developed at birth, grew minimally after puberty despite other masculinizing changes. It was this observation, which is directly tied to the deficiency in 5α-reductase activity, that led researchers to consider the possibility of therapeutic inhibition of 5α-reductase enzymes in the treatment of symptomatic BPH.

DEVELOPMENT OF 5α-REDUCTASE INHIBITORS

As discussed, although other approaches to androgen ablation and androgen inhibition (antiandrogens) have been evaluated in the past, these methods produced only a moderate desired impact and had many side effects, thus limiting their use (14). Typical antiandrogen (e.g., flutamide) side effects include onset of erectile dysfunction, impairment in libido and ejaculation, gastrointestinal distress, nausea, flatulence, gynecomastia, breast pain, diminished energy levels, impairment in spermatogenesis, and decreased muscle mass. In contrast, because mature (postpubertal) patients with 5α-reductase deficiency did not appear to have impaired sexual function or diminished external masculinization, the 5α-reductase enzyme was a logical target for treating men with clinically significant BPH. The potential blockade of 5α-reductase seemed to provide hope for decreasing prostate growth and minimizing side effects.

Investigators began to work to create an effective 5α-reductase inhibitor to treat BPH. Early research included the development of 3-oxosteroid compounds. Unfortunately, these agents were rapidly inactivated or metabolized, thus limiting their clinical usefulness (15). Subsequently, 4-aza-3-oxosteroid derivatives of testosterone were developed. However, in addition to their effective 5α-reductase inhibition properties, many of the early agents also demonstrated partial antiandrogenic effects such as those described previously, thus diminishing their clinical usefulness. In 1994 researchers developed finasteride (MK-906), a 4-azasteroid compound that showed great promise for clinical efficacy with minimal side effects. A critical feature of finasteride was its stable A-ring that resembled the transition state between T and DHT (Fig. 3). This stable A-ring permits finasteride to bind with high affinity to the active site of the 5α-reductase enzyme, thus preventing the enzyme from acting on T. Finasteride treatment was subsequently found to decrease 5α-reductase activity in prostate tissue by 100-fold in comparison to tissue from placebo-treated control patients (16). Furthermore, finasteride was shown to be capable of

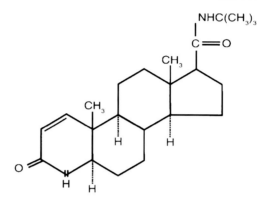

Fig. 3. Molecular formula of finasteride. Permission obtained from Proscar®
product monograph. Rahway, NJ: Merck & Co, 1993.

blocking 5α-reductase without affecting the binding of T to the androgen receptor (17). These features are critical to the potential maintenance of fertility, libido, erectile function, and secondary sexual
characteristics.

Stoner reported in 1992 that men taking finasteride 5 mg/day had a
25% decrease in ejaculate volume, but no changes were noted in total
sperm count, motility, or sperm morphology (18). Other studies have
shown that finasteride at doses 543 times human exposure did not negatively affect fertility, sperm concentration, or ejaculate volume in sexually mature male rabbits (19). Finally, finasteride was found not to exert
any estrogenic or other steroid hormone effects, which had been a problem with some of the earlier investigational compounds (17).

FINASTERIDE MOLECULAR KINETICS

In humans, a single oral dose of 5 mg of finasteride leads to rapid
absorption, with peak plasma concentrations seen 1–2 h after administration. Ninety percent of circulating finasteride is bound to plasma
proteins; in a study of 15 young, healthy subjects, the bioavailability
was 63% (19). Finasteride ingestion leads to a rapid drop in serum DHT
concentration, with the maximal effect seen within 8 h of administration
and persisting throughout the 24-h dosing-interval (19).

The finasteride 5α-reductase complex is highly stable, and its turn-
over is quite slow, with a half-life of approx 30 d. The elimination half-
life of finasteride is 6 h, and metabolism is achieved by means of the
cytochrome P450 system within the liver. Excretion occurs primarily
through the bile (20). No clinically significant drug interactions have

been identified, and specific testing has been conducted with digoxin, propanolol, theophylline, warfarin, and antipyrine. As a result of 5α-reductase inhibition, the mean serum concentration of testosterone increases by 10–20%. However, these levels typically remain within normal physiologic limits *(19)*.

USE OF FINASTERIDE IN THE TREATMENT OF BPH

BPH is an extremely common condition that affects most men age 55 yr and older. BPH develops almost exclusively in the periurethral and transition zone tissues within the prostate gland. The cause of BPH is not known; androgens are necessary but not sufficient to initiate and maintain subsequent growth. Histologically, hyperplastic nodules develop in part as a result of prolonged exposure of prostatic tissue to androgens *(1,21)*. Clinical symptoms compatible with BPH are present in most men over 60 yr of age. These lower urinary tract symptoms often include obstructive symptoms such as diminished force of stream, hesitancy, and postvoid dribbling *(22)*. Over time, these obstructive changes can lead to bladder dysfunction, with related symptoms such as urgency, straining, and urgency incontinence. In severe cases, hydronephrosis and chronic renal impairment may develop.

Urinary tract symptoms and urinary flow rates tend to worsen over time, although there is not a direct correlation between an individual's prostate size and his symptoms *(23)*. This is logical because a patient may have profound enlargement of the transition zone without accompanying urethral obstruction. Conversely, obstruction is seen in some men without much overall change in their prostate volume. The topographic arrangement and possibly the capsular tone of the gland seem to be more important than the actual prostate volume in determining onset of secondary urinary tract symptoms.

Three clinical parameters that are commonly measured in patients with BPH at baseline and after initiation of treatment include prostate size, urinary flow rate, and symptom scores. Prostate size and flow rate are objective variables that can be readily assessed by the physician during routine office visits. Patient symptom scores and other questionnaires are also widely used to delineate symptoms. Many of these are modified versions of the symptom index survey designed by Boyarsky and associates *(24)*. Obtaining baseline measurements before initiating therapy allows longitudinal tracking of specific symptoms. The decision to actively treat the patient is often based on the degree of bother that the patient experiences. As described in the following section, these symptom questionnaires are an important component of patient follow-up and have been routinely used in finasteride clinical trials, along with assessment of change in prostate size and uroflow rate.

FINASTERIDE PHASE III CLINICAL TRIALS

Two separate phase III clinical trials studying symptomatic patients with palpably enlarged prostates were conducted to evaluate the safety and efficacy of finasteride in treating symptomatic BPH. These 12-mo studies of men receiving either 5 mg of finasteride or placebo daily were performed in a randomized, double-blind, placebo-controlled fashion. In the first trial, the North American Study, men who received finasteride 5 mg/d ($n = 297$ patients) had a decrease in prostate volume of 19% vs a 3% drop noted in men taking placebo ($n = 300$ patients) *(25)*. In the International Study, also known as the Finasteride Study Group, men receiving 5 mg/d of finasteride experienced a 22% drop in prostate volume, compared to a 5% drop in the placebo group *(26)*. Regarding maximum urinary flow rate, men in the North American Study group treated with 5 mg/d of finasteride had a statistically significant but clinically limited increase in maximum flow rate of 1.6 mL/s; men receiving placebo were found to have a gain of only 0.2 mL/s. Similar results of 3.7 mL/s mean difference in maximum urinary flow rate with finasteride 5 mg/day compared with placebo were observed after initiation of treatment in the International Study. A significant but limited improvement in urinary symptoms on a modified Boyarsky questionnaire accompanied these changes *(24–26)*.

In both phase III trials, adverse side effects associated with finasteride were evaluated. On the basis of these studies, finasteride was shown to be clinically safe. The incidence of adverse side effects for finasteride patients in both studies was limited and was generally quite similar to the incidence in placebo patients. Exceptions to this included a higher incidence of decreased libido, erectile dysfunction, and diminished ejaculate volume in patients receiving finasteride.

The phase III trials were extended in an open-label fashion for up to 7 yr. No increase in adverse events was noted over the course of the open-label component, and the total incidence of study drop-outs as a result of sexual adverse events was 2–3 % over the 5- to 7-yr extension period *(27,28)*. More importantly, the decrease in prostate volume seen at the end of the first 12 mo of treatment was maintained throughout the next 5 yr of open-label study, and gains in urinary flow rate and symptom score were maintained and even increased during the 4-yr extension. The issue of patient selection for these open-label studies is obviously a possible confounding variable. However, the results suggested that long-term use of finasteride effectively sustained the limited gains seen after 12 mo in prostate volume, urinary flow rate, and symptom score, with an excellent safety and tolerability profile.

PROSCAR LONG-TERM EFFICACY AND SAFETY STUDY

After the phase III studies, finasteride was further evaluated in a 4-yr, multicenter, double-blind, placebo-controlled, randomized study called PLESS or Proscar Long-Term Efficacy and Safety Study *(29)*. The goals of this study were to compare long-term (4-yr) treatment with finasteride 5 mg vs placebo in the following parameters: urinary symptoms, urinary flow rates, incidence of surgery for BPH, and acute urinary retention. There were 3040 men enrolled, with a mean age of 64 yr. To be eligible for randomization, subjects had to exhibit moderate-to-severe urinary symptoms, enlarged prostate gland on digital rectal exam (DRE), serum prostate specific antigen (PSA) concentration < 10 ng/mL, and peak urinary flow rate < 15 mL/s. Furthermore, men with PSA concentrations greater than or equal to 4 mg/mL and < 10 mg/mL had to undergo screening prostate biopsies to rule out the presence of prostate cancer before undergoing randomization.

In this study, 1524 men were randomized to finasteride, and 1516 were randomized to placebo. A total of 1833 patients completed the study, 1000 in the finasteride group and 833 in the placebo group. Differences between the two groups were evident within 4 mo of the start of the study and continued to increase throughout the study. Specifically, 152 patients in the placebo group (10%) and 69 patients in the finasteride group (5%) underwent surgical procedures for BPH. This represented a risk reduction of 55% with finasteride ($p < 0.001$). Acute urinary retention developed in 99 men in the placebo group (6.5%) and 42 men in the finasteride group (2.8%), a risk reduction of 57% for the finasteride group ($p < 0.001$). When the issue of retention was examined more closely, patients taking finasteride were found to have a statistically significant decreased risk for both spontaneous and precipitated acute urinary retention. Despite the large risk reduction, it should be noted that the overall risk for retention in both the placebo and finasteride arms of the study was relatively low.

Men in both the finasteride and placebo groups experienced a reduction in symptom scores over the first 8 mo of the study. However, from that point on, only the finasteride group had a continued decline in symptom scores. The mean decrease in symptom scores for men in the finasteride group was 2.6 and 1.0 for men in the placebo group. For men completing PLESS, the finasteride group mean symptom score dropped by 3.3 points, and the mean symptom score for the placebo group dropped by 1.3 points.

Throughout PLESS, the prostate volume for the placebo group progressively increased. In contrast, the patients taking finasteride had a drop in prostate volume during the first year of the study, with no subsequent increase in prostate volume during the remaining years. Among men who completed the study, the mean change in prostate volume was a drop of 18% for patients taking finasteride and a gain of 14% for men on placebo. The mean difference between the two groups was 32% and was statistically significant ($p < 0.001$).

Men in both the finasteride and placebo groups attained an improvement in maximal urinary flow rate, with a mean increase in the finasteride group of 1.9 mL/s and 0.2 mL/s in the placebo group. This difference was also statistically significant (mean difference = 1.7 mL/s; $p < 0.001$) but limited. This disparity in improvement in flow rates between the two groups was evident within the first 4 mo and was maintained throughout the study.

No difference in the incidence of serious adverse events between the two groups was observed. In fact, the only adverse effects that were drug-related and for which the incidence was greater than or equal to 1% and greater than placebo were symptoms of sexual dysfunction (impotence, decreased libido, decreased ejaculate volume, ejaculation disorder), breast enlargement/tenderness, and rash. Interestingly, two cases of breast cancer were diagnosed in the placebo group; neither man had an antecedent history of gynecomastia. No cases of breast cancer were detected in the finasteride group during the study.

Serum PSA levels and DREs were closely followed throughout the course of the study. During this time, prostate biopsies were performed in 325 men in the finasteride group and in 320 men in the placebo group. The incidence of prostate cancer was 5% in each group; no difference was observed between those taking finasteride and those taking placebo.

The key result from the PLESS study was that finasteride therapy diminished the risk of both acute urinary retention and the need for prostatic surgery. These findings were observed within the first 4 mo of the study and persisted for the rest of the 4-yr investigational period. The investigators noted that to prevent one event of acute urinary retention or surgery, 15 men would need to be treated for 4 yr (29). Although α-adrenergic antagonists clearly improve urinary symptoms for BPH patients, this class of drugs has not yet been shown to diminish the incidence of acute urinary retention or need for surgical therapy (30,31). The PLESS investigators noted that the decrease in need for surgery is important from a public health and financial standpoint, especially given that TURP is the second most commonly performed operative procedure in men over 65 yr of age *(29)*. However, whereas the drop in relative risk for surgery is notable (55%), the percentage of men confronted with the need for surgery was fairly low (only 10% in the placebo group). Furthermore, when reviewing the PLESS data, it is critical to consider this study's entry criteria. All enrolled subjects had moderate-to-severe symptoms and an enlarged prostate on DRE. The findings of diminished risk of acute urinary retention and decreased likelihood for surgical procedures may not be applicable to patients who do not also have these characteristics.

ADDITIONAL CLINICAL TRIALS

Three other double-blind, placebo-controlled, randomized, multicenter studies were conducted to evaluate finasteride vs placebo in terms of onset of urinary retention, need for catheterization, and need for surgical procedure. These studies included the Scandinavian Study on Reduction of the Prostate by Andersen et al. *(32)*, Proscar Safety Plus Efficacy Canadian 2-Year Study by Nickel *(33)*, and the Proscar Worldwide Efficacy and Safety Study *(33a)*.

Andersen and associates performed a post-hoc analysis of 4477 patients with moderate symptoms who participated in the above three studies *(34,35)*. Acute urinary retention developed in 55 patients in the placebo arm and 19 in the finasteride group. Additionally, 146 patients in the placebo group underwent surgical intervention, whereas only 95 patients taking finasteride had operative procedures performed. Statistically, patients taking finasteride were three times less likely to have acute urinary retention ($p < 0.001$) and 1 1/2 times less likely to require surgery than patients taking placebo ($p < 0.001$). The results of these three previously published trials were thus quite similar to those of the PLESS data.

Tempany and associates performed a 1-yr study evaluating the impact of finasteride on prostate volume as measured by magnetic resonance imaging (MRI) *(36)*. Patients given 1- and 5-mg doses of finasteride were grouped together because there was not a significant difference in their results. After 12 mo of treatment, patients receiving finasteride had a significant decline in their total prostate volume (11.5 ± 3.2 mL; $p < 0.02$). Additionally, the change in periurethral zone volume (6.2 ± 3.0 mL; $p < 0.03$) was statistically significant. This was the first study to demonstrate that androgen deprivation leads to a significant decrease in the size of the periurethral zone in men with BPH, and the investigators postulated that it was this effect that led to improvement in clinical symptoms of BPH.

HISTOLOGIC EFFECTS OF FINASTERIDE THERAPY

Rittmaster et al. evaluated the effects of finasteride from a histologic perspective in their 1996 study *(7)*. Tissue was collected from men with BPH who were 52–82 yr old at the time of prostatectomy. Patient groups included controls not taking finasteride, patients taking finasteride 5 mg/d for 6–18 days, patients taking finasteride 5 mg/d for 23–73 days, and patients taking finasteride 5 mg/d for 3 mo–4 yr. Epithelial cell width and ductal width were measured. Apoptosis was determined by immunostaining for double-strand DNA breaks and tissue transglutaminase. The investigators found that, compared with controls, patients treated with finasteride had diminished intraprostatic DHT levels and elevated intraprostatic T levels. Additionally, finasteride-treated patients had diminished epithelial cell width and diminished ductal width. For each parameter assessed (epithelial cell width and ductal width), increased length of finasteride treatment led to more pronounced histologic atrophic change. Maximal decline in epithelial cell width and ductal width occurred at 4 mo after initiation of finasteride therapy. On inspection of stromal cells, the investigators found that little overall histologic change had occurred. However, some of the patients on longer courses of finasteride exhibited increased stromal positive staining for DNA breaks and tissue transglutaminase, signs of increased apoptotic activity in the stromal tissue. The investigators concluded that a combination of atrophic changes and frank apoptosis, primarily in the epithelial cells, together lead to the diminishment in prostatic volume with finasteride therapy.

Fenley and associates performed a 6-mo randomized, placebo-controlled study to determine the biochemical and histologic effects of finasteride therapy and their clinical correlates in terms of symptomatic response *(37)*. The researchers determined that type 2,5α-reductase was severely inhibited by finasteride, with the resultant drop in type 2:type 1 activity from 2.7 to 0.07 ($p = 0.001$). The maximal volume change occurred in the transition zone, again with greater change seen in the epithelial component. For the first time, this study also demonstrated that finasteride therapy does lead to a drop in human prostatic type 2,5α-reductase activity.

In an attempt to identify factors predictive of a response to finasteride, Marks and associates studied 40 men with symptomatic BPH for 6 mo in a randomized, placebo-controlled, prospective trial *(38)*. MRI was used to follow prostate volume changes. The investigators found that finasteride-induced prostate volume change was correlated in a positive linear fashion with inner gland epithelial cell volume assessed at the start of the study ($p = 0.01$). Thus, the researchers concluded that finasteride caused a selective inhibition of periurethral and transition zone epithelium.

Finally, Montironi et al. examined prostatectomy specimens from six patients who had symptomatic BPH but whose disease did not respond adequately to finasteride (representative of 5% of the patients treated with finasteride) *(39)*. These patients underwent prostate adenoma removal during finasteride therapy. Twenty untreated age-matched controls were also evaluated. The investigators found that finasteride diminished the transition zone lobules but not the periurethral stroma in patients whose disease did not respond to long-term finasteride therapy. Specifically, compared with untreated BPH controls, those whose disease did not respond to finasteride demonstrated an increase in the stroma:epithelial and stroma:lumen ratios. The researchers concluded that lack of clinical efficacy of finasteride on stroma cells (including smooth muscle cells) might be the primary reason for finasteride failure, independent of the patient's epithelial cell response to treatment.

LONG-TERM URODYNAMIC CHANGES WITH FINASTERIDE THERAPY

Urodynamic studies have been used by urologists as a tool to study lower urinary tract function for over 50 years. In patients with BPH, several changes can occur when the hyperplastic prostate tissue obstructs the urethral orifice. Specifically, urethral resistance to flow rises, urinary flow rate drops, and detrusor pressure rises.

Kirby and associates found a mean increase in urinary flow rates of 2.7 mL/s after 1 yr when comparing patients taking 5 or 10 mg of finasteride per day with patients taking placebo *(40)*. Furthermore, patients who continued in the study taking 5 mg/d for 3 yr (open extension) demonstrated improved maximal urinary flow rates from 8.7 mL/s to 13.8 mL/s and decreased mean maximal subtracted voiding pressure from 72 cm H2O to 49 cm H2O. However, the authors concluded that the maximal therapeutic effects are not seen until after 1 yr of therapy.

In 1996, Lepor and the Veterans Affairs Cooperative Studies Benign Prostatic Hyperplasia Study Group published a manuscript detailing the efficacy of terazosin, finasteride, or both in treating BPH. Placebo, terazosin (10 mg/d), finasteride (5 mg/d), and combination finasteride/terazosin therapy were compared after 1 yr of treatment. The investigators found that peak urinary flow rates were equally affected by finasteride and placebo. Furthermore, finasteride and terazosin combination therapy was no more effective than terazosin alone in improving flow rates. They concluded that in BPH, terazosin was effective therapy, whereas finasteride was not, and that the combination of terazosin/finasteride treatment was no more effective than terazosin alone.

In 1999, Schafer and associates in the Finasteride Urodynamics Study Group found that, compared with placebo-treated patients, finasteride-treated patients experienced a significant decrease in detrusor pressure at maximum flow and a significant increase in maximum flow rate *(41)*. Patients in this study who had enlarged prostate glands (> 40 mL volume) demonstrated greater improvement in urodynamic parameters.

Additionally, Roehrborn and associates evaluated the PLESS data in 1999 and found that baseline PSA and prostate volume were both good predictors of posttreatment changes in symptom scores and flow rates *(42)*. Baseline PSA levels > 1.4 ng/mL and enlarged prostate glands were parameters predictive of effective patient response to long-term finasteride treatment.

Collectively, these studies suggest that careful patient evaluation is essential in properly selecting individuals who will demonstrate urodynamic improvement as a result of finasteride therapy. Patients with small prostate glands (< 40 mL volume) and low baseline PSA (< 1.4 ng/mL) display marginal urodynamic improvement with the same treatment.

FINASTERIDE TREATMENT
AND PSA CONCENTRATION

PSA is impacted by finasteride administration. After 12 mo of treatment with finasteride 5 mg/day, Narayan and colleagues found a mean 43.27% decrease in PSA from baseline values *(43)*. Guess' group in the North American clinical trial found a 50% median decline in PSA values after 12 mo of treatment *(44)*. Moore and associates determined that patients had a 53.76% decline in mean PSA level after 5 yr of finasteride therapy *(45)*.

The decrease in serum PSA levels are generally predictable over the entire range of PSA values, even in those patients with prostate cancer *(19)*. In numerous clinical trials where elevated PSA was closely monitored with serial repeat testing and prostate biopsies, finasteride did not appear to affect the rate of detection of prostate cancer. In fact, in these studies, there was no significant difference in the detection of prostate cancer for patients taking finasteride vs those taking placebo. The PLESS study group, which included 3000 patients, confirmed that in men treated with finasteride for 6 mo or more, PSA results should be doubled for comparison with ranges from untreated men *(29)*.

FUTURE DIRECTIONS IN FINASTERIDE THERAPY

The National Institutes of Health-funded Medical Therapy of Prostate Symptoms trial, which recently concluded, compared treatment with doxazosin, finasteride, and combination therapy *(46)*. Both doxazosin-treated and finasteride-treated individuals had equivalent reductions in risk of BPH progression. Combination treatment with doxazosin and finasteride was more effective than monotherapy with either agent in preventing progression of clinical BPH. All treatments reduced the risk of acute urinary retention, with doxazosin yielding a short-term risk reduction and finasteride and combination therapy resulting in long-term risk reduction. Regarding AUA symptom score and maximal urinary flow rate, combination therapy was more effective than either agent alone. In summary, combination treatment with doxazosin and finasteride was more effective than either alone in producing improvements in AUA symptom score and maximal voiding pressure, whereas finasteride monotherapy and combination therapy both reduced the long-term risks of acute urinary retention and surgical intervention.

Recently, combination, type 1 and type 2,5α-reductase inhibitor therapy, dutasteride, has been approved for use. In initial pharmacokinetic studies, dutasteride was found to be three times more potent than finasteride in blocking the type 2,5α-reductase enzyme. Nearly full blockade of both isoenzymes is achieved at 10-mg doses *(47)*. At this time, it is unclear whether dual blockade offers increased efficacy in treatment of BPH.

REFERENCES

1. Isaacs JT, Coffey DS. Etiology and disease process of benign prostatic hyperplasia. Prostate 1989;2(suppl):33–50.
2. Guinan P, Didomenico D, Brown J, et al. The effect of androgen deprivation on malignant and benign prostate tissue. Med Oncol 1997;14(3–4):145–152.
3. Stegmayr B, Johansson JE, Schnurer LB. Flutamide-an antiandrogen inhibiting prostatic cancer and prostatic secretion with retention of potency. Med Oncol & Tumor Pharmacother 1998;5(1):61–65.
4. Huggins C, Stevens RA. The effect of castration on benign hypertrophy of the prostate in man. J Urol 1940;43:705.
5. Marks LS, Partin AW, Gormley GJ, et al. Prostate tissue composition and response to finasteride in men with symptomatic benign prostatic hyperplasia. J Urol 1997;157:2171–2178.
6. Marks LS, Partin AW, Dorey FJ, et al. Long-term effects of finasteride on prostate tissue composition. Urology 1999;53:574–580.

7. Rittmaster RS, Norman RW, Thomas LN, Rowden G. Evidence for atrophy and apoptosis in the prostates of men given finasteride. J Clin Endocrinol Metab 1996;81:814–819.
8. Sells SF, Wood DP Jr, Joshi-Barve SS, et al. Commonality of the gene programs induced by effectors of apoptosis in androgen-dependent and -independent prostate cells. Cell Growth Differ 1994;5(4):457–466.
9. Bruchovsky N, Lesser B, Van Doorn E, Craven S. Hormonal effects on cell proliferation in rat prostate. Vit Horm 1975;33:61–102.
10. Wilson JD, Gloyna RE. The intranuclear metabolism of testosterone in the accessory organs of reproduction. Recent Prog Horm Res 1970;26:309–336.
11. Siiteri PK, Wilson JD. Dihydrotestosterone in prostatic hypertrophy. I. The formation and content of dihydrotestosterone in the hypertrophic prostate of man. J Clin Invest 1970;49(9):1737–1745.
12. Walsh PC, Madden JD, Harrod MJ, et al. Familial incomplete male pseudohermaphroditism, type 2. Decreased dihydrotestosterone formation in pseudovaginal perineoscrotal hypospadias. N Engl J Med 1974;291(18):944–999.
13. Imperato-McGinley J. 5 alpha-metabolism in finasteride-treated subjects and male pseudohermaphrodites with inherited 5 alpha-reductase deficiency. A review. Eur Urol 1991;20 (suppl 1):78–81.
14. Steers WD, Zorn B. Benign prostatic hyperplasia. Dis Mon 1995;41(7):439–497.
15. Rittmaster RS. Drug therapy: finasteride. N Engl J Med 1994;330(2):120–125.
16. Span PN, Voller MC, Smals AG, et al. Selectivity of finasteride as an in vivo inhibitor of 5 alpha reductase isozyme enzymatic activity in the human prostate. J Urol 1999;161:332–337.
17. Stoner E. The clinical development of a 5α-reductase inhibitor, finasteride. J Steroid Biochem Molec Biol 1990;37(3):375–378.
18. Stoner E. Proceedings of the Food and Drug Administration Endocrinologic & Metabolic Drug Products Advisory Committee Meeting, Bethesda, MD, February 4, 1992. Fairfax, Va.: CASET Associates, 1992:354.
19. Proscar(r) product monograph. Rahway, NJ: Merck & Co, 1993.
20. Ohtawa M, Morikawa H, Shimazaki J. Pharmacokinetics and biochemical efficacy after single and multiple oral administration of N-(2-methyl-2-propyl)-3-oxo-4-aza-5alpha-androst-1-ene-17beta-carboxamide, a new type of specific competitive inhibitor of testosterone 5alpha-reductase, in volunteers. Eur J Drug Metab Pharmacokinet 1991;16:15–21.
21. Wilson JD. The pathogenesis of benign prostatic hyperplasia. Am J Med 1980;68:745–56.
22. Chute CG, Panser LA, Girman CJ, et al. The prevalence of prostatism: a population-based survey of urinary symptoms. J Urol 1993;150:85–89.
23. Hald T. Urodynamics in benign prostatic hyperplasia: a survey. Prostate 1989;2(suppl):69–77.
24. Boyarsky S, Jones G, Paulson DF, Prout GR Jr. A new look at bladder neck obstruction by the Food and Drug Administration regulators: guidelines for investigation of benign prostatic hypertrophy. Trans Am Assoc Genito-Urinary Surg 1976;68:29–32.
25. Gormley GJ, Stoner E, Bruskewitz RC, et al. The effect of finasteride in men with benign prostatic hyperplasia. The Finasteride Study Group. N Engl J Med 1992; 327(17):1185–1191.
26. Stoner E. The clinical effects of a 5alpha-reductase inhibitor, finasteride, on benign prostatic hyperplasia: the Finasteride Study Group. J Urol 1992; 147:1298–1302.

27. Hudson PB, Boake R, Trachtenberg J. Efficacy of finasteride is maintained in patients with benign prostatic hyperplasia treated for 5 years. Urology 1999;53(4):690–695.

28. McConnell JD. Long-term 5- to 7-year experience with finasteride in men with benign prostatic hyperplasia. J Urol 2001;165(5 suppl):261.

29. McConnell JD, Bruskewitz R, Walsh P, et al. The effect of finasteride on the risk of acute urinary retention and the need for surgical treatment among men with benign prostatic hyperplasia. Finasteride Long-Term Efficacy and Safety Study Group. N Engl J Med 1998;338(9):557–563.

30. Somers WJ, Mora MJ, Mason MF, Padley RJ. The natural history of benign prostatic hypertrophy: incidence of urinary retention and significance of AUA symptom score. J Urol 1996;155(5):586A.

31. Roehrborn CG, Oesterling JE, Auerbach S, et al. The Hytrin Community Assessment Trial study: a one-year study of terazosin versus placebo in the treatment of men with symptomatic benign prostatic hyperplasia. HYCAT Investigator Group. Urology 1996;47(2):159–68.

32. Andersen JT, Ekman P, Wolf H, et al. Can finasteride reverse the progress of benign prostatic hyperplasia? A two-year placebo-controlled study. The Scandinavian BPH Study Group. Urology 1995;46(5):631–637.

33. Nickel JC. Long-term implications of medical therapy on benign prostatic hyperplasia end points. Urology 1998;51(S 4A):50–57.

33a. McConnell JD, Bruskewitz R, Walsh P, et al. The effect of finasteride on the risk of acute urinary retention and the need for surgical treatment among men with benign prostatic hyperplasia. NEJM 1998;338(9):557–563.

34. Andersen JT, Nickel JC, Marshall VR. Finasteride significantly reduces the occurrence of acute urinary retention and surgical interventions in patients with symptomatic benign prostatic hyperplasia. J Urol 1997;157:523.

35. Andersen JT, Nickel JC, Marshall VR, Schulman CC, Boyle P. Finasteride significantly reduces acute urinary retention and need for surgery in patients with symptomatic benign prostatic hyperplasia. Urology 1997;49(6):839–45.

36. Tempany CM, Partin AW, Zerhouni EA, Zinreich SJ, Walsh PC. The influence of finasteride on the volume of the peripheral and periurethral zones of the prostate in men with benign prostatic hyperplasia. Prostate 1993;22(1):39–42.

37. Feneley MR, Schalken J, Horsfall DJ, et al. Tissue effects of finasteride in patients with benign prostatic hyperplasia: a controlled randomised study. J Urol 1997;157:134.

38. Marks LS, Partin AW, Gormley GJ, et al. Prostate tissue composition and response to finasteride men with symptomatic benign prostatic hyperplasia. J Urol 1997;157:2171–2178.

39. Montironi R, Valli M, Fabris G. Treatment of benign hyperplasia with 5-α-reductase inhibitor: morphological changes in patients who fail to respond. J Clin Pathol 1996;49:324–328.

40. Kirby RS, Vale J, Bryan J, Holmes K, Webb JAW. Long-term urodynamic effects of finasteride in benign prostatic hyperplasia: a pilot study. Eur Urol 1993;24:20–26.

41. Schafer W, Tammela TL, Barrett DM, et al. Continued improvement in pressure-flow parameters in men receiving finasteride for two years. Urology 1999;54(2):278–283.

42. Roehrborn CG, Boyle P, Berger D, et al. Serum prostate-specific antigen and prostate volume predict long-term changes in symptoms and flow rate: results of a four-year, randomized trial comparing finasteride versus placebo. Urology 1999;54(4):662–669.

43. Narayan P, Tewari A, Jacob G, et al. Differential suppression of serum prostatic acid phosphatase and prostate-specific antigen by 5-alpha-reductase inhibitor. Br J Urol 1995;75:642–646.

44. Guess HA, Heyse JF, Gormley GJ. The effect of finasteride on prostate-specific antigen in men with benign prostatic hyperplasia. Prostate 1993;22:31–37.

45. Moore E, Bracken B, Bremner W, et al. Proscar: five-year experience. Eur Urol 1995;28:304–309.

46. McConnell JD. The long term effects of medical therapy on the progression of BPH: results from the MTOPS trial. J Urol 2002;167(suppl 4):265.

47. Olsson Gisleskog P, Hermann D, Hammarlund-Udenaes M, Karlsson MO. Validation of a population pharmacokinetic/pharmacodynamic model for 5 alpha-reductase inhibitors. Eur J Pharm Sci. 1999;8(4):291–299.

7

Transurethral Needle Ablation of the Prostate

Timothy F. Donahue, MD
and Joseph A. Costa, DO

Contents

INTRODUCTION
TUNA PRINCIPLES AND BACKGROUND
TUNA PROCEDURE
CLINICAL TRIALS
TUNA COMPLICATIONS
CONCLUSION
REFERENCES

INTRODUCTION

There has been considerable interest over the past decade in the development of nonsurgical and minimally invasive therapies for benign prostatic hyperplasia (BPH), especially for patients who do not desire surgery or for those who are poor surgical candidates. Transurethral resection of the prostate (TURP) remains the most effective and durable endoscopic therapy for symptomatic BPH, but it has been associated with potentially significant morbidity *(1)*. A meta-analysis of patients undergoing TURP estimated that 30.7% of patients experienced some morbidity or complication *(2)*. Borboroglu et al. reported on a series of 520 patients who underwent TURP from 1990 to 1998 and had immediate and late complication rates of 10.8% and 8.5%, respectively *(3)*. Approximately 15% of patients require a second intervention within 10 yr of undergoing TURP *(4)*. The combination of patient demands and socioeconomic concerns has spurred the increased interest in less

From: *Management of Benign Prostatic Hypertrophy*
Edited by: K. T. McVary © Humana Press Inc., Totowa, NJ

invasive, less morbid treatment options for BPH. Medical therapies such as α-blockers and 5α-reductase inhibitors as well as balloon dilation, urethral stents, and thermal therapies have been the focus of attention. Various thermal strategies have been investigated as minimally invasive procedures for BPH, including the use of microwave, laser, high-intensity focused ultrasound, and radiofrequency (RF) energy to deliver heat to the interstitium of the prostate. All thermotherapies, regardless of the form of energy used, achieve necrosis of the prostate by raising the temperature of the tissue to above 60° C *(5)*. Transurethral needle ablation of the prostate (TUNA) uses low-energy RF delivered directly into the prostate to produce controlled necrosis of the obstructing adenoma. RF has been used successfully in other medical applications such as to ablate accessory atrioventricular bundles in Wolff-Parkinson-White syndrome and to destroy neoplastic hepatocellular tumors and anomalous neural tissue *(6–8)*. For the past decade, TUNA has been investigated as a minimally invasive alterative to TURP for the management of symptomatic BPH. The precision of the RF delivery and the reproducible necrosis have made TUNA an attractive alternative to more invasive surgery.

TUNA PRINCIPLES AND BACKGROUND

The TUNA system requires the use of a specially designed cystoscope that contains two independent energy delivery needles and a low-level RF generator. TUNA uses low-level RF waves (490 kHz) that allow a deeper and more uniform penetration than microwave thermotherapy. The RF energy is delivered by two independent 22-mm needles placed at the end of the specially designed 22-Fr rigid cystoscope. The needles and protective sheaths advance and retract by controls on the catheter handle and are put into the prostate tissue at an acute angle to the catheter and at 40° to each other. The sheaths can be placed over the needles to protect the urethral lining. Thermocouples at the tip of each protective sheath and at the side of the catheter tip monitor the temperature at the intra-adenoma region and prostatic urothelium, respectively. The catheter tip can be rotated manually to direct the needles into either lateral lobe of the prostate. The RF energy can only be delivered to the tissues by direct contact, and its effects are dissipated quickly over a distance of approx 6 mm *(9)*. The dimensions of the thermal lesion correspond to the geometry of the needles, the length of time of the energy delivery, the temperature core that is achieved, and the tissue impedance. Increased impedance such as that caused by tissue desiccation can result in tissue self-insulation and arrest thermal propagation.

The tissue effects of RF are also dramatically influenced by heat loss caused by convection (i.e., vascularity) (9). Thus, a balance must be struck: enough energy must be delivered to cause tissue necrosis, but not such a high level of energy that tissue charring is produced, leading to increased tissue impedance. In addition, the vascularity of the prostate adenoma can serve as a heat sink to draw thermal energy away from the target area (1).

Two major studies were performed to measure the feasibility of TUNA before its application in humans. Goldwasser et al. performed TUNA in dogs and demonstrated that 1-cm necrotic lesions could be created in the gland with no concurrent injury to the rectum, bladder base, or distal prostatic urethra (10). This success was replicated in studies performed by Ramon et al., who also created 1-cm necrotic lesions in ex vivo prostates (11).

Schulman et al. reported on the safety, tolerance, and efficacy of lesions created by TUNA in 25 patients undergoing radical prostatectomy (5). Patients were treated with TUNA anywhere from 1 d to 3 mo before undergoing radical retropubic prostatectomy. Macroscopic evaluation of the glands at the time of prostatectomy demonstrated the presence of defined necrotic lesions that were sharply demarcated from areas of untreated prostate (5). These investigators found hemorrhagic lesions in specimens recovered within 48 h of TUNA and discovered that necrotic lesions were maximal at 1 wk after treatment. Lesions ranged in size from 10×7 mm to 20×10 mm. Pathologic survey of the necrotic lesions by both visual inspection and immunohistochemical staining demonstrated destruction of all tissue components. Correlating the lesion size to the parameters recorded at the time of TUNA, these researchers discovered that when temperatures at the sheath (the lowest temperature of the lesion) were below 47°C, the size of the necrotic lesion was dramatically reduced (5). Rasor et al. performed mapping studies of the lesions produced by TUNA using an infrared temperature monitor and a specially designed TUNA catheter (12). They found that the lesion at the tip of the needle reached 90–100° C in an ex vivo animal model. In a study of patients undergoing TUNA before prostatectomy, temperatures of 50° C corresponded to core temperatures of 85–100°C within the target area. The extent of the lesion created by TUNA depends on the length of the needle that is used, the wattage used, the duration of treatment, the temperature achieved at the core of the lesion, and the temperature recorded at the tip of the protective sheath (12).

One of the appealing aspects of TUNA is the ability to spare the prostatic urothelium from injury at the time of therapy. Zlotta and colleagues performed neurohistochemical staining of prostate specimens treated with TUNA before radical prostatectomy *(9)*. They found that the lesions were located 0.3–1 cm beneath the preserved urothelium, that nerve destruction was complete within the necrotic lesion, and that the normal nerve fibers were located typically within 0.5–1 cm of the urothelial lining *(9)*. There is a higher density of innervation in the stromal portions of the prostate, under the capsule, adjacent to epithelial nodules, and just under the prostate urothelium. Sparing of these pain-sensitive areas adjacent to the prostatic urothelium and the rapid destruction of the nerve fibers within the necrotic lesions are the presumed major reasons why this procedure can usually be performed without the use of general or spinal anesthesia. Urethral sparing also may account for the low incidence of postprocedure voiding symptoms and the decreased risk of urinary retention following treatment *(9)*.

TUNA PROCEDURE

The optimal candidate for TUNA is a patient with mild-to-moderate obstructive voiding symptoms attributable to BPH, who has no evidence of neurologic bladder dysfunction and no significant obstruction caused by median lobe hypertrophy. Cystoscopy is useful preoperatively to rule out urethral stricture disease and bladder neck contracture and to evaluate for median lobe hypertrophy. Transrectal ultrasound is necessary for volume estimation of the prostate and to plan the needle placement. The transverse diameter of the gland should be measured at the base, at midgland, and at the apex to accurately map out the desired necrotic lesions within the gland *(13)*. TUNA is most successful in patients with predominant lateral lobe enlargement and an estimated gland size of < 60 g *(14)*. For those patients with either large glands (> 100 g) or isolated median lobe hypertrophy, TUNA has not had equal success *(14)*. Traditionally, the median lobe and bladder neck have been avoided during TUNA because of concerns about causing retrograde ejaculation. Preoperative assessment of the patient's voiding symptoms using the International Prostate Symptoms Score (I-PSS) and measuring peak urinary flow rates and residual urine volume is useful to allow postoperative comparison to assess the efficacy of the procedure *(13)*.

The TUNA procedure is generally well tolerated with the use of intraurethral lidocaine supplemented as needed with intravenous sedation. Some investigators have advocated the use of oral narcotics administered in the preoperative holding area. Antibiotics, either oral or intravenous, are administered before the procedure *(15)*. Approximately 10 to 20 mL of 2% lidocaine is instilled per urethra for 5–15 min before the procedure. Some investigators have used a prostatic block by either transperineal or transrectal infiltration of local anesthesia around the prostate gland, as described by Nash and co-workers *(16)*.

There is rarely a need for general or spinal anesthesia during TUNA, and it can be performed as an outpatient procedure *(5,9,16)*.

The TUNA device is a specially designed cystoscopic instrument connected to an RF generator. The design of the instrument has been modified over the past decade, and the model most commonly used these days is the ProVu (Vida Med) system. This system has reusable parts and improved optics to allow for direct visualization as the needles are deployed. Two 22-mm needles with protective Teflon sheaths that diverge at 40° angles to each other and at an acute angle to the cystoscope tip are independently deployable by the use of handles at the base of the catheter. The sheaths are deployed over the needle to protect this area from thermal ablation. Thermal sensors at the tip of the protective sheath and at the tip of the catheter monitor prostate and urethral temperatures during the procedure. The generator has a cut-off safety feature that is activated when the urethral temperature exceeds 46°C to protect the urethra from thermal injury. The length of needle insertion within the prostate is calculated based on the ultrasound estimate of the gland size. Thermal injury can occur up to 6 mm beyond the tip of the inserted needle. Therefore, the needle should not be inserted more than half the diameter of the prostate minus 6 mm (L = 1/2TD – 6, where L = length of needle deployment and TD = transverse diameter of the gland) *(9)*. In addition, the protective Teflon sheaths should be deployed 5–6 mm within the gland to protect the prostatic urethra. The number of treatment planes is based on the estimated length of the prostatic urethra, typically starting 1 cm distal to the bladder neck and extending to 1 cm proximal to the verumontanum. For patients with a prostatic urethral length of 3 cm, one treatment plane is used; 2 planes for 3–4 cm; 3 planes for > 4 cm. The treatment planes should be equidistant to each other, and the procedure should start proximally and move distally with successive treatment planes. Another guideline for the number of treatment planes is one pair of lesions per 20 g of prostate *(17)*. The instrument is rotated to visualize the lateral lobe of the gland, and the pair of needles is inserted into the tissue using direct visualization.

Once the needles are placed within the prostate, RF energy beginning at 2 watts and increasing up to 15 watts is delivered for approx 5 min per lesion. The power is gradually increased to avoid desiccating the tissue surrounding the needles and to prevent charring of the needles. Both of these will interfere with energy propagation and heat generation *(5)*. The RF energy is delivered slowly to achieve a temperature of 50°C at the tip of the protective sheath. This temperature corresponds to a temperature of 85–100° C at the core of the necrotic lesion. Advances in RF generator technology have allowed for more accurate delivery of energy to achieve and maintain a minimum temperature of 50° C for at least 2 min to ensure that necrotic lesions are as large as possible *(9)*.

At the conclusion of the procedure, the instrument is removed, the bladder is drained, and the patient is observed. No Foley catheter is required at the end of the treatment, and patients can be discharged once they have voided. If the patient is unable to spontaneously void, a catheter is placed for 1–7 d. Discharge medications include antibiotics and antiinflammatory agents, both of which are continued for several days after the procedure *(13,18)*.

CLINICAL TRIALS

The first clinical trial to report early experience with TUNA for the treatment of BPH was performed by Schulman and Zlotta *(13)*. Their experience treating 20 patients with TUNA and describing the results demonstrated that TUNA could provide improvement in peak flow rate, quality of life, and I-PSS at 6 mo after treatment. The initial United States trial evaluated 12 patients and also demonstrated significant improvement in both peak flow rates and quality of life parameters at 6 mo; patients in this study also experienced a significant decline in maximum detrusor pressures and detrusor opening pressures *(18)*. Roehrborn et al. described the results of a prospective, 12-mo, multicenter trial of 130 patients undergoing TUNA. At the 12-mo evaluation, I-PSS had decreased from 23.7 to 11.9 ($p < 0.0001$), peak flow rates had increased from 8.7 mL/s to 14.6 mL/s ($p < 0.0001$), and quality of life had improved significantly. One treatment plane was used for 38% of patients, two planes were used in 51%, and three planes were used in 14%. All patients received intraurethral lidocaine; 8.5% also received oral anxiolytics, 84.5% also received parenteral sedation, and 7% also received parenteral analgesics. Nearly 60% of patients did not require a urinary catheter at the time of discharge; the remainder received either a catheter or instruction on intermittent catheterization. The mean duration of catheterization was 3.1 d (range 0.5–35 d) *(19)*. A prospective, multicenter trial of 76 patients from seven centers in Europe and Israel demonstrated similar efficacy: significant improvements in I-PSS, urinary flow rate, and quality of life at 1-yr follow-up *(20)*. Namiki et al. reported the 12-mo follow-up of 30 patients undergoing TUNA and found similar success, with significant improvements in I-PSS, quality of life, and peak flow rates *(21)*. Table 1 summarizes the results of clinical trials for TUNA.

Table 1
Summary of TUNA Clinical Trials

Clinical Trial	Number of Patients	Follow-up (months)	IPSS Baseline	IPSS Postoperative	Qmax (mL/sec) Baseline	Qmax (mL/sec) Postoperative
Schulman and Zlotta	20	3	21.9	10.2	9.5	14.7
	20	6	21.9	6.7	9.5	15.0
Issa	12	6	25.6	9.8	7.8	13.5
Bruskewitz et al.	65	12	24.7	11.1	8.7	15.0
Roehrborn et al.	93	12	23.7	11.9	8.7	14.6
Rosario et al.	58	12	23.0	10.6	9.0	11.3
Ramon et al.	60	12	22.0	7.5	8.7	11.6
Giannakopoulos et al.	50	12	22.4	9.1	7.6	16.8
Namiki et al.	30	12	20.7	11.2	8.0	11.0
Kahn et al.	45	3	20.9	16.1	8.3	13.4
	45	6	20.9	10.7	8.3	13.1
	45	12	20.9	9.9	8.3	14.9
Campo et al.	72	12	20.8	6.2	8.2	15.9
	42	18	20.8	6.7	8.2	14.9
Steele and Sleep	41	12	22.4	7.0	6.6	10.2
	38	24	22.4	9.5	6.6	11.0
Schatzl et al.	15	6	17.7	8.7	9.3	13.6
	15	12	17.7	6.5	9.3	11.9
	15	18	17.7	7.9	9.3	10.7
	15	24	17.7	7.7	9.3	11.6
Schulman and Zlotta	36	12	21.6	7.8	9.9	16.8
	17	36	21.6	7.6	9.9	16.2
Virdi et al.	71	36	22.3	7.4	7.0	16.1

Sustained results have been shown 2 and 3 yr after TUNA. Steele and Sleep reported data on 47 patients 2 yr after TUNA and found that I-PSS, quality of life, and peak flow rates remained significantly improved over baseline at 2 yr after treatment *(22)*. Campo et al. described similar findings at 18 mo after therapy *(23)*. Minardi et al. confirmed the durability of TUNA at 2 yr, although they found a slight increase in I-PSS and quality of life parameters in patients older than 70 yr and in those with a higher baseline quality of life score *(24)*. Three-year data reported by Virdi et al. describing the results of 140 patients undergoing TUNA showed significant improvement in I-PSS, quality of life, peak flow rate, and residual urine volume *(25)*. Schulman and Zlotta reported sustained improvements in these same parameters at 3-yr follow-up *(26)*.

A large-scale, prospective, randomized trial was performed to compare TUNA and TURP for the treatment of BPH. In this trial, 65 men underwent TUNA and 56 received TURP. I-PSS and quality-of-life parameters were each significantly improved over baseline but were equivalent for TUNA and TURP at 1-yr follow-up. Peak flow rates were greater for patients who underwent TURP compared with TUNA (20.8 mL/s vs 15.0 mL/s, respectively). The incidence of complications was less with TUNA, especially with respect to sexual dysfunction, retrograde ejaculation, and need for postoperative urinary catheter *(27)*. Schatzl and colleagues compared the efficacy of TURP with that of less-invasive treatment options during a 2-yr follow-up. Patients who underwent TURP ($n = 28$) were compared with those who received TUNA ($n = 15$). During the period of the study, one patient (4%) in the TURP group required a second TURP, whereas three patients (20%) in the TUNA arm required another procedure. For those patients who did not require a second intervention, the I-PSS decreased a mean of 13.9 after TURP compared with 9.8 after TUNA. The mean increase in peak flow rate after TURP was 11.5 mL/s; the mean improvement for patients in the TUNA arm was 2.3 mL/s *(28)*. Because of its minimally invasive nature, TUNA has been explored as a treatment modality for patients with urinary retention who were felt to be poor surgical candidates. Zlotta et al. described the results of TUNA in 38 patients whose indication for treatment was urinary retention. Nearly 80% of patients resumed voiding within 8.7 d after receiving treatment There were no complications, and none of the patients had subsequent retention *(29)*.

Although TUNA has been traditionally reserved for patients with an estimated gland weight of < 60 g, results of a short-term study of patients with larger prostates are encouraging. Sullivan and colleagues performed TUNA in 10 patients with a mean estimated prostate weight of

76.9 g (range 62–98 g) *(30)*. They found that at 6 mo patients showed mean improvements in I-PSS (19.9 to 12.1), peak flow rate (8.6 mL/s to 12.75 mL/s), and quality of life (4.2 to 2.3). Urinary retention developed in one patient and required TURP, and one patient was retreated with TUNA approx 13 mo after initial therapy *(30)*.

The ability of perform TUNA without general or spinal anesthesia has been an attractive quality for both patients and urologists. Although most studies confirm that TUNA is generally well tolerated with intra-urethral lidocaine and intravenous sedation, Kahn et al. reported that, of 45 patients undergoing TUNA, 10 received general anesthesia, 2 had epidural anesthesia, and 4 received spinal anesthesia *(15)*. Three patients had managed anesthesia care. In an attempt to maximize patient comfort and minimize the need for greater anesthesia, Issa et al. investigated the effectiveness of transperineal prostatic nerve blockade *(16)*. They used an equal mixture of 1% lidocaine and 0.25% marcaine with epinephrine (1:1000 concentration) and instilled an average of 40 mL of local anesthetic transperineally around the base of the prostate gland. They found that this was well tolerated and provided adequate analgesia for the procedure *(16)*.

TUNA COMPLICATIONS

The appeal of minimally invasive therapies for the treatment of BPH is the ability to achieve efficacy similar to that of TURP but with significantly lower morbidity. Mortality has not been described in patients undergoing TUNA. The most common complications experienced by these patients are urinary retention, hematuria, and irritative voiding symptoms. In most cases, patients are able to void spontaneously shortly after treatment, but urinary retention has been described in 13.3–41.6% of patients *(27,31–33)*. Most commonly, retention is transient and resolves within 1 wk. Hematuria, although common within the first days after treatment, has never been reported to require a blood transfusion. Rosario et al. reported no increased incidence of bleeding complications, even in patients receiving warfarin at the time of TUNA *(34)*. The presumed ability of TUNA to spare the prostatic urethra from thermal injury accounts for the incidence of irritative voiding symptoms, dysuria, frequency, and urethral sloughing. These irritative symptoms are usually mild and transient and can be managed successfully with anti-inflammatory agents *(5)*. Retrograde ejaculation was reported only in the initial U.S. trial by Issa *(18)*. One patient experienced retrograde ejaculation, but this has been an isolated event and has not been found in any other trial *(18)*. The degree to which patients were queried regarding this event is not clear. No urinary incontinence has been reported after TUNA, and the incidence of urethral stricture is estimated to be less than 1% *(13,19,22,23,27)*. Bladder neck contracture has not been described. The re-operation rate for patients undergoing TUNA has been reported to be approx 10 to 15% of patients *(22)*.

CONCLUSION

TUNA of the prostate has been investigated over the past decade as a minimally invasive approach to the management of BPH and has been shown to have some promise. For those patients who do not desire TURP or who have been found to be poor surgical candidates, TUNA provides an opportunity for improvement in I-PSS, quality-of-life parameters, and peak urinary flow rates, even up to 3 yr after treatment. It can usually be performed without general or spinal anesthesia, and patients can be treated as an outpatient. The rates of sexual dysfunction are not clear but are thought to be low; and incontinence has described infrequently. Potential disadvantages of TUNA are its questionable efficacy in patients with larger prostate glands, the lack of any tissue for pathologic evaluation, and the lack of any extensive long-term follow-up data. Although the long-term efficacy remains unknown, TUNA has emerged as an attractive alternative choice for patients with symptomatic BPH.

REFERENCES

1. Mebust WK, Holtgrewe HL, Cockett AT, et al. Transurethral prostatectomy: immediate and postoperative complications. A cooperative study of 13 participating institutions evaluating 3, 885 patients. J Urol 1989;143:243.
2. McConnel JD, Barry MJ, Bruskewitz RC, et al. Benign prostatic hyperplasia: diagnosis and treatment. Clinical practice guidelines, number 8. Agency for Health Care Policy and Research Publication No. 94-0582. Rockville, Maryland: Public Health Service, United States Department of Health and Human Services, February, 1994.
3. Borboroglu PG, Kane CJ, Ward JF, et al. Immediate and postoperative complications of transurethral prostatectomy in the 1990s. J Urol 1999;162:1307.
4. Roos NP, Wennberg JE, Malenka DJ, et al. Mortality and reoperation after open and transurethral resection of the prostate for benign prostatic hyperplasia. N Engl J Med 1989;320:1120.
5. Schulman CC, Zlotta AR, Rasor JS, et al. Transurethral needle ablation (TUNA): safety, feasibility, and tolerance of a new office procedure for treatment of benign prostatic hyperplasia. Eur Urol 1993;24:415.
6. Calkins H, Langberg J, Sousa J, et al. Radiofrequency catheter ablation of accessory atrioventricular connections in 250 patients. Circulation 1992;85:1337.
7. Rossi S, Di Stasi M, Buscarini E, et al. Percutaneous radiofrequency interstitial thermal ablation in the treatment of small hepatocellular carcinoma. Cancer J Sci Am 1995;1:73.

8. Zlotta AR, Kiss R, De Decker R, et al. MXT mammary tumor treatment with a high temperature radiofrequency ablation device. Int J Oncol 1995;7:863.

9. Zlotta AR, Raviv G, Peny MO, et al Possible mechanisms of action of transurethral needle ablation of the prostate on benign prostatic hyperplasia symptoms: a neurohistochemical study. J Urol 1997;157:894.

10. Goldwasser B, Ramon J, Engelberg S, et al. Transurethral needle ablation (TUNA) of the prostate using low-level radiofrequency energy: an animal experimental study. Eur Urol 1993;24:400.

11. Ramon J, Goldwasser B, Stenfeld B, et al. Needle ablation using radiofrequency current as a treatment for benign prostatic hyperplasia: experimental results in ex vivo human prostate. Eur Urol 1993;24:406.

12. Rasor JS, Zlotta AR, Edwards SD, et al. Transurethral needle ablation (TUNA): thermal gradient mapping and comparison of lesion size in a tissue model and in patients with benign prostatic hyperplasia. Eur Urol 1993;24:411.

13. Schulman CC, Zlotta AR. Transurethral needle ablation of the prostate for treatment of benign prostatic hyperplasia: early clinical experience. Urology 1995;45:28.

14. Naslund MJ. Transurethral needle ablation of the prostate. Urology 1997;50:167.

15. Kahn SA, Alphonse P, Tewari A, et al. An open study on the efficacy and safety of transurethral needle ablation of the prostate treating symptomatic benign prostatic hyperplasia. The University of Florida experience. J Urol 1998;160:1695.

16. Issa MM, Perez-Brayfield M, Petros JA, et al. A prospective study of transperineal prostatic block for transurethral needle ablation for benign prostatic hyperplasia: the Emory University experience. J Urol 1999;162:1636.

17. Roehrborn CG, Fiona C, Burkhard RC, et al. The effects of transurethral needle ablation and resection of the prostate on pressure flow urodynamic parameters: analysis of the United States randomized study. J Urol 1999;162:92.

18. Issa MM. Transurethral needle ablation of the prostate: report of the initial United States clinical trial. J Urol 1996;156:413.

19. Roehrborn CG, Issa MM, Bruskewitz RC, et al. Transurethral needle ablation for benign prostatic hyperplasia: 12-month results of a prospective, multicenter U.S. study. Urology 1998;51:415.

20. Ramon J, Lynch TH, Eardley I, et al. Transurethral needle ablation of the prostate for benign hyperplasia: a collaborative multicenter study. Br J Urol 1997;80:128.

21. Namiki K, Shiozawa H, Tsuzuki M, et al. Efficacy of transurethral needle ablation of the prostate for the treatment of benign prostatic hyperplasia. Int J Urol 1999;6:341.

22. Steele GS, Sleep DJ. Transurethral needle ablation of the prostate: a urodynamic based study with 2-year follow-up. J Urol 1997;158:1834.

23. Campo B, Bergamaschi F, Corrada P, et al. Transurethral needle ablation (TUNA) of the prostate: a clinical and urodynamic evaluation. Urology 1997;49:847.

24. Minardi D, Garofalo F, Yehia M, et al. Pressure-flow studies in men with benign prostatic hypertrophy before and after treatment with transurethral needle ablation. Urol Int 2001;66:89.

25. Virdi J, Pandit A, Sriram R. Transurethral needle ablation of the prostate (TUNA). A prospective study, three year follow-up. Eur Urol 1998;33(suppl 1):A9.

26. Schulman CC, Zlotta AR. Transurethral needle ablation (TUNA) of the prostate: clinical experience with three years follow-up in patients with benign prostatic hyperplasia (BPH). Eur Urol 1998;33(suppl 1):A586.

27. Bruskewitz R, Issa MM, Roehrborn CG, et al. A prospective, randomized 1-year clinical trial comparing transurethral needle ablation to transurethral resection of the prostate for the treatment of symptomatic benign prostatic hyperplasia. J Urol 1998;159:1588.
28. Schatzl G, Madersbacher S, Djavan B, et al. Two-year results of transurethral resection of the prostate versus four 'less-invasive' treatment options. Eur Urol 2000;37:695.
29. Zlotta AR, Peny MO, Matos C, et al. Transurethral needle ablation of the prostate: clinical experience in patients in urinary retention. Br J Urol 1996;77:391.
30. Sullivan LD, Paterson RF, Gleave ME, et al. Early experience with transurethral needle ablation of large prostates. Can J Urol 1999;6:686.
31. Schulman CC, Zlotta AR. Transurethral needle ablation of the prostate (TUNA): pathological, radiological, and clinical study of a new office procedure for treatment of benign prostatic hyperplasia using low-level radiofrequency energy. Semin Urol 1994;13:205.
32. Schulman CC, Zlotta AR. Transurethral needle ablation of the prostate: a new treatment of benign prostatic hyperplasia using interstitial low-level radiofrequency energy. Curr Opin Urol 1995;5:35.
33. Issa MM, Oesterling JE. Transurethral needle ablation (TUNA): an overview of radiofrequency thermal therapy for the treatment of benign prostatic hyperplasia. Curr Opin Urol 1996;6:20.
34. Rosario DJ, Woo H, Potts KL, et al. Safety and efficacy of transurethral needle ablation of the prostate for symptomatic outlet obstruction. Br J Urol 1997;80:579.

8 Transurethral Microwave Thermotherapy

Jonathan N. Rubenstein, MD
and Kevin T. McVary, MD

CONTENTS

INTRODUCTION
HISTORY OF THE PROCEDURE
MECHANISM OF ACTION
INDICATIONS FOR TUMT
PREOPERATIVE CONSIDERATIONS
HISTOLOGIC FINDINGS
CONTRAINDICATIONS
PREOPERATIVE DETAILS
INTRAOPERATIVE DETAILS
POSTOPERATIVE DETAILS
RESULTS
OTHER USES AND FUTURE DIRECTIONS
CONCLUSIONS
REFERENCES

INTRODUCTION

Transurethral resection of the prostate (TURP) remains the gold standard for treatment of benign prostatic hyperplasia (BPH). Although this procedure is generally safe, patients require a spinal, epidural, or general anesthesia and often need several days of hospital stay. In addition, potential morbidity limits the use of TURP in high-risk patients. Pharmacotherapy has been recommended as a first line therapy for all patients

From: *Management of Benign Prostatic Hypertrophy*
Edited by: K. T. McVary © Humana Press Inc., Totowa, NJ

with mild-to-moderate symptoms. Unfortunately, the long-term outcomes of such therapy have not been fully elucidated. Patients must adhere to a strict medication schedule, and outcome indicators for pharmacotherapy are not reached as well or as reliably as outcome indicators for TURP. Patients choose pharmacotherapy because of the perceived reduced risk of adverse events and the desire to avoid surgery. This trade-off of risk for efficacy is a common thread running through all elective treatments for BPH. Newer modalities have been aimed at providing alternatives to pharmacotherapy or watchful waiting. Patients prefer a one-time treatment for lower urinary tract symptoms (LUTS) resulting from BPH, provided the method offers reduced risk and allows efficacy equal to that of medical therapy. One such method is transurethral microwave thermotherapy (TUMT). Heat in the form of microwaves is used for the destruction of hyperplastic prostate tissue. Early results show excellent symptomatic relief, with one outpatient encounter using minimal anesthesia. Clinical indications and treatment parameters for TUMT are still evolving as technology advances and more experience is gained. This chapter summarizes current knowledge regarding the indications and efficacy of microwave therapy of the prostate.

HISTORY OF THE PROCEDURE

Applying heat to the prostate gland is not new. In 1921, McCaskey used heat in the form of ultraviolet lamps to treat prostatism, and Corbus used diathermy probes for the same purpose in 1929 *(1,2)*. These therapies were never clinically accepted. In the 1980s, the use of heat to treat BPH regained clinical interest as alternatives to TURP and open prostatectomy were being explored. The modern use of microwaves has been credited to Yerushalmi and associates *(3)*. In 1982, they performed microwave therapy on a patient with prostatic adenocarcinoma and later reported the therapeutic use of microwaves by the transrectal route to treat patients with BPH who were poor operative candidates *(3,4)*.

The first machines studied in clinical trials used the transurethral route in a series of 10 1-hr sessions. These machines used software and instrumentation that allowed only limited and often interrupted delivery of energy to the prostate. Intraprostatic temperatures reached 40–45°C. Patients reported a subjective improvement in symptoms, although an objective improvement of voiding parameters was not observed *(5)*. Histologic studies revealed that prostatic cells were not destroyed, but symptomatic improvement was proposed to be the result of destruction

of the α-adrenergic nerve fibers around the prostate, leading to a change
in the voiding reflex.

Further research revealed that temperatures greater than 45°C were
necessary to cause coagulative necrosis, protein denaturation, and tissue ablation to reliably destroy prostate cells. These cells would slough
away over a period of weeks to months. Increasing the temperature to
47°C further enhanced apoptosis. The introduction of urethral cooling
reduced the pain threshold and allowed higher energy to be used, resulting in higher intraprostatic temperatures and tissue destruction. The
term hyperthermia was coined to describe treatment using temperatures
<45°C, and thermotherapy was used to describe therapy with tempera-
tures >45°C.

As prostate tissue was destroyed more reliably, the time of therapy
was decreased. Antennae were improved to provide concentric distribution of heat. Heat distribution now generally follows the anatomic
borders of the transition zone, the main source of adenomatous tissue.
The use of thermotherapy resulted in significant improvement in both
objective and subjective measures. Histologic examination of specimens revealed cell destruction but no reliable cavitations. Patients
invariably had severe prostatic edema and urinary retention requiring the
use of a urinary catheter, which became standard practice after TUMT.

To further improve outcomes, high-energy thermotherapy was introduced. Temperatures greater than 70°C were reached, causing thermoablation of prostatic tissue. Unlike with thermotherapy, prostatic cavities
were observed on histologic sections with high-energy thermotherapy,
resulting in greater improvement in symptom and objective parameters.
However, patients did not notice an immediate improvement after high-
energy thermotherapy but rather had a gradual change over a period of
months.

MECHANISM OF ACTION

Normal prostate cells undergo necrosis when exposed to temperatures of 44–45°C for 30 min (6). Microwaves, which fall within 300–
3000-MHz wavelengths, are absorbed as they propagate through tissue,
causing local changes that produce heat. TUMT is performed by the
transurethral route, using an external power source to create microwaves at a frequency of 900–1100 MHz. Tissue penetration leads to
electromagnetic oscillations of free charges and the polarization of small
molecules such as water, resulting in the release of kinetic energy and
increasing the temperature of the tissue. Finally, cell necrosis, vascular
injury, and apoptosis ensue.

INDICATIONS FOR TUMT

Patients who should be considered for TUMT include those with obstructive or irritative voiding symptoms, those in whom medical therapy has failed, or those who choose not to be managed medically. When a patient wishes to undergo a therapeutic intervention, the type of intervention must be carefully evaluated. As the standard, TURP is offered to most patients. The potential advantages of microwave therapy over TURP include the relief of LUTS with an in-office procedure, the use of minimal anesthesia, and the potential for rapid recovery. TUMT is considered for patients who prefer an outpatient setting rather than a hospital stay and for those who are at an increased surgical or anesthetic risk.

PREOPERATIVE CONSIDERATIONS

Patient Selection

For all eligible patients, a thorough medical history should be taken and a physical examination performed. The presence and degree of voiding dysfunction and/or the role played by BPH should be evaluated clinically. Medical history should include the presence, onset, progression, and severity of urinary symptoms of nocturia, hematuria, urgency, frequency, hesitancy, intermittency, and incomplete emptying. Focus should be placed on questions regarding prior treatments for BPH such as α-blockade, herbal therapy, or previous surgical attempts.

A medical history should focus on the patient's urologic history along with surgical risks and concomitant medical problems. Urologic history should include a history of sexually transmitted diseases, kidney stones, trauma, previous catheterizations, genitourinary cancer, renal insufficiency, neurologic disease, and neurogenic bladder. Medical conditions that may influence bladder functioning include diabetes and neurologic diseases. Surgical risks predominantly are the result of renal failure, coronary artery disease, and cerebrovascular disease. Medicines containing α-sympathomimetics, including over-the-counter cold remedies, enhance bladder outlet obstruction. A family history should focus on a history of urologic cancer, and a social history should focus on risks for cancer such as smoking and occupational exposure.

The physical examination should be systematic and meticulous, focusing on the presence or absence of distended bladder, urethral stenosis, meatal stenosis, and anal area and rectal tone. The prostate is evaluated for size and presence or absence of nodularity, laterality, consistency, and landmarks.

Laboratory Studies

Patients should be evaluated for renal insufficiency and electrolyte abnormalities before undergoing TUMT. A reversible cause for renal insufficiency should be sought before performing TUMT.

A determination of serum prostate-specific antigen (PSA) level may be important in the screening for prostate cancer. If clinically suggested, transrectal biopsies should be performed and may lead to alternative therapies. Patients with an increased PSA at baseline respond more favorably to TUMT than those with lower PSA, possibly because of the heterogeneous nature of prostatic hyperplasia and the different response of cell types to microwaves *(7,8)*.

To decrease the risk of urosepsis, all patients should undergo testing and have a documented negative culture before any urethral instrumentation is used.

Imaging Studies

A transrectal ultrasound (TRUS) is suggested before performing TUMT to evaluate the size of the prostate gland. Patients with prostate volumes estimated to be <25 mL or >100 mL respond poorly to TUMT. In addition, this allows the evaluation of prostatic cysts and seminal vesicle disease.

Patients should undergo renal ultrasound to rule out hydronephrosis if they have a history of urinary retention or an increased creatinine level.

A cystourethroscopy is mandatory for all patients before TUMT. The urethra should be evaluated for evidence of stricture disease, especially in patients with a history of urethritis or sexually transmitted diseases. In addition, this allows for the evaluation of prostate length and determines the degree of obstruction. Patients with lateral lobe hypertrophy respond much better to TUMT than those with middle lobe hypertrophy or a median bar. The presence of a middle lobe should be excluded before performing TUMT because this structure will alter the way in which the projected microwave pattern overlaps the obstructive tissue. The urethra and bladder urothelium should also be evaluated for evidence of tumors, stones, and other problems. The location of the ureteral orifices should be noted.

Symptom Score

A variety of symptom indices are available and are commonly used to evaluate the causes of a patient's urinary symptoms. The indices are not meant to be used to diagnose or screen for the presence or absence of BPH or bladder outlet obstruction. Rather, they are used to confirm the components of the patient's history, quantify the patient's response to treatment, and compare the results of research protocols. Studies have failed to document a strong correlation between symptom scores and physiologic changes caused by BPH. Patients may have minimal voiding symptoms that may severely interfere with the quality of life and vice versa. Scores that are used commonly include the American Urological Association (AUA) Symptom Score and the International Prostate Symptom Score (I-PSS), which is identical to the AUA score but contains an additional category for quality of life. The Madsen quality of life score evaluates the effect of the symptoms on the patient's quality of life.

The flow rate (Qmax) or voiding velocity is a noninvasive but nonspecific electronic recording of urinary flow rate. Voiding velocity can be used to monitor response to treatment. For accuracy, the patient should void at least 125 to 150 mL, and a minimum of two voids should be recorded because of inherent variations between voids. False-negative results occur with a weak urinary stream because of inadequate detrusor contraction rather than as a result of bladder outlet obstruction. It has been suggested that patients with initially lower flow rates may respond better to TUMT.

The postvoid residual (PVR) is the volume of urine remaining immediately after micturition. It may be measured by the insertion of a urinary catheter into the bladder or may be estimated by transabdominal ultrasound. Usually, patients void to completion; however, those with neurogenic bladder or bladder decompensation caused by chronic outlet obstruction may retain significant quantities of urine. This test does not correlate with the signs and symptoms of prostatism and does not predict surgical outcome, but it does determine how closely patients need to be followed. Patients with high PVR have slightly higher rates of failure of watchful waiting and are at increased risk for complications such as urinary tract infections and renal failure.

HISTOLOGIC FINDINGS

Unlike TURP, no specimen is submitted for pathologic evaluation after TUMT. Even with a normal PSA and negative biopsies, patients are at risk for prostate cancer. Few studies in vivo have evaluated the histologic effect of TUMT on prostatic tissue. Khair performed radical prostatectomy on nine patients with prostate cancer after performing microwave therapy on seven patients within 7 d of TUMT and on two patients 1 yr after TUMT (9). The early pathologic studies revealed hemorrhagic necrosis and devitalized tissues without inflammation. Necrosis was observed in benign areas, in stromal areas, and in cancer areas without skips. The mean volume of necrosis was 8.8 mL (range 1.4–17.8 mL), and the average amount of necrosis was 22% (3–39%). In six of seven patients, there was symmetric necrosis with mean radial distance of 1.4 cm. However, in the two patients who underwent prostatectomy 1 yr later, only nonspecific chronic inflammation and desquamous metaplasia with evidence of periurethral fibrosis was found. The mean volume of necrosis remaining was 0.2 mL, which was less than 1%, implying that cells were sloughed away. No other histologic differences were observed between BPH and cancerous elements.

CONTRAINDICATIONS

All patients undergoing transurethral procedures must have a documented sterile urine culture and must be evaluated for prostate or urothelial cancer if it is clinically suspected. The underlying neurogenic problem should be evaluated and treated in patients with neurogenic bladder voiding dysfunction.

Contraindications specific to TUMT are evolving as the technology changes and outcomes are studied further. Patients with a history of TURP or pelvic trauma should not undergo TUMT because of potential alterations in pelvic anatomy. Patients with glands <25 gm or with a prostatic urethral length <2.0 cm respond poorly to TUMT, as do patients with glands >100 gm or patients with a prominent median bar or middle lobe. Other contraindications include the presence of a penile prosthesis, severe urethral stricture disease, Leriche syndrome/severe peripheral vascular disease, or an artificial urinary sphincter. Patients with pacemakers should consult their cardiologist concerning pacemaker management during therapy. Hip replacement is no longer a contraindication. Acute urinary retention was previously thought to be a contraindication to TUMT; however, high-energy TUMT has shown promise in this population, although efficacy has yet to be determined.

PREOPERATIVE DETAILS

In preparation for TUMT, patients need to be counseled about the risks and benefits of therapy, alternatives to TUMT, and what to expect from therapy. Patients who have a urinary catheter in place or had recent urinary tract manipulation should be placed on appropriate antibiotic therapy. An appropriate oral analgesic (such as ibuprofen, ketorolac, or morphine) and an anxiolytic (benzodiazepine) may be administered before the procedure.

The patient is brought to the therapy suite and asked to void to completion. The bladder is emptied by straight catheterization, and 40 mL of sterile water is placed within the bladder. For anesthesia, 10–20 mL of 1–2% xylocaine gel is inserted within the urethra. Our recent experiences with periprostatic blocks using 1% lidocaine are encouraging but require further study before formal recommendations can be made. The treatment catheter is then placed within the urethra, confirmed by return of the sterile water and by ultrasound, and the balloon is inflated. This catheter has a Coude tip with a temperature sensor and microwave unit near the tip. The distal ports include those for balloon inflation, urine drainage, coolant, microwave cable, and fiberoptic connector. The rectal probe, if used, continuously monitors the rectal temperature.

When the preparations are completed, the program is started. Current reliable pretreatment identification of patient characteristics that consistently predict a successful outcome after TUMT is not possible. There appears to be no difference in outcome based on the preoperative American Society of Anesthesiologists' (ASA) Score *(10)*.

INTRAOPERATIVE DETAILS

A variety of thermotherapy machines exist, each with its own intraoperative mechanism and specifics. The two most commonly used machines are the Targis and the Prostatron, and therefore they will be discussed here.

The Targis system is a small portable machine with treatment times ranging from 28.5 to 60 min. The power ranges from 0 to 60 watts, and it uses a frequency of 902 to 928 MHz. After placing the 21-Fr catheter with either a 2.8- or 3.5-cm antennae and confirming its placement, the rectal thermosensing unit is placed. The rectal thermosensing unit is a balloon with five anteriorly placed thermosensors that continuously monitor rectal temperature and automatically shut down the machine if rectal temperature reaches 42.5°C. The antenna is a helical bipolar antenna that provides impedance matching with the prostatic tissue so that thermal energy is delivered with minimal antennae self-heating. The shape allows preferential heating at the anteriolateral prostate, resulting in fewer automatic shut-downs as a result of increased rectal temperatures. High prostate tissue temperatures of 60–80°C persist throughout therapy while the urethral coolant circulates at 8°C. This results in a uniform area of coagulative necrosis of 3.2 cm in diameter without damage to the urethra and rectum.

The Prostatron device uses a monopolar antenna. This antennae design has been found by experimental observation to lack the capability for impedance matching. The Prostatron uses different software that has differing energy and heating parameters. Prostasoft 2.0 is a low-energy protocol with maximum energy of 60 watts. Treatment takes 60 min. The high-energy Prostasoft 2.5 allows a stepwise increase in energy without interruption to allow intraprostatic temperatures to reach 75°C. The treatment takes 60 min, and the urethral cooling device circulates water at 20°C. The newest protocol, Prostasoft 3.5, is the most powerful of the three. It provides a maximum 80 watts of power at the very start of therapy, and intraprostatic temperatures of up to 75°C are reached.

During the procedure, patients commonly experience mild perineal warmth, mild pain, and a sense of urinary urgency. However, only 5% of patients reported severe pain during TUMT therapy. Despite this, more than half of these patients required substantial oral analgesics during treatment.

POSTOPERATIVE DETAILS

Most centers performing TUMT routinely catheterize patients following treatment. Clear intermittent catheterization is an alternate procedure. Patients return to the clinic for a trial of decatheterization, which varies according to the protocol used. As prostatic edema is nearly universal after microwave therapy, the initial decatheterization trial fails in most patients if the trial is performed too early.

Posttreatment convalescence is relatively rapid, and most patients are able to void in less than 3 d at home, with a mean recovery time of 5 d at home. With low-energy protocols, 12–36% of patients require catheterizations for up to 1 mo, whereas 10% of patients undergoing high-energy protocols require catheterization for more than 3 mo. Patients with larger prostates are more prone to catheterization because of increased edema. Studies of the Prostatron 2.0 have shown that 34% of patients are unable to void 2 h after the procedure, and an additional 6% of patients require a catheter after initially voiding. In comparison, with the Prostatron 3.5, urinary retention is expected in all patients. The average length of catheterization is 1–2 wk. With the Targis system, patients are catheterized routinely for 2 d.

A slow process of LUTS improvement is characteristic of high-energy transurethral microwave thermotherapy. Coagulated tissue must be absorbed, and the treated area must be reorganized before sufficient voiding is achieved. Patients may notice an improvement over a period of many months. If they are able to void, they proceed home and are advised to watch for the inability to void, painful voiding, high fevers, abdominal pain, or other problems.

To decrease the risk of acute urinary retention after TUMT, many patients are maintained on α-blockade therapy. Studies have shown that these patients have improved symptomatology earlier than those who do not receive α-blockade therapy and to have a lower incidence of retention *(11)*. Djavan et al. reported the use of a novel temporary prostatic bridge catheter for 1 mo after TUMT. The catheter provides an effective and well-tolerated option for preventing prostatic obstruction in the immediate posttreatment period *(12)* and avoids the use of a standard indwelling catheter or intermittent self-catheterization. Of 54 patients, 88.9% tolerated the bridge catheter and had significant improvement in peak flow, I-PSS, and quality of life compared to a similar group without the stent.

RESULTS
Efficacy
TUMT ALONE AND VS SHAM

Several small studies of randomized, controlled trials comparing TUMT and sham treatments are available. One of largest TUMT studies (220 men) revealed a decrease in AUA index score from 23.6 to 12.7 points, whereas the sham treatment scores dropped only 5 points after 6 mo *(16)*. Studies in selected groups undergoing treatment with the Targis system have reported a decrease in I-PSS from 23 to 3 at 6 mo, which was maintained through 24 mo *(17)*. Mean maximum flow increased from 6.0 mL/s to 13 mL/s at 6 mo and to 13.9 remained stable at 12 mo *(17)*. Mean PVR decreased from 170 to 17 and 27 at 6 and 24 mo, respectively. Prostatic volume decreased from 57 mL to 40 mL. A substantial decrease in voiding pressures occurred, and only 13% of patients required retreatment within 1 yr and 229 at 2 yr *(17)*.

The low-energy Prostasoft 2.0 has been in use long enough to provide both short-term and long-term results. A remarkable symptomatic improvement, with an average decrease in Madsen Symptom Score from 13 to 4, has been reported *(18)*. However, a complementary objective improvement did not occur with the maximal flow rate, which only increased by 35%. In addition, the results were not durable over a 4-yr period. At 12 mo, 62% of patients said they were satisfied with their treatment, but this fell to 34% at 24 mo and to 23% at 48 mo. During this same time, the Madsen score rose accordingly. Nearly two-thirds of these patients required supplemental treatment *(18)*. Preprocedure urine flow >10 mL/s and an irritative score <5 were factors related to a favorable outcome. Neither prostate volume nor energy delivered influenced the results.

In comparison, higher-energy protocols using the Prostatron device resulted in symptomatic improvement similar to that of lower-energy protocols, whereas improvement in uroflowmetry was much more pronounced. De la Rosette reported an average decrease in I-PSS from 20.0 to 9.3, an increase in flow rate from 9.4 mL/s to 14.6 mL/s, an average catheter time of 18 d, and no serious complications 6 mo after treatment with the Prostasoft 3.5 *(14)*. Benefits of this high-energy protocol include a treatment time of only 30 min, but a disadvantage is the higher rate of urinary retention because of more intense prostatic edema. Compared with the Prostasoft 2.5, the Prostasoft 3.5 resulted in patients reporting a slightly higher level of pain early in treatment because of the initial higher power, but the level is lowered during treatment to the same level as its predecessor *(15)*.

TUMT vs α-BLOCKERS

When compared with α-blockade over the short term, TUMT is associated with an initially poorer outcome. However, by 12 wk, those undergoing TUMT have a better outcome by most measures A prospective, randomized study of 51 patients undergoing high-energy TUMT and 52 patients receiving terazosin therapy revealed much better I-PSS, peak flow, and quality of life levels in the terazosin group at 2 wk. However, at intervals up to 6 mo, all patients did better with TUMT. Terazosin had a more rapid onset of action, with maximal effects reached by 6 wk, whereas the maximal effect of TUMT was not observed until 6 mo after therapy. More adverse events occurred with α-blockade therapy (17/52) than with TUMT (7/51). Three of the seven adverse events in the TUMT group were urinary tract infections. Patients on α-blockade (5.5%) complained of dizziness, asthenia, headaches, and lack of effectiveness of therapy, prompting discontinuation in 11.5% of patients *(18)*. In the same cohort at 6 mo, there was significant improvement in I-PSS, urine flow parameters, and quality of life, although the magnitude was greater in the TUMT group. However, by 18 mo, I-PSS, Qmax, and quality of life were 35%, 22%, and 43% better in the TUMT group. In addition, there was a seven-fold greater treatment failure rate seen in the terazosin group *(19)*.

TUMT vs TURP

There have been three prospective, randomized trials comparing TUMT and TURP to date, and the results have shown that TUMT is effective but inferior to TURP in terms of objective and subjective treatment parameters. Ahmed et al. reported that 60% of a cohort of 30 patients had symptomatic improvement after TUMT but had no relief of obstruction after 6 mo. Of patients who underwent TURP, 100% had symptomatic improvement, and 27 of 30 had resolution of obstruction *(20)*. At a longer follow-up of 2.5 years, d'Ancona et al. reported that flow rates increased by 62% using TUMT (compared to 105% using TURP), and Madsen score improved by 56% (vs 76%) *(21)*. Patients reported as completely unobstructed included 50% using TUMT vs 82% using TURP. Floratos et al. revealed an improvement in Qmax from a baseline of 9.2 mL/s to 15.1 mL/s at 1 yr, 14.5 mL/s at 2 yr, and 11.9 mL/s at 3 yr in patients undergoing TUMT. A similar group undergoing TURP had a better and more durable improvement to 24.5, 23, and 24.7 mL/s at 1, 2, and 3 yr, respectively *(22)*. In the same cohort, the I-PSS improved from 20 to 8, 9, and 12 at 1, 2 and 3 yr using TUMT compared with an improvement from 20 to 3, 4, and 3 in the TURP group. Of patients undergoing TUMT, 19.8% required further procedures compared to 12.9% of the TURP group at 33 mo.

TUMT in Patients With Urinary Retention

The recommended treatment for patients with acute urinary retention caused by BPH is transurethral or open prostatectomy, which is used to relieve urinary outflow and minimize the risk of new retention episodes. This population is generally older and has poorer health, larger prostates, and more impaired renal function and are, therefore, at a higher risk of perioperative morbidity and complications. TUMT was originally believed to be contraindicated because of a high failure rate. However, with the advent of high-energy TUMT, patients are now offered this less-invasive therapy with moderate success. Many patients deemed too risky to undergo TURP or open prostatectomy are able to void spontaneously after TUMT *(23)*. Djavan et al. reported that 29 of 31 (94%) patients treated were able to void spontaneously after 4 wk *(24)*.

Complications

Overall

Although relatively safe, TUMT is associated with a number of complications, and a variety of other rare but reported complications may occur. This includes, but is not limited to, urethrorectal fistula, bladder perforation, and emphysematous prostatic abscess *(25,26)*. Proper monitoring by both physicians and nurses during treatment and accurate catheter placement are vital to decrease these risks.

Complications Compared with TURP

TUMT and TURP are associated with a similar complication rate, although the types of complications differ. Acute urinary retention and postoperative voiding dysfunction are more common after TUMT, and bleeding, retrograde ejaculation, and urethral strictures are more common after TURP. After TURP, patients are catheterized for an average of 2–4 d, whereas many patients undergoing TUMT have prolonged catheterization because of prostatic edema. There is an increased risk of urinary tract infection after TUMT because of the longer duration of catheterization and the remaining *in situ* necrotic tissue. Retrograde ejaculation has been reported to occur in 48–90% of patients after TURP compared with 0–29% after TUMT *(27)*.

Erectile dysfunction after TURP or TUMT is rare if a patient is previously normal but is commonly observed in patients with prior erectile difficulties. Although the cause has not been fully elucidated, psychogenic factors, bladder neck trauma, and neurogenic voiding dysfunction probably play a role. Lower-energy TUMT protocols have a lower incidence of erectile dysfunction *(28)* reported an incidence of erectile dysfunction in 18.2% of patients undergoing high-energy TUMT, compared with 26.5% for TURP.

Overall, satisfaction with sex life seems to be higher in patients who have had TUMT than in patients who have had TURP, with 55% of patients undergoing microwave thermotherapy reported as very satisfied vs 21% of those who underwent TURP. However, only 27% of this population were satisfied with their urinary flow after TUMT compared with 74% of patients after TURP.

The risk of acute myocardial infarction in the posttreatment period is not negligible with TUMT. There is a higher risk of myocardial infarction after both TURP and TUMT, especially more than 2 yr after therapy *(29)*. More patients died from cardiovascular disease from both therapies than would be expected in the general population. The explanation for this finding is not understood.

OTHER USES AND FUTURE DIRECTIONS

In the future, because of the risk factors for symptomatic BPH, patients may be better stratified to determine the optimal choice of therapies (i.e., pharmacotherapy vs TURP vs TUMT vs other methods). Responders and nonresponders may be differentiated better by prostatic biopsy, and the optimal combination of preoperative medicines may allow for increased comfort, with the optimal time and energy requirements for therapy decreasing morbidity. The long-term results of the balance between patient tolerability and efficacy need to be evaluated adequately in a controlled setting.

Microwave therapy may be of value to treat other types of prostate disease. Microwave therapy is known to be lethal to many microorganisms because microwaves are used to sterilize urinary catheters and surgical scalpels. Microwave thermotherapy may have a role in the treatment for selected patients with nonbacterial prostatitis who are unresponsive to traditional therapies *(30)*.

CONCLUSIONS

TUMT is a safe and effective minimally invasive alternative for the treatment of symptomatic BPH. TUMT can be performed during a short office visit without using intravenous sedation. This is a good alternative for patients who are at high surgical and anesthetic risk. It is not effective for patients with a large median lobe or a very large prostate and results in less vigorous urinary flow patterns than TURP.

Enthusiastic reassessment of procedures that may reduce local and overall morbidity and maintain or improve immediate and long-term physiologic results is understandable and laudable. Currently, the limited number of patients and the evolving selection and technical approaches as well as limited follow-up information make this difficult. In summary, this minimally invasive therapy appears to balance efficacy and tolerability, although this balance might be tenuous for patients long term.

REFERENCES

1. McCaskey D. Ultra-violet light as a medical adjuvant. Am J Electrother Radiol 1921;39:152–154.
2. Corbus BC. Carcinoma of penis treated by thermoelectrocagulation. Am J Surg 1929;6:816.
3. Yerushalmi A, Servadio C, Leib Z, et al. Local hyperthermia for the treatment of carcinoma of the prostate: a preliminary report. Prostate. 1982;3(6):623–630.
4. Yerushalmi A, Fishelovitz Y, Singer D. Localized deep microwave hyperthermia in the treatment of poor operative risk patients with benign prostatic hyperplasia. J Urol 1985;133(5):873–876.
5. Sapozink MD, Boyd SD, Astrahan MA. Transurethral hyperthermia for benign prostatic hyperplasia: preliminary clinical results. J Urol 1990;143(5):944–949.
6. Brehmer M, Svensson I. Heat-induced apoptosis in human prostatic stromal cells. BJU Int 2000;85(4):535–541.
7. Djavan B, Bursa B, Basharkhah A. Pretreatment prostate-specific antigen as an outcome predictor of targeted transurethral microwave thermotherapy. Urology 2000;55(1):51–57.
8. d'Ancona FC, Albers YH, Kiemeney LA. Can histopathology predict treatment outcome following high-energy transurethral microwave thermotherapy of the prostate? Results of a biopsy study. Prostate 1999;40(1):28–36.
9. Khair AA, Pacelli A, Iczkowski KA. Does transurethral microwave thermotherapy have a different effect on prostate cancer than on benign or hyperplastic tissue? Urology 1999;54(1):67–72.

10. d'Ancona FC, van der Bij AK, Francisca EA. Results of high-energy transure-thral microwave thermotherapy in patients categorized according to the American Society of Anesthesiologists operative risk classification. Urology 1999;53(2):322–328.

11. Djavan B, Shariat S, Fakhari M. Neoadjuvant and adjuvant α-blockade improves early results of high-energy transurethral microwave thermotherapy for lower urinary tract symptoms of benign prostatic hyperplasia: a randomized, prospective clinical trial. Urology 1999;53(2):251–259.

12. Djavan B, Fakhari M, Shahrokh S, Keywan G, Marberger M. A novel intraurethral prostatic bridge catheter for prevention of temporary prostatic obstruction following high energy transurethral microwave thermotherapy in patients with benign prostatic hyperplasia. J Urol 1999;161(1):144–151.

13. Hallin A, Berlin T. Transurethral microwave thermotherapy for benign prostatic hyperplasia: clinical outcome after 4 years. J Urol 1998;159(2):459–464.

14. de la Rosette JJ, Francisca EA, Kortmann BB. Clinical efficacy of a new 30-min algorithm for transurethral microwave thermotherapy: initial results. BJU Int 2000;86(1):47–51.

15. Francisca EA, Kortmann BB, Floratos DL. Tolerability of 3.5 versus 2.5 high-energy transurethral microwave thermotherapy. Eur Urol 2000;38(1):59–63.

16. Roehrborn CG, Preminger G, Newhall P, et al. Microwave thermotherapy for benign porstatic hyperplasia with the Dornier Urowave: results of a randomized, double-blind, multicenter, sham-controlled trial. Urology 1998;51(1):19–28.

17. Thalmann GN, Mattei A, Threuthardt C, Burkhard FC, Studer UE. Transurethral microwave therapy in 200 patients with a minimum followup of 2 years: urodynamic and clinical results. J Urol 2002;167(6):2496–2501.

18. Djavan B, Roehrborn CG, Shariat S. Prospective randomized comparison of high energy transurethral microwave thermotherapy versus α-blocker treatment of patients with benign prostatic hyperplasia. J Urol 1999;161(1):139–143.

19. Djavan B, Seitz C, Roehrborn CG, et al. Targeted transurethral microwave thermotherapy versus alpha-blockade in benign prostatic hyperplasia: outcomes at 18 months. Urology 2001;57(1):66–70.

20. Ahmed M, Bell T, Lawrence WT, et al. Transurethral microwave thermotherapy (Prostatron version 2.5) compared to transurethral resection of the prostate for the treatment of benign prostatic hyperplasic: a randomized, controlled, parallel study. BJ Urol 1997;79:181–185.

21. d'Ancona FC, Francisca EA, Eitjes EP, et al. Transurethral resection of the prostate versus high-energy thermotherapy of the prostate in patients with benign prostatic hyperplasia: long-term results. BJ Urol 1998;81:259.

22. Floratos SL, Kiemeney LA, Rossi C, et al. Long-term followup of randomized transurethral microwave thermotherapy versus transurethral prostatic resection. J Urol 2001;165(5):1533–1538.

23. Floratos DL, Sonke GS, Francisca EA. High energy transurethral microwave thermotherapy for the treatment of patients in urinary retention. J Urol 2000;163(5):1457–1460.

24. Djavan B, Seitz C, Ghawidel K, et al. High-energy transurethral microwave thermotherapy in patients with acute urinary retention due to benign prostatic hyperplasia. Urology 1999;54(1):18–22.

25. Norby B, Frimodt-Moller PC. Development of a urethrorectal fistula after transurethral microwave thermotherapy for benign prostatic hyperplasia. BJU Int 2000;85(4):554–555.

26. Lin DC, Lin TM, Tong YC. Emphysematous prostatic abscess after transurethral microwave thermotherapy. J Urol 2001;166(2):625.

27. Francisca EAE, d'Ancona FCH, Mueleman ESH, et al. Sexual function following high energy microwave thermotherapy: results of a randomized controlled study comparing transurethral microwave thermotherapy to transurethral prostatic resection. J Urol 1999;161(2):486–490.

28. Arai Y, Aoki Y, Okubo K. Impact of interventional therapy for benign prostatic hyperplasia on quality of life and sexual function: a prospective study. J Urol 2000;164(4):1206–1211.

29. Hahn RG, Farahmand BY, Hallin A. Incidence of acute myocardial infarction and cause-specific mortality after transurethral treatments of prostatic hypertrophy. Urology 2000;55(2):236–240.

30. Liatsikos EN, Dinlenc CZ, Kapoor R, Smith AD. Transurethral microwave thermotherapy for the treatment of prostatitis. J Endourol 2000;14(8):689–692.

9 Transurethral Incision of the Prostate

Robert F. Donnell, MD, FACS

Contents

INTRODUCTION
BACKGROUND
PATIENT SELECTION
METHODS
RESULTS
TREATMENT SIDE EFFECTS
DISCUSSION
REFERENCES

INTRODUCTION

Men often report increasing irritative and obstructive voiding symptoms with advancing age and believe this to be a normal process of aging. Whereas these urinary symptoms are common, they should not be viewed as normal. Fortunately, although the age-related processes that produce the changes in urinary symptoms may have significant impact on quality of life, there is little risk to the quantity of life. Many of these patients seek medical evaluation out of fear of prostate cancer. However, it is the patient bother caused by these symptoms that justifies the decision to pursue therapy. Transurethral incision of the prostate (TUIP) can provide excellent relief in a select group of patients with a lower side-effect profile than transurethral resection of the prostate (TURP).

BACKGROUND

Historically, the development of lower urinary tract symptoms (LUTS) was attributed to age-associated benign prostate enlargement.

From: *Management of Benign Prostatic Hypertrophy*
Edited by: K. T. McVary © Humana Press Inc., Totowa, NJ

As early as the 1800s, physicians attempted surgical relief of lower urinary tract obstruction caused by prostate enlargement. Initial attempts focused on sharp curetting or urinary tract incisions. In the early 1900s, McCarthy incorporated a fenestrated tube, a high-frequency current delivered by means of a Tungsten wire loop to resect tissue, and the foroblique lens by Wappler to provide the basis for the modern resectoscope. Further improvements such as the fiberoptic lighting systems; a wide-angle lens; a constant-flow, low-pressure resectoscope; and endoscopic cameras provide us with the modern-day resectoscope. Today, TURP and the requisite patient outcomes are a reflection of a technology developed over the past 125 years. TURP remains the gold standard of treatment despite all advances in health care. However, the complication rate, including blood loss requiring transfusion, retrograde ejaculation, impotence, stricture formation, and rate of re-operation remains high. Further, TURP is reported to have greater perioperative mortality than open prostatectomy, and higher retreatment rates, which increases the long-term cost. The side effect profile of TURP and failure of the procedure to provide symptomatic relief in a significant number of men justifies the search for less invasive therapies.

The development of TUIP parallels the development of TURP. Credit for the first transurethral procedure is often given to Guthrie in 1834 and Bottini in 1897. Keitzer incorporated these techniques for the surgical relief of obstructive symptoms from bladder neck contracture. Realization that individuals with LUTS attributed to benign prostate enlargement may benefit from these techniques, Orandi popularized the application of TUIP to this condition in the United States (1–4). Transurethral prostatic incision is a simpler and less invasive procedure than transurethral prostatic resection, but it is underused. It has been suggested that at least half of the patients who currently undergo transurethral prostatic resection would be treated effectively with transurethral prostatic incision, thereby avoiding many of the risks of the former procedure.

PATIENT SELECTION

Patient indications for treatment are similar to patient indications for TURP. Patients should meet absolute indicators (recurrent urinary tract infections, bladder calculi, impairment of renal function caused by bladder outlet obstruction, urinary retention) or relative indicators (significant impairment of quality of life) for selection. Because many of these patients are younger than patients considered for TURP, proper patient selection is imperative to prevent the need for repeated therapy. Prostate tissue is not removed during TUIP and therefore no tissue is obtained for pathologic analysis. Thus, all patients undergoing TUIP should be evaluated preoperatively with both a serum prostate specific antigen (PSA) determination and a digital rectal examination (5).

The majority of physicians consider prostate size important when selecting a therapy for benign prostate obstruction. Physicians performed TURP in 79% of patients, with only 15% undergoing TUIP (typically those patients with a mean prostate volume of ≤ 25 mL) (6). Yet, the majority of individuals undergoing TURP have less than 30 g of tissue resected, and therefore, many would have been good candidates for TUIP. Today, transrectal ultrasound provides an accurate assessment of prostate volume and improves patient triage based on gland size (7). Adequate volume assessment avoids the use of TUIP in those men whose gland is too large for TUIP. The deep incisions increase risk of transfusion, result in both surgical and sexual complications, and may fuse by adhesions with return of symptoms (4).

The use of urodynamics for the male with LUTS remains controversial. Current Agency for Health Care Policy Research guidelines support urodynamics as an optional test, the use of urodynamics in the younger man being considered for TUIP often provides additional guidance. Relatively young, symptomatic men without video fluoroscopic evidence of elevated voiding pressures (mean pressures 60–106 cm H_2O) (8,9); men with poor peak urinary flow rates, and poor funneling of the bladder neck do not benefit from invasive therapy to disrupt the bladder neck (10). Finally, cystoscopy is useful to rule out other urethral, prostatic, and bladder disease as the source of symptoms. However, cystoscopic findings of a high or tight bladder neck are nonspecific and should not be considered diagnostic of primary bladder neck obstruction. Because the cause of LUTS in these men is not clear and may have a psychological component, it is recommended that empiric surgical treatment be avoided (11).

Trapped Prostate

Turner-Warwick introduced the term trapped prostate to describe the small obstructing prostate trapped between the bladder neck and the external sphincter (12). Today, this poorly understood cause of LUTS in men is termed primary bladder neck obstruction, Marion's disease, (13) dysfunctional bladder neck, (14) or bladder neck dyssynergia (15,16). Often, these men are young (age 20–50 yr), with long-standing obstructive and irritative voiding symptoms, and often they have been misdiagnosed with chronic nonbacterial prostatitis, neurogenic bladder dysfunction, or psychogenic voiding dysfunction (8–10,14). Video urodynamics and pressure-flow studies demonstrate elevated detrusor pressures, decreased urine flow rates, and obstruction at the bladder neck as noted previously. Although the cause of this disorder is not clear, abnormalities of the bladder neck musculature and sympathetic nervous dysfunction have been implicated, providing the rationale for use of α-blocking agents *(9,12,16,17)*. Although most patients initially choose α-blocker therapy, few realize adequate long-term relief *(8)*. In contrast, 87% of men report adequate relief of symptoms after transurethral incision *(18)*. Transurethral incision of the bladder neck is the standard treatment for primary bladder neck obstruction and is effective at improving urinary flow rates and lower urinary tract symptoms *(8–10,14)*.

Urinary Obstruction After Brachytherapy

Significant LUTS following brachytherapy for prostate cancer remains a significant clinical issue. Often, these patients are younger and are selected for brachytherapy based on the desire to minimize the risks associated with radical surgery or external beam radiation. It is tempting to believe that the less invasive nature of TUIP will translate into improved outcomes and a lower complication rate in men with retention after permanent brachytherapy. Furthermore, TURP could compromise full-dose effective radiation delivery to the prostate. The unacceptable complication rate has prompted the recommendation for nonsurgical alternatives *(19)*. A report on a small series of patients who underwent TUIP to relieve obstruction after brachytherapy identified some degree of permanent incontinence in 70% of patients *(20)*. However, there was no obvious relationship between the degree of incontinence and the use of TURP vs TUIP, the amount of tissue resected, or the time between brachytherapy and TURP or TUIP.

METHODS

Surgical planning for TUIP follows the same planning procedure used for TURP. Many physicians would recommend performing a cystoscopic examination at the beginning of the procedure. The feasibility of the planned procedure can be confirmed, and if required, local anesthesia administered to the surgical area. Lidocaine or bupivacaine local anesthesia can be administered transurethrally using an endoscopic needle or transperineal periprostatic infiltration *(21–24)*. The majority of TUIP patients given local anesthesia in reported series (>80%) felt that it provided satisfactory pain prevention, and 90% would agree to undergo the procedure again after receiving only local anesthesia

(21,22,25). Patient premedication with an opioid and a benzodiazepine in addition to lidocaine was an option in some series *(21)*. Although the use of local anesthesia is possible, we use a regional anesthetic such as spinal anesthesia most commonly at our institution.

Therapy should begin with the smallest resectoscope sheath to reduce risk of stricture formation. The table setup should include a Collin's knife or resectoscope loop based on the surgeon's preference. After anesthesia is administered, the urethra is sounded and the resectoscope sheath with obturator is inserted atraumatically. The obturator is replaced with the Iglasius working element and surgical incisions are made according to surgeon preference, extent of anesthesia field, and real-time relief bladder outlet obstruction. One or two incisions can be made in assorted locations, or some physicians would create a trough to relieve outflow obstruction. The details of each technique are detailed in the following.

One-Incision Technique

The one-incision technique has been described with the incision located at the 5, 6, 7, or 12 o'clock position. When the physician selects a posterior or a lateral incision, the incision is created from the area approx 1 cm distal to the ureteral orifice (or the intraureteric ridge with a 6 o'clock incision) and continued to the cephalad extent of the verumontanum. There are no studies comparing patient outcomes with variations in the single-incision technique; however, incisions at the 6 o'clock position may be associated with a greater potential for injury to the rectum and lateral posterior incisions may increase the risk of injury to the neurovascular bundles. Incisions at the 12 o'clock position may increase the risk of hemorrhage from the dorsal vein. Initial reports comparing the outcomes of TUIP and TURP confirm the effectiveness and reduced complication rate with TUIP. In a large series of 700 men (transurethral resection = 388; bladder neck incision = 312), the catheterization period was shorter and there was less infection and a significantly reduced need for blood transfusion with TUIP, in addition to satisfactory outcome in terms of symptom relief and need for further surgery. This technically simpler procedure was easier to teach and worked well for patients with acute retention as well as for those treated electively *(26)*. Long-term follow up in early series confirmed the durability of the technique. The mean symptom scores decreased significantly from 9.66 preoperatively to 4.59 at a mean follow-up of 2.24 yr, and peak urinary flow rates increased from 7.4 to 14.7 mL/s ($p < 0.0001$). A total of 87% of men were satisfied with their clinical improvement, and only 7.6% of men required subsequent TURP, which compares with historic results for TURP *(27)*. Notably, the incidence of retrograde ejaculation was markedly less at 16%, although 52.5% of patients noted a reduction in the volume of ejaculate *(28)*.

Two-Incision Technique

The two-incision approach creates incisions at the 5 and 7 o'clock positions from approx 1 cm distal to each ureteral orifice through the bladder neck to just proximal to the verumontanum. The incisions are deepened until no ridge is visible at the bladder neck and fat is visualized through the distracted capsular fibers *(23)*. Some surgeons make an incision down to the circular fibers but not through the fibers to reduce the risk of hemorrhage. The absence of prostate tissue for histologic analysis represented a valid argument against TUIP in the pre-PSA era, prompting the suggestion for prostate grooving. Simsek used a standard resectoscope loop to create grooves at 5 and 7 o'clock and submitted the prostate chips for pathologic examination. In his series of 25 patients, the outcomes and re-operation rate were similar to those of the standard two-incision technique *(29)*. However, in the post-PSA era, there is probably no advantage to the grooving technique. Still others describe full resection of the prostate floor between the 5 and 7 o'clock positions. This approach is more correctly labeled a limited TURP and is not considered here.

Postoperative Care

In the immediate postoperative period, two patient care decisions are required. In reality, the response to the first decision often influences the second decision. The first decision is whether it is feasible to treat the patient as an outpatient. The second decision concerning catheter removal is often dictated by the response to the first decision. In the late 1980s, hospital stays were typically 4.4 to 6.2 and 4.4 to 8.4 days for incision and resection, respectively *(30–32)*. Subsequent studies have reported hospital stays that vary from a few hours *(23,33)* to 4 or more days *(26)* after removal of Foley catheter. The average hospital stay is 2 d for TURP *(34,35)* and 1 d for TUIP *(36)*. Economic pressures played a key role in decreasing length of stay after these procedures, and presently, most studies report a catheterization interval of 24–48 h postoperatively *(4,23,32,36–40)*. Today, the catheter is removed and the patient is discharged home the morning after surgery or the transurethral incision is performed on an outpatient basis with the catheters removed the next day in the office *(40)*. Because patient comfort immediately after surgery is often related to the catheterization period, the patient is usually very willing to return to the clinic for catheter removal. Whereas a decreased catheterization time is theoretically associated with a decreased complication rate (stricture and infection), early catheter removal does not appear to influence complications *(34)*. When choosing a patient for early catheter removal, the physician and the patient should be cautioned that the need for recatheterization is greatest in men with diabetes and in those with a history of urinary tract distention. Interestingly, the choice of anesthesia, history of urinary tract infection, size of the prostate gland, and patient age do not significantly influence the risk for recatheterization *(37)*.

Outpatient follow-up after surgery should include short-term assessment for retention as well as intermediate follow-up for adequate relief of symptoms. Four weeks after transurethral surgery, approx 60% of patients experience one or more significant symptoms, and 12% of patients complain of persistence of symptoms 3 mo after TURP, which justifies the follow-up of all patients *(41)*.

Laser TUIP

The use of lasers for TUIP represented efforts to further decrease the risk of transfusion, catheterization time, and establish TUIP as an outpatient procedure *(42–44)*. Investigators have described the use of both the neodymium:yttrium-aluminum-garnet and Holmium lasers. In one series of 100 men, a single transmural incision out to the fat was made from the ureteral orifice to the verumontanum using holmium:yttrium-aluminum-garnet laser energy (transmitted through a 400-nm fiber sheathed in a ureteral catheter). The patients reported rapid improvements in symptom scores (International Prostate Symptom Score decreased from 19.2 to 3.7 at 6 wk), urine flow rates (peak urinary flow rate decreased from 9.79 to 19.23), and postvoid residuals (decreased from 133.6 mL preoperatively to 27 mL after the procedure). All of these values were unchanged after 2-yr follow-up. Finally, laser TUIP was performed without the need for postoperative catheterization, and erectile dysfunction did not develop as a result of the procedure in any patient *(45)*.

RESULTS

There are few large, randomized studies that compare the one-incision technique with the two-incision or the trough technique. A prospective comparison of the single-incision with the two-incision technique (44 unilateral vs 60 bilateral) failed to find a significant difference between the unilateral and bilateral incision groups. The improvement in subjective parameters (indirect parameters) postoperatively seemed to be similar; however, TURP was needed more often after unilateral incision than after bilateral incision. Postoperative complications were reported only in the bilateral incision group *(46)*. Turner-Warwick noted similar subjective and objective improvements in patients who were treated with incisions at the 4 and 8 o'clock positions and in those treated with a single full-thickness incision. He reported results in 50 patients who were treated with a single full-thickness incision that were as satisfactory as those of patients treated with a bilateral incision *(47)*.

Defining patient outcomes after therapy for LUTS has undergone significant change over time. One can change the paradigms to measure the outcome, putting emphasis on cost, need to retreat, and quality of life *(48)*. The advent of the Agency for Health Care Policy Research Guidelines for BPH brought to light that a successful outcome defined by the physician might differ from the patient's definition of success. This is most evident in the literature when direct vs indirect endpoints are compared. Physicians have used direct endpoints because they are measurable. Available direct measures include the AUA symptom index, urine flow rates, postvoid residuals, and pressure flow studies. However, the degree of improvement in urodynamic parameters does not correlate with the degree of symptomatic improvement reported by the patient after TURP *(23,49)* transurethral incision *(23)*, and laser prostatectomy *(49–52)*.

Because patient perception of success often centers on improvement in quality of life, treatment outcomes need to be evaluated in light of this changing endpoint. This observation becomes critical when one realizes that therapies associated with a decreased urine flow rate, voided volumes, or increased postvoid residuals are unlikely to be accepted by either physician or patient. However, a therapy associated with minimal improvement in urine flow rate, voided volume, or postvoid residual may not be rejected by the patient if the bother attributed to the urinary tract decreases and the risk profile is more acceptable.

Direct Outcome Measures

Direct outcome measures such as urinary flow rates, detrusor pressures at maximum flow, and postvoid residuals are common historic measures used to evaluate the efficacy of therapy for LUTS. Improvement in urodynamic parameters after TURP compared with TUIP are typically slightly in favor of TURP, but the clinical significance when a difference is demonstrated is controversial. The improvement in urinary flow rate is typically greater after TURP, in the range of 0 to 4.1 mL/s greater than after TUIP. In two studies, detrusor pressure at maximum flow rate decreased more in the TURP group than in the TUIP

group, and the urethral pressure profile was shorter after the operation
(6,30). Urodynamic improvements remained at a mean follow-up of 53
mo. At that time, the reported mean detrusor pressure at peak flow had
decreased from 85 to 44 cm H2O, the maximum detrusor pressure had
decreased from 114 to 55 cm H_2O, and the mean maximum flow rate
increased from 10.3 to 15.3 mL/s *(23)*. The average urethral resistance
factor value decreased from 41 cm H_2O to the unobstructed range (16 cm
H_2O) *(53)*. The size of the prostate was an important selection criterion in
these studies (prostate volume ≤ 30 cm) *(23,30,54,55)*.

Of note, although urodynamic testing is helpful in many men preoperatively, postoperative urodynamic data do not correlate with patient
reported improvement. A reported 80% of all patients participating in
urodynamic studies of transurethral resection, transurethral incision,
and laser prostatectomy had obstruction before treatment, but the number of men who did not have obstruction after treatment was low (transurethral resection 51%; laser prostatectomy 41%, and transurethral
incision 29%) *(23,50–52,56)*.

Indirect Outcome Measures

Improvement in indirect parameters after TUIP and TURP would
suggest that both procedures produce similar improvement in quality of
life, as both procedures report an 85% success rate judged by patients'
personal evaluation *(57)*. Symptom scores 12 mo after randomization
were improved in 63–85% of patients undergoing incision and in 63–
88% of those undergoing resection.

Given the similarity of improvement in indirect parameters, the lower
risk profile associated with TUIP has become a major criterion for pro-
motion of TUIP. These factors include the cost related to operative and
hospitalization time, patient comfort related to catheterization time, risk
of blood transfusion, stricture or bladder neck contracture, impotence,
and retrograde ejaculation. The mean intervention time required for
TUIP was 14–18 min compared with 32–44 min for the transurethral
resection group *(30,32,37,39,58)*.

TREATMENT SIDE EFFECTS

Sexual Function

Preservation of sexual function after transurethral surgery for LUTS
includes both antegrade ejaculation and erectile function. Retrograde
ejaculation after TURP is reported in 62–100% of men but in only 0–
35% of men after TUIP *(8–10,30,47,57,59,60)*. The successful preservation of antegrade ejaculation after transurethral surgery is most likely

related to the quantity of residual tissue. Studies have noted that preservation of antegrade ejaculation is more likely in those men treated with a single incision than in those treated by the two-incision technique (46,61). The risk of erectile dysfunction after TUIP is estimated at 3.9–24.4 %. Other investigators have reported a 100% potency preservation rate when TUIP was performed with the holmium:yttrium-aluminum-garnet laser (45).

Bladder Neck Contracture

There is a significant incidence of bladder neck contracture after TURP, particularly when treating smaller prostates (62). Fortunately, the bladder neck contracture rate is dramatically less after TUIP, and some series would suggest that contracture of the bladder neck and urinary incontinence do not occur with transurethral incision. These same studies also indicate that the incidence of epididymo-orchitis and stricture is lower with TUIP than with resection (3).

Re-Operation

Studies indicate that BPH is progressive. Primary success rates for TURP, TUIP, and open prostatectomy are good, but in long-term follow-up studies, 10–25% of patients undergo secondary procedures after 5–10 yr (7). Therapies for LUTS attributed to BPH may fail because of continued growth of the prostate, failure to adequately relieve obstruction, or patient selection. Cystoscopy 24 mo after surgery showed adhesions between the lateral lobes, closed incisions, or obstructing prostatic lobes in most of the patients who were treated by incision, but not in those treated with TURP (39). Initial reports indicated a retreatment rate for TUIP that was similar to or lower than that of TURP during the first 5 yr of follow-up (4,62,63). However, others have reported a re-operation rate of 7–23% at 2–5 yr (27,28,59).Overall, the durability of TUIP is probably slightly less than that of open prostatectomy and TURP, and patients who are treated with a unilateral incision may be more likely to require a secondary operation (transurethral prostatic resection) than those who undergo a bilateral incision (46,64).

Transfusion of Blood Products

The historic risk of blood transfusion associated with TURP and TUIP must be evaluated in light of the stricter standards for transfusion in the era of the Acquired Immune Deficiency Syndrome virus. Transfusion rates today are lower than historic models because of higher standards for transfusion. Many studies support the greater risk for blood transfusion when patients are treated with TURP compared with TUIP;

however, a review by Madsen and Bruskewitz identified a relatively small difference in the two treatment groups *(26,32,34,39,57,58,65,66,70)*.

DISCUSSION

In 1999, American urologists performed 2482 transurethral prostatic incisions (CPT 52450) vs 88,517 transurethral prostatic resections (CPT 52601) within the Medicare program *(67)*.

Roehrborn reported the following order of magnitude of symptomatic improvement attributed to therapies for LUTS: transurethral resection, open prostatectomy, transurethral incision, balloon dilation, α-blocker therapy, placebo, and finasteride *(68)*. Long-term outcome data from randomized trials revealed no statistically significant difference in total, irritative, or obstructive symptom improvement at all follow-up intervals for either the TURP or TUIP group *(59)*. Operating time, estimated blood loss, time to catheter removal postoperatively, and duration of postoperative hospital stay were all significantly better with TUIP *(59)*. The cost associated with TUIP may be reduced because of decreased operative time, decreased hospital stay, and the ability to perform the surgery using local anesthesia *(69)*. Further, sexual function, including erectile function and ejaculation, are better preserved after TUIP. Finally, long-term success rates are probably less than with TURP or open prostatectomy, but are greater than with medical therapy.

TUIP is relatively easy to learn and perform. TUIP has been shown to be a safe and effective method of relieving urinary outflow obstruction caused by BPH when prostatic size is 30 g or less. This may be the situation for approx 80% of patients undergoing TURP. However, TUIP is not effective for patients with a prominent median lobe or those with a markedly enlarged prostate gland (>30 g). As the management of LUTS continues to evolve, studies evaluating the new minimally invasive techniques should probably compare those techniques with TUIP instead of with TURP, given the safety and efficacy of TUIP *(70)*.

REFERENCES

1. Orandi A. Transurethral incision of the prostrate. J Urol 1973;110(2):229–231.
2. Orandi A. Transurethral incision of prostate. Seven-year follow-up. Urology 1978;12(2):187–189.
3. Orandi A. A new method for treating prostatic hypertrophy. Geriatrics 1978;33(6):58–60,64,65.
4. Orandi A. Transurethral incision of prostate (TUIP): 646 cases in 15 years— a chronological appraisal. Br J Urol 1985;57(6):703–707.
5. Kletscher BA, Oesterling JE. Transurethral incision of the prostate: a viable alternative to transurethral resection. Sem Urol 1992;10(4):265–272.

6. Yang Q, Abrams P, Donovan J, Mulligan S, Williams G. Transurethral resection or incision of the prostate and other therapies: a survey of treatments for benign prostatic obstruction in the UK. BJU Int. 1999;84(6):640–645.

7. Janknegt RA. Surgical management for benign prostatic hyperplasia: indications, techniques, and results. Prostate 1989;2(suppl):79–93.

8. Kaplan SA, Te AE, Jacobs B Z. Urodynamics evidence of vesical neck obstruction in men with misdiagnosed chronic bacterial prostatitis and the therapeutic role of endoscopic incision of the bladder neck. J Urol 1994;152:2063–2065.

9. Webster GD, Lockhart JL, Older RA. The evaluation of bladder neck dysfunction. J Urol 1980;123:196–198.

10. Norlen LJ, Blaivas JG. Unsuspected proximal urethral obstruction in young and middle-aged men. J Urol 1986;135:972–976.

11. George NJR, Slade N. Hesitancy and poor stream in younger men without outflow tract obstruction—the anxious bladder. Br J Urol 1979;51:506–509.

12. Turner-Warwick R, Whiteside CG, Worth PH, Milroy EJ, Bates CP. A urodynamic view of the clinical problems associated with bladder neck dysfunction and its treatment by endoscopic incision and trans-trigonal posterior prostatectomy. Br J Urol 1973;45:44–59.

13. Marion G. Surgery of the neck of the bladder. Br J Urol 1933;5:351.

14. Woodside JR. Urodynamic evaluation of dysfunctional bladder neck obstruction in men. J Urol 1980;124:673–677.

15. Turner-Warwick R. Bladder outflow obstruction in the male. In Mundy AR, Stephenson TP, Wein AJ, eds., Urodynamics. Principles, Practice and Application, Edinburgh: Churchill Livingstone, 1984, pp. 183–204.

16. Crowe R, Noble J, Robson T, et al. An increase of neuropeptide Y but not nitric oxide synthase-immunoreactive nerves in the bladder neck from male patients with bladder neck dyssynergia. J Urol 1995;154:1231–1236.

17. Awad SA, Downie JW, Lywood DW, Young RA, Jarzylo SV. Sympathetic activity in the proximal urethra in patients with urinary obstruction. J Urol 1976;115:545–547.

18. Trockman BA, Gerspach J, Dmochowski R, et al. Primary bladder neck obstruction: urodynamic findings and treatment results in 36 men. J Urol 1996; 156(4):1418–1420.

19. Konety BR, Phelan MW, O'Donnell WF, Antiles L, Chancellor MB. Urolume stent placement for the treatment of postbrachytherapy bladder outlet obstruction. Urology 2000;55(5):721–724.

20. Hu K, Wallner K. Urinary incontinence in patients who have a TURP/TUIP following prostate brachytherapy. Int J Radiat Oncol Biol Phys 1998;40(4):783–786.

21. Irani I, Bon D, Fournier F, Dore B, Aubert J. Patient acceptability of transurethral incision of the prostate under local anaesthesia. Br J Urol 1996;78(6):904–906.

22. Hugosson J, Bergdahl S, Norlen L, Ortengren T. Outpatient transurethral incision of the prostate under local anesthesia: operative results, patient security and cost effectiveness. Scand J Urol Nephrol 1993;27(3):381–385.

23. Sirls LT, Ganabathi K, Zimmern PE, et al. Transurethral incision of the prostate: an objective and subjective evaluation of long-term efficacy. J. Urol 1993; 150(part 2):1615–1621.

24. Sinha B, Haikel G, Lange PH, Moon PD, Narayan P. Transurethral resection of the prostate with local anesthesia in 100 patients. J Urol 1986;135:719–721.

25. Graversen PH, Gasser TC, Larsen EH, Dorflinger T, Bruskewitz RC. Transurethral incisions of the prostate under local anaesthesia in high-risk patients: a pilot study. Scand J Urol Nephrol. 1987;104(suppl):87–90.

26. Edwards LE, Bucknall TE, Pittam MR, Richardson DR, Stanek J. Transurethral resection of the prostate and bladder neck incision: a review of 700 cases. Br J Urol 1985;57(2):168–171.

27. Katz PG, Greenstein A, Ratliff JE, Marks S, Guice J. Transurethral incision of the bladder neck and prostate. J Urol 1990;144(3):694–696.

28. Mobb GE, Moisey CU. Long-term follow-up of unilateral bladder neck incision. Br J Urol 1988;62(2):160–162.

29. Simsek F, Turkeri LN, Ilker YN, Akdas A. Transurethral grooving of the prostate in the treatment of patients with benign prostatic hyperplasia. An alternative to transurethral incision. Br J Urol 1993;72(1):84–87.

30. Hellstrom P, Lukkarinen O, Kontturi M. Bladder neck incision or transurethral electroresection for the treatment of urinary obstruction caused by a small benign prostate? A randomized urodynamic study. Scand J Urol Nephrol 1986;20:187–192.

31. Li MK, Ng ASM. Bladder neck resection and transurethral resection of the prostate; a randomized prospective trial. J Urol 1987;138:807–809.

32. Dorflinger T, Jensen FS, Krarup T, et al. Transurethral prostatectomy compared with incision of the prostate in the treatment of prostatism caused by small benign prostate glands. Scand J Urol Nephrol 1992;26:333–338.

33. McLoughlin MG, Kinahan TJ. Transurethral resection of the prostate in the outpatient setting. J Urol 1990;143:951–952.

34. Mebust WK, Holtgrewe HL, Cockett ATK, Peters PC, and Writing Committee: Transurethral prostatectomy: immediate and postoperative complications. A cooperative study of 13 participating institutions evaluating 3,885 patients. J Urol 1989;141:243–247.

35. American Urological Association. Guidelines for Urologic Patient Care, Baltimore: American Urological Association, 1987, p. 13.

36. Kelly MJ, Roskamp D, Leach GE. Transurethral incision of the prostate: a preoperative and postoperative analysis of symptoms and urodynamic findings. J Urol 1989;142:1507–1509.

37. Hedlund H, Ek A. Ejaculation and sexual function after endoscopic bladder neck incision. Br J Urol 1985;57:164–167.

38. Irani J, Fauchery A, Dore B, et al. Systematic removal of catheter 48 hours following transurethral resection and 24 hours following transurethral incision of prostate: a prospective randomized analysis of 213 patients. J Urol 1995;153(5):1537–1539.

39. Jahnson S, Dalen M, Gustavsson G, et al. Transurethral incision versus resection of the prostate for small to medium benign prostatic hyperplasia. Br J Urol 1998;81;276–281.

40. Drago JR. Transurethral incision of prostate. Urology 1991;38(4):305–306.

41. Puri R, Smaling A, Lloyd SN. How is follow-up after transurethral prostatectomy best performed? BJU Int. 1999;84(7):795–798.

42. Kabalin JN, Gilling PJ, Fraundorfer MR. Holmium:yttrium-aluminum-garnet laser prostatectomy. Mayo Clin Proc. 1998;73(8):792–797.

43. Perkash I. Use of contact laser crystal tip firing Nd:YAG to relieve urinary outflow obstruction in male neurogenic bladder patients. J Clin Laser Med Surg 1998;16(1):33–38.

44. Cornford PA, Biyani CS, Brough SJ, Powell CS. Daycase transurethral incision of the prostate using the holmium: YAG laser: initial experience. Br J Urol 1997;79(3):383–384.

45. Cornford PA, Biyani CS, Powell CS. Transurethral incision of the prostate using the holmium:YAG laser: a catheterless procedure. J Urol 1998;159(4):1229–1231.

46. Hellstrom P, Tammela T, Mehik A, Lukkarinen O, Kontturi M. Efficacy and safety of bladder neck incision in patients with benign prostatic hyperplasia. Ann Chir Gynaecol 1993;206(suppl):19–23.
47. Turner-Warwick RT. A urodynamic review of bladder outlet obstruction in the male and its clinical implications. Urol Clin N Am 1979;6:171–192.
48. Altwein JE. Obstructive benign prostatic hyperplasia: therapeutical aspects. Eur Urol 1998;34(suppl 1):31–37.
49. Kabalin JN, Gill HS, Bite G, Wolfe V. Comparative study of laser versus electrocautery prostate resection: 18-month followup with complex urodynamic assessment. J Urol 1995;153:94–97.
50. Bosch JL, Groen J, Schroder FH. Treatment of benign prostatic hyperplasia by transurethral ultrasound-guided laser-induced prostatectomy (TULIP): effects on urodynamic parameters and symptoms. Urology 1994;44:507–511.
51. Te Slaa E, de Wildt MJ, Rosier PF, et al. Urodynamic assessment in the laser treatment of benign prostatic enlargement. Br J Urol 1995;76:604–610.
52. Devonec MA. Transurethral thermotherapy. In: Kirby R, McConnell JD, Fitzpatrick JM, Roehrborn CG, Boyle P, eds., Textbook of Benign Prostatic Hyperplasia, Oxford: Isis Medical Media Ltd., 1996, pp. 413–421.
53. Rollema HJ, Van Mastrigt R. Improved indication and followup in transurethral resection of the prostate using the computer program CLIM: a prospective study. J Urol 1992;148:111–115.
54. Holtgrewe HL. Guidance for clinical investigation of devices used for the treatment of benign prostatic hyperplasia. J Urol 1993;150:1588–1590.
55. Edwards L, Powell C. An objective comparison of transurethral resection and bladder neck incision in the treatment of prostatic hypertrophy. J Urol 1982;128:325–327.
56. Kabalin JN, Gill HS, Bite G, Wolfe V. Comparative study of laser versus electrocautery prostate resection: 18-month followup with complex urodynamic assessment. J Urol 1995;153:94–97.
57. Larsen EH, Dorflinger T, Gasser TC, Graversen PH, Bruskewitz RC. Transurethral incision versus transurethral resection of the prostate for the treatment of benign prostatic hypertrophy. A preliminary report. Scand J Urol Nephrol 1987;104(suppl):83–86.
58. Li MK, Ng ASM. Bladder neck resection and transurethral resection of the prostate; a randomized prospective trial. J Urol 1987;138:807–809.
59. Christensen MM, Aagaard J, Madsen PO. Transurethral resection versus transurethral incision of the prostate. A prospective randomized study. Urol Clin N Am 1990;17(3):621–630.
60. Riehmann M, Knes JM, Heisey D, Madsen PO, Bruskewitz RC. Transurethral resection versus incision of the prostate: a randomized, prospective study. Urology 1995;45(5):768–775.
61. Ronzoni G, De Vecchis M. Preservation of anterograde ejaculation after transurethral resection of both the prostate and bladder neck. Br J Urol 1998;81(6):830–833.
62. Orandi A. Transurethral incision of prostate compared with transurethral resection of prostate in 132 matching cases. J Urol 1987;138(4):810–815.
63. Yang Q, Peters TJ, Donovan JL, Wilt TJ, Abrams P. Transurethral incision compared with transurethral resection of the prostate for bladder outlet obstruction: a systematic review and meta-analysis of randomized controlled trials. J Urol 2001;165(5):1526–1532.

64. Roehrborn CG. Treatment outcomes and their interpretation in benign prostatic hyperplasia. In: Kirby R, McConnell JD, Fitzpatrick JM, Roehrborn CG, Boyle P, eds., Textbook of Benign Prostatic Hyperplasia, Oxford: Isis Medical Media Ltd, 1996, pp. 473–506.

65. McConnell JD, Barry MJ, Bruskewitz RE, et al. Benign Prostatic Hyperplasia: Diagnosis and Treatment. Clinical Practice Guideline, No 8. AHCPR Publication No 94-0582. Agency for Health Care Policy and Research, Public Health Service, U. S. Department of Health and Human Services, 1994.

66. Soonawalla PF, Pardanani DS. Transurethral incision versus transurethral resection of the prostate. A subjective and objective analysis. Br J Urol 1992;70:174–177.

67. Holtgrew HL. American Urological Association survey of transurethral prostatectomy and the impact of changing medicare reimbursement. Urol Clin N Amer 1990;17(3):587–593.

68. Roehrborn CG. Treatment outcomes and their interpretation in benign prostatic hyperplasia. In: Kirby R, McConnell JD, Fitzpatrick J, Roehrborn C, Boyle P, eds., Textbook of Benign Prostatic Hyperplasia, Oxford: Isis Medical Media Ltd, 1996, pp. 473.

69. Riehmann M, Bruskewitz R. Transurethral incision of the prostate and bladder neck. J Androl 1991;12(6):415–422.

70. Madsen FA, Bruskewitz RC. Transurethral incision of the prostate. Urol Clin N Am 1995;22(2):369–373.

10 Interstitial Laser Coagulation and High-Intensity Focused Ultrasound for the Treatment of Benign Prostatic Hyperplasia

Christopher M. Dixon, MD

CONTENTS

INTRODUCTION
INTERSTITIAL LASER COAGULATION
HIGH-INTENSITY FOCUSED ULTRASOUND
REFERENCES

INTRODUCTION

Medical therapies for benign prostatic hyperplasia (BPH) have been critically investigated by well-designed clinical trials, which is the current model for assessing the safety and efficacy of any treatment for BPH. Pivotal medical studies for BPH are prospective, multicenter, randomized, double-blind, and placebo-controlled *(1,2)*. This study design is the accepted standard to assess clinical safety and efficacy. For ethical and practical reasons, it is often more difficult to design surgical studies that meet all of these criteria. Many of the sponsoring companies do not have adequate financial resources to perform multicenter clinical trials. Designing a trial to minimize bias is essential, particularly because of the public's somewhat automatic acceptance of new technology, in particular laser therapy, as state-of-the-art treatment. Many patients enroll in clinical trials specifically because of the favorable perception that new technology conveys, and this bias is likely to influence subjective outcome parameters. Few studies control for

From: *Management of Benign Prostatic Hypertrophy*
Edited by: K. T. McVary © Humana Press Inc., Totowa, NJ

these important biases. There is not a single device trial that is equivalent in design when compared with the pivotal medical trials.

The development of minimally invasive therapies for the treatment of BPH has seen many innovations during the past 10 years. None were more enthusiastically received than the side-firing laser delivery systems of the early 1990s. Unfortunately, many of these were compared with transurethral resection of the prostate (TURP) and were reported to have equivalent efficacy. Widespread clinical use led to discouraging results, usually with less effectiveness and more irritative symptoms than with TURP, and consequently this approach is rarely used today. The continued development of laser systems has increased the variety of available devices for BPH, but each system has significant differences and each should be assessed independently.

Minimally invasive treatments for BPH should be considered treatment alternatives, not replacements for TURP. In general, minimally invasive devices are less effective than transurethral surgery unless the visual result immediately following treatment is similar to TURP. The role of minimally invasive treatments is becoming established largely because of reasonable symptom improvement, improved safety, reduced risk of adverse sexual effects, outpatient nature of these procedures, and favorable reimbursement policies.

The chapter will focus on interstitial laser coagulation (ILC) and high-intensity focused ultrasound (HIFU) for the treatment of BPH. The clinical data regarding the use of ILC and HIFU are limited. Interpreting the available clinical data must be done in view of the limits of study design, the lack of direct comparative data with other therapeutic choices, and the frequent improvements of these technologies during the evolution of treatment techniques to optimize clinical outcomes. Currently, ILC is widely used, whereas HIFU is not available.

INTERSTITIAL LASER COAGULATION

Laser delivery systems for BPH have continued to evolve over the past 10 years. Even though most of the early delivery systems used neodymium:yttrium-aluminum-garnet (Nd:YAG) as the laser energy source, the delivery devices and lasing techniques were quite different. More recently, diode and holmium:YAG laser sources have been added to the list. Currently there are five categories of delivery systems that have been used for the treatment of BPH: 1) transurethral ultrasound-guided laser prostatectomy, 2) visual laser ablation of the prostate using free-beam side-fire fibers, 3) contact tip laser ablation, 4) ILC, and 5) holmium:YAG prostate resection. All laser delivery systems for the prostate are not the same, and it is important to understand the differences in these systems. Currently, only holmium resection and ILC are used with any regularity.

ILC represents the evolution of laser technology to minimize various problems seen with other laser techniques. For example, a major criticism of visual laser ablation of the prostate was the irritative symptoms often associated with it. This may have been caused by ablation of the urethral lining and exposure of coagulated tissue. The interstitial approach attempts to preserve the urothelium by creating the thermal lesion within the transition zone. Energy loss seen with earlier free-beam systems is eliminated by using a diffuser-tip laser fiber. The fiber is inserted into the prostate, depositing all of the energy into the tissue. Many of the other minimally invasive techniques require specialized equipment and are more difficult to learn. The technique currently recommended involves little more than the endoscopic skills required for rigid cystoscopy. The use of a temperature feedback system and automated treatment cycle makes this minimally invasive approach the fastest available procedure.

Equipment

One of the advantages of this minimally invasive device is the sophisticated yet user-friendly system that has been developed. In addition to the necessary equipment to perform rigid cystoscopy, the Indigo Laser Optic System (Ethicon Endosurgery, Cincinnati, OH) consists of the laser generator, the quartz fiber, and wavelength-specific eye protection.

The laser generator is a 20-watt, 830-nm diode laser that is about the size of a typical computer tower (Fig. 1). It is designed to be portable and does not require any external cooling mechanism. It operates on standard voltage without any special electrical considerations. The generator provides readouts to monitor power delivery, interstitial temperature at the tip of the laser fiber, and a countdown of the treatment time. Total energy delivered (joules) is also recorded. The device is activated by a foot pedal control and has audio notification of both active laser therapy and completion of the energy cycle.

The energy cycle can be controlled manually, but typically the automated feedback cycle is used. This computer-controlled feedback loop optimizes the energy delivery, controlling the laser power delivery based on continued temperature monitoring from the tip of the laser fiber. The target temperature is 85°C, and the treatment cycle lasts for 3 min. Refinements in the system will soon allow the treatment time to be shortened to only 90 s. Built-in safety features monitor the function of the laser generator and the integrity of the laser fiber.

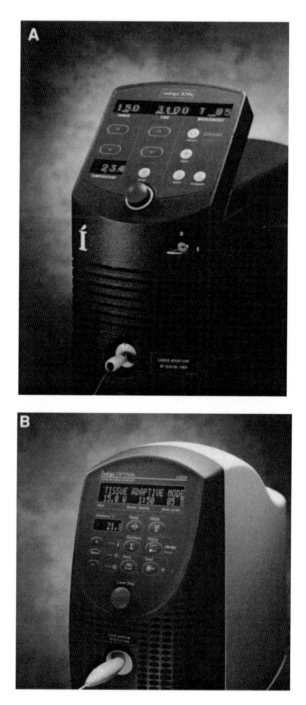

Fig. 1. (A) Laser generator with instrument display. **(B)** The newest generation of the Indigo Laser Optic System, which shortens the treatment cycle to 90 s.

144

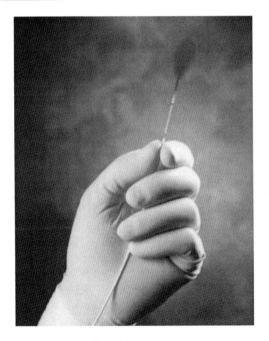

Fig. 2. Diffuser tip illustrating the pattern of laser energy distribution.

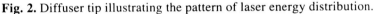

The quartz fiber consists of a coupling mechanism at the proximal end and a diffuser tip with an internal alexandrite crystal to provide interstitial thermal monitoring at the distal end. As the name implies, the diffuser tip dissipates the laser energy in an ellipsoid pattern along the axis of the fiber (Fig. 2). The diffuser portion of the fiber is 1 cm long. The tip of the fiber is sharpened to a point to allow transurethral insertion into the prostate. Fibers are used once per patient.

Procedure

Preprocedure antibiotics are administered. The choice of anesthesia includes general, regional, or local. Issa and others have detailed an office technique using a periprostatic block to allow office-based treatment with ILC in many patients *(3–6)*. The patient is placed in the low lithotomy position as for rigid cystoscopy. A 21-Fr cystoscope is passed into the bladder, and the laser fiber is passed through the working channel of the scope. Fiber position has taken several approaches. One approach involves positioning the scope at the level of the verumontanum, angling the fiber into the right or left side of the prostate. The fiber is advanced deep into the prostate such that two thermal treatments can be performed with one puncture. After the first treatment, the fiber is partially withdrawn to the untreated area of the prostate and a second treatment is performed. A second approach involves multiple punctures along the prostatic urethra. With either approach, the scope is angled 30° to the right or left of the midline. This places the thermal lesion within the prostate and minimizes the chances of thermal damage to the urethral lining. The median lobe is treated directly by one ore more punctures, depending on its size. After the treatment is completed, an indwelling catheter is placed.

Clinical Data

Initially, ILC was performed with Nd:YAG (1064 nm) laser energy and various diffuser fibers. Transperineal and transurethral approaches were also used. Currently, a diode laser (830 nm), a diffuser tip fiber with a temperature feedback system, and a transurethral approach are universally used (Laser Optic System).

In 1995, Muschter and Hofstetter reported on 239 patients treated with an Nd:YAG system *(7)*. Eight patients had retention, and 59 had previous urinary retention. The mean prostate volume was 47.7 mL (range 15–175 mL). Most patients were treated transurethrally (164), but 75 were treated transperineally or by both routes. Multiple different laser fibers were used. An average of 6.2 fiber placements (2–15) were performed. Improvement in symptom score, flow rate, and urinary residuals was significant (Table 1). The retreatment rate within 1 yr was 9.6%.

This uncontrolled series represented the developing experience with this technology and suggested promising results with this device. Treatment became more aggressive as familiarity with the device was gained. Outcomes compared favorably with those of TURP and other laser techniques.

In 1996, Mueller-Lisse et al. reported a series of 18 patients studied with magnetic resonance imaging (MRI) to determine the thermal effects of ILC on the prostate *(8)*. All patients were treated using an Nd:YAG interstitial system. MRI evaluation was performed before and after treatment. All 18 patients were examined 2–3 wk and/or 6–8 wk after treatment. One patient was examined 6 mo after laser treatment. T2-weighted images and image evaluation software were used to measure total prostate, transition zone, and laser-induced necrotic volumes. Intraobserver and interobserver variability was 3% and 4.5%, respectively. For the final measurements, two observers evaluated the images and came to a consensus.

Total prostate volume averaged 68.5 mL (range 28.9–144.4 mL). Transition zone volume averaged 45.2 mL (range 18.2–100.2 mL).

Table 1
Clinical Outcomes for Interstitial Laser Coagulation

Author	Study design	Baseline N	Follow-up (months)	AUA Symptom Scores			Mean Qmax (cc/sec)			Comments
				N	Baseline	Follow-up	N	Baseline	Follow-up	
Muschter 1996 (9)	Multicenter, Prospective	112	3	86	20.9	9.6	86	8	15.2	Diode
Muschter 1995 (7)	Prospective	239	12	127	25.4	6.2	127	7.7	17.6	Nd:Yag
Martenson 1999 (12)	Prospective, Randomized	30	26	NR	21.7	12		7.3	10.3	ILC vs TURP, ILC data shown
Martenson 1999 (12)	Prospective	34	26	NR	19.8	6.4	NR	7.8	12.3	ILCe
Williams 1998 (10)	Prospective	25	12	24	23.2	7.2	24	8.4	16.8	
Greenberger 1998 (11)	Prospective	25	3	15	20.2	10.4	15	8.3	12.7	Interim

147

Laser-induced lesions were clearly visualized within the prostate as low-intensity, well-demarcated areas on T2-weighted images. Periprostatic edema was seen in all patients at 48 h after treatment but had resolved in patients who underwent imaging after several weeks. Prostatic swelling was evident by the significant transient increase in total and central prostate volumes 48 h after treatment (43% and 41%, respectively). Mean total lesion size was 16.4 mL, averaging 24% of the total prostate and 36% of the central gland. In the five patients followed 6–8 wk or more, the coagulated areas decreased in size, but overall prostate volume did not decrease.

This well-conducted study confirms the ability of MRI to define thermal areas based on the lack of signal compared with pretreatment images. It also suggests that interstitial laser energy can be accurately placed within the central prostate. No specific correlation between energy delivered and thermal lesion volumes or clinical outcome was presented. A significant tissue response was suggested by the presence of transient periprostatic and presacral edema.

In 1996, Muschter et al. presented the initial results using the Indigo 830e diode laser system (9). They studied 112 men with BPH at six centers. Inclusion criteria were American Urological Association (AUA) system score >12, peak urinary flow rate (Qmax) <13 mL/s, and residual volume <300 mL. All patients were screened to exclude prostate cancer. Transrectal ultrasound was used for prostate volume measurement. Interstitial treatment was carried out using a 17 to 21.5 Fr rigid cystoscope. The mean prostate volume was 56 mL, and 25% of patients received treatment to the median lobe.

Results were reported for 86 patients at 3 mo postprocedure and for 40 patients at 6 mo postprocedure. Symptom score improvements decreased from 20.9 to 9.6 at 3 mo (54%). Flow rates improved from 8.0 mL/s to 15.2 mL/s at 3 mo (90%). Postoperatively, 11% experienced transient dysuria. Retrograde ejaculation occurred in 2.7%, but impotence or incontinence did not occur. Three patients had undergone TURP by 7 mo postprocedure (2.7%).

This report showed excellent short-term results, with no serious adverse effects. Obviously, long-term data are important, but this initial report includes the early experience of six centers and suggests that the learning curve with this technique is brief.

Treatment strategies for ILC therapy have been based on treating a high or low volume of tissue (10). William presented his experience treating 25 patients with the low-volume approach using the Indigo 830e Laser Optic system. The number of lesions was standardized by the formula 0.5 × total prostate volume/8 mL and rounded to the nearest even whole number. The number of lesions was distributed equally between the right and left prostatic lobes. If needed, the median lobe was treated in addition to the lateral lobes.

The mean prostate volume was 38 mL (range 25–90 mL). Three patients had treatment of the median lobe. At 12 mo, the AUA symptom score improved from 23.2 to 7.2, and Qmax improved from 8.4 mL/s to 16.8 mL/s. No procedural or severe adverse experiences occurred. Retrograde ejaculation, incontinence, or worsening erectile dysfunction did not occur. One patient underwent TURP at 6 mo post-ILC treatment.

This study addresses the issue of standardizing the amount of tissue based on prostate volume. Assuming that each thermal lesion is approximately 8 mL and is reproducible, the formula represents the maximal amount of tissue that is treated. It does not account for the possibility of treatment overlap or that subsequent thermal lesions may vary based on changes in prostate blood flow or prostate temperature. With a limited number of patients, it is difficult to assess the outcome of a volume-based treatment approach because a significant number of patients with varying prostate volumes were not treated. Nonetheless, the clinical outcome in this small, single-center experience using this formula was good. With most current thermal treatments, symptom improvement seems to be indifferent to the volume of tissue treated, whereas flow rates improve more significantly with increasing energy delivery.

In 1998, Greenberger and Steiner reported their interim experience using the Indigo 830e Laser Optic System in 25 men with BPH who were followed for an average of 6 mo (11). Inclusion criteria were >40 yr old, AUA score >12, Qmax <13 mL/s, or residual urine volume >100 mL. Medical therapy had failed in all patients, and two patients had previously undergone TURP.

The first 15 patients were treated using general or regional anesthesia, whereas the last eight were treated using local periprostatic block with or without sedation. The mean prostate volume was 42 mL (range 25–80 mL). Symptom scores improved from 20.2 to 9.8, and flow rates improved from 8.3 mL/s to 12.0 mL/s at 9 mo.

Patients were catheterized for 3 d; retention developed in five patients (21%) after initial catheter removal. Postoperative complications were minimal. No new onset of erectile dysfunction or incontinence occurred. One patient reported loss of ejaculatory volume. Transient frequency and urgency was reported in 35% and 20%, respectively. One patient required TURP within the follow-up interval.

This single-center, uncontrolled small series showed good symptom improvement and reasonable flow improvement with no significant adverse outcomes during the limited follow-up period. Conclusions are limited given the obvious study design limitations.

Martenson and de la Rosette presented 44 patients randomized in a 2:1 ratio, ILC vs TURP (14 TURP and 30 ILC). An additional 34 patients were treated using ILC alone in a second study *(12)*. In the randomized trial, a low-energy protocol was used for ILC. The nonrandomized trial used the feedback cycle based on the temperature recorded from the tip of the laser fiber to optimize energy delivery.

For both studies, standard assessments included symptom scores, quality of life, sexual function, flow rate, residual urine measurement, and prostate ultrasonography for volume determination. Patients also underwent pressure-flow urodynamic studies and were followed for 2 yr.

In the randomized trial, ILC showed significant improvements in symptom and flow rate parameters; however, TURP out-performed ILC. Specifically, ILC showed a 45% reduction in symptom score at 2 yr compared with a 77 % reduction in the TURP group. Similarly, flow improvement at 2 yr was greater in the TURP group (41% vs 116%). Prostate volume decreased from 50 mL + 16 mL to 28 mL + 11 mL in the TURP group, but little change was seen in the ILC group (46 + 20 mL to 40 + 21 mL).

Irritative symptoms were rated in both groups but persisted slightly longer in the ILC group. Hematuria was more pronounced in the TURP group. Three patients in the TURP group reported erectile dysfunction at 1 yr. Retrograde ejaculation was reported in 75% of TURP patients and in 42% of ILC patients. No incontinence or transfusion requirement was seen in either group. One patient in the TURP group required a urethrotomy, and six in the ILC group required TURP.

Prolonged urinary retention in the group was anticipated in this trial. A suprapubic catheter was removed on average at 27 d (range 4–102 d) in the ILC group compared with 3 d in the TURP group. In the ILC-treated patients, the suprapubic tube was removed at scheduled visits if adequate voiding was demonstrated (1, 2, or 4 wk).

This is one of the few reports that includes pressure-flow urodynamics. Six months after treatment, improvement in the urethral resistance factor was 29% in the ILC group and 61% in the TURP group. Using the Shafer classification, ILC improved almost 1 class, whereas TURP improved more than 2 classes at an equivalent follow-up interval.

In the nonrandomized trial, greater improvements in outcome parameters were seen compared with ILC therapy without the temperature feedback system. The 830e Laser Optic System provided an improved clinical outcome, presumably because more consistent thermal ablation was provided by the feedback system. This represented a therapeutic improvement, although the magnitude of those improvements did not surpass or equal those seen in the TURP cohort.

This report provides the only comparison of ILC and TURP. The most significant advantages of ILC over TURP in this report were the lower occurrences of erectile dysfunction (TURP 3/14, 21% vs ILC 0/64) and retrograde ejaculation (ILC 42% vs TURP 75%). The disadvantages of ILC compared with TURP included longer catheter times and less clinical or urodynamic improvement. From this report, the clinical efficacy of ILC treatment represents an alternative approach to TURP, although not an equivalent one.

Safety and Morbidity

The safety of any device is of obvious importance. Mebust et al. reviewed the immediate and postoperative complications of TURP, which serves as a benchmark for comparison *(13)*. Immediate complications occurred in 18% of patients, with the most common being failure to void (6.5%), bleeding requiring transfusion (3.9%), clot retention (3.3%), and infection (2.3%). Intraoperative complications occurred in 6.9% of patients, with the most common complication being bleeding requiring transfusion (2.5%). Dilutional hyponatremia caused by TUR syndrome occurred in 2% of patients. Late complications after TURP included bladder neck contracture (2.7%), urethral stricture (2.5%), mild stress incontinence (1.2%), and significant incontinence (0.5%). The reported incidence of impotence was variable and ranged from 4% to 13%. These complication rates were reported from a national survey of American urologists conducted by the AUA in 1987.

Comparative trials are designed to enroll an adequate number of patients to assess efficacy and not highlight adverse events. Compared with TURP, the use of ILC has minimized the major complications of bleeding and incontinence associated with TURP and has eliminated TUR syndrome. Irritative symptoms after ILC appear to be less frequent than after other laser methods, presumably because of urethral preservation, but symptoms are probably not more improved than with TURP. Catheter times are generally longer with ILC. Re-operation rates after ILC have been reported to be from 2.7% to 9.6%, usually requiring TURP. Safety appears to be the most consistent advantage of laser devices at a cost of decreased efficacy compared with TURP.

With more experience, more aggressive laser treatment has been possible, which may increase the complication rate. As techniques are modified, adverse events need to be closely monitored.

Summary

The ILC procedure is intended for symptomatic men with LUTS caused by BPH. Although there are few contraindications to using this approach for BPH, appropriate patient selection will provide a better outcome (14,15).

ILC is best reserved for patients with bothersome symptoms and prostate volumes of 35–75 mL. Patients with elevated urinary residuals (>300 mL), urinary retention, or poor bladder function have been treated, but better outcomes are likely with more conventional treatment such as TURP (16).

Preoperative patient education should include appropriate patient expectations with regard to transient symptom worsening, possible irritative symptoms, and catheter management after treatment. Various approaches have been used, including suprapubic tube placement, urethral catheterization, or clean intermittent catheterization until satisfactory voiding resumes. This decision is best determined on a case-by-case basis. Although not required, preoperative transrectal ultrasound volume measurement is recommended to determine size limitations and the configuration of the median lobe.

Preoperative issues related to sexual function must be discussed, particularly because this is often one of the deciding issues between minimally invasive therapy and TURP. The literature indicates that the likelihood of erectile dysfunction is less with ILC than with TURP. The issue of retrograde ejaculation is more uncertain and probably depends on several issues. These include the aggressiveness of the ILC treatment and whether treatment of a prominent median lobe is necessary. Treatment of the median lobe jeopardizes bladder neck function and presumably increases the likelihood of retrograde ejaculation. The literature does not address this issue in detail, although it is clear that retrograde ejaculation is much less likely than with TURP.

Another issue that is uncertain is the need for continued medical therapy after minimally invasive treatments, including ILC. No reliable data exist to adequately answer this question, but some practical recommendations can be considered. If pretreatment medical therapy is ongoing, generally this is continued posttreatment at least until any treatment-related symptom worsening has resolved. Usually this is approximately 1 mo. Eventual withdrawal of medical therapy would seem reasonable; however, the long-term issues related to prevention of BPH sequelae after minimally invasive therapy are unknown. With recent medical studies concluding that long-term medical therapy can prevent the progression of BPH (defined as worsening symptoms and urinary retention) and the relatively insignificant changes in prostate volume with most minimally invasive approaches, continued medical therapy after these treatments deserves consideration.

ILC has been performed using various anesthetic approaches. Little attention was paid to this issue until office-based treatment became the favored treatment for reimbursement. General or regional anesthesia is obviously adequate for ILC, but the procedure can also be performed using local and/or intravenous sedation. Patient selection and prostate volume are important in making this choice. Prostate block-infiltrating short- and/or long-acting local anesthetics such as lidocaine and marcaine have been recommended when using either the perineal approach or transrectal ultrasound guidance. Adequate anesthesia can usually be achieved by combining intraurethral lidocaine and oral or intravenous sedation, particularly because of the short procedure time of ILC.

ILC represents an accepted minimally invasive option for men with symptomatic BPH. It is the fastest procedure currently available, with recent improvements further shortening the energy cycle to only 90 s per treatment. It is an easy technique to learn, and ongoing clinical trials will further define its role in the treatment of BPH.

HIGH-INTENSITY FOCUSED ULTRASOUND

Another heat-based approach for tissue ablation has been developed using HIFU. As the name implies, this novel technique targets high-energy ultrasound and is guided by standard ultrasound imaging. The focused energy creates heat within the tissue, resulting in irreversible thermal injury. The obvious advantage of this approach is that there are no invasive procedures associated with it as there are with most other minimally invasive therapies.

The development and use of focused ultrasound dates back to the 1940s and 1950s, when it was used primarily for destruction of selected tissue within the brain. In more recent times, its clinical use has been expanded into ophthalmology, oncology, and urology (17).

Technology

The technology of high-intensity ultrasound has been reviewed elsewhere but will be summarized briefly (17). Diagnostic ultrasound imaging and focused ultrasound surgery differ primarily in the way sound energy is delivered and in the acoustic power that is used. Ultrasound imaging uses very short pulses (1–10 ms) and low power of about 200 milliwatt. Focused physiotherapy uses longer pulses (10–100 ms) and power levels of about 1 watt. Focused ultrasound surgery, however, uses much longer pulses (1–3 s) and powers of 100 watts and higher. The purpose of physiotherapy ultrasound is to stimulate tissue repair without irreversible tissue damage, whereas focused ultrasound surgery results in cell death and tissue ablation.

Ultrasound energy interacts with tissue by being absorbed, which results in heating, and by passage of a pressure wave through tissue, creating a phenomenon known as acoustic cavitation. This latter effect can give rise to the formation of gas bubbles by drawing the gas out of solution in the tissue. If the proper acoustic conditions exist, this may lead to very high local temperatures and pressures, resulting in tissue tears and cavitation. In focused ultrasound surgery, cavitation is generally undesirable. As the ultrasound energy travels through tissue, energy loss results by backward scatter (which is used in ultrasound imaging) and absorption by tissue located between the transducer and target organ.

The basic principle of this technique is the delivery of a high-energy pulse of ultrasound in a short time, rapidly raising tissue temperature before organ cooling mechanisms can effectively respond. To avoid damage to intervening tissue (nontarget tissue) and cavitation problems, treatment cycles consist of several seconds of energy delivery for tissue heating, followed by an energy-off interval, allowing some tissue cooling. During the energy-off cycle, imaging of the target occurs to monitor the treatment.

Medical applications use piezo-electric crystals to produce the ultrasound energy after applying an oscillating voltage. Similar to shock-wave lithotripsy, the ultrasound energy can be focused, resulting in a high-intensity focal zone. Extracorporeal systems use a spherical bowl, but this results in a fixed focal length. More flexible systems use a series of lenses or phased-array systems to allow variable focal distances. For the purposes of prostate therapy, most systems use a transrectal approach, which combines the imaging and therapeutic elements into a single probe.

As with any technology, there are various physical impediments to effective tissue ablation. One of the major problems has been the relatively small volume of tissue ablated per unit of time. Efforts to shorten treatment times include the simultaneous use of multiple focused probes, in effect overlapping the focal zones and rotation of the transducer to paint a volume of tissue for ablation. As with diagnostic ultrasound, an air interface severely impedes the transmission of ultrasound energy. A coupling media such as an aqueous gel or water bath/balloon interface is needed. Tissue such as bone or gas in the acoustic path generally limit ultrasound use; however, phased-array techniques may allow therapy to be performed through bone.

Beam intensity refers to the amount of energy reaching a given area in a given time and is measured in Wcm2.

Focal intensity refers to the highest temperature achieved in the treatment zone, whereas *in situ* intensity refers to the actual temperature achieved in the tissue. The latter accounts for loss of energy from scatter, coupling interfaces, and absorption by intervening tissue. The optimal frequency varies depending on the target depth and the volume of tissue to be treated. Higher frequencies generally have smaller focal zones and are better used superficially. For prostate therapy, generally 4 MHz is used.

There is no question that focused ultrasound technology is capable of ablating tissue, including human prostate tissue. Numerous studies, including canine prostate studies, human benign prostatic hyperplasia studies, and prostate cancer studies confirm permanent tissue destruction *(18–37)*. Clinical studies have demonstrated tissue injury by direct histologic evidence or by indirect findings, including MRI or color Doppler changes compatible with devascularization, transient rises in prostate-specific antigen level, and clinical outcomes such as transient posttreatment urinary retention and eventual improved urinary flow rates.

Foster et al. provided a detailed description of canine prostates treated transrectally with a 4-MHz high-intensity ultrasound transducer *(18)*. Twenty-six dogs were treated and killed at various intervals posttreatment (immediately to 12 wk). These authors confirmed histologic tissue ablation that progressed from coagulative necrosis acutely to well-defined zones of coagulative necrosis at 72 h to progressive cystic cavity formation with resolution of the inflammatory response and urothelial regeneration by 12 wk. For smaller lesions, fibrosis occurred instead of formation of cystic cavities.

Histologic studies of HIFU for treating various nonurologic solid tumors also confirm coagulative necrosis and tumor cell death *(17)*. Similarly, HIFU before radical prostatectomy or as a primary treatment for prostate cancer has been reported *(28,29,31)*. These studies confirm the use of this technology to ablate human prostate tissue and cause morphologic changes of cell death seen by conventional light microscopy as well as more subtle changes noted by electron microscopy and immunohistochemistry. Typically, there is a well-demarcated line between treated tissue and normal tissue.

Procedure

The procedure is performed using a transrectal probe that combines ultrasound imaging and focused ultrasound ablation capability. Patient preparation includes a cleansing enema. As is usual with the initial investigation of new technology, most patients were treated using a regional or general anesthesia, but as experience increased, the use of sedation or local anesthesia was reported. A Foley catheter is placed to more confidently visualize the bladder neck and verumontanum. Initially, the catheter was removed before active treatment, but later it was left in place to enhance ablation. After the probe is placed transrectally, a coupling balloon filled with degassed water is inflated.

The prostate is visualized by ultrasound and the treatment zone is defined using the computer cursors. Different focal length probes are used, depending on the prostate size. The probe is then locked relative to the treatment table. The computer controls the treatment cycles, treating an area $2 \times 2 \times 10$ mm. After the treatment cycles are completed (9–17 cycles), therapy is complete.

Clinical Experience in BPH

Bihrle et al. reported their initial human experience using HIFU for BPH in 1994 (23). This initial experience used a 4-MHz transducer. The power cycle was 25 watts for 4 s followed by a 12-s interval to allow heat dissipation (Sonoblate, Focal Surgery, M. Ipitas, CA). The group studied 15 patients with BPH patients who were selected based on symptom scores (AUA > 12), peak urinary flow rate (Qmax $\leq$ 2 mL/s), voided volume (>125 mL), postvoid residual volume (<300 mL), prostate volume measured by ultrasound (<80 mL), and an anteroposterior diameter $\geq$ 26mm. In addition to prostate therapy, the first ten patients underwent invasive transperineal thermometry for safety monitoring. Therapy was directed at the transition zone between the bladder neck and the verumontanum and was computer controlled to allow treatment of multiple sectors. Safety assessment included proctoscopy immediately after treatment, cystoscopy, and renal ultrasound 3 mo after treatment.

The series is too small and too short to make conclusions regarding efficacy but serves as an excellent initial trial to provide insight into possible clinical efficacy and safety information. The mean symptom score decreased from 31.2 to 15.8 at 90 d. All but two patients had a reduction in baseline symptom score by 3 mo. Average urinary flow rates improved by 51% at 3 mo. All but two patients showed improvement in flow rates. Postvoid residual volumes did not change significantly (mean 154 mL to 123 mL at 3 mo).

The most frequent complication was urinary retention, which occurred in 11 of 15 patients. The high rate of transient urinary retention was likely related to invasive thermometry; 9 of the first 10 patients undergoing thermometry experienced retention, whereas only 2 of 5 who did not have thermometry required catheterization. There were minor and transient effects such as hematuria and hematospermia, but minimal irritative symptoms were noted. No erectile dysfunction, transfusions, incontinence, or changes in sexual function were noted. Injury to the rectum or periprostatic tissue did not occur with the exception of insignificant subtrigonal extension in one patient seen on cystoscopy.

This initial experience showed promising clinical efficacy as measured by standard outcome parameters used in BPH clinical trials. More importantly, the thermometry and safety assessment confirmed the ability to use focused ultrasound technology to specifically target the transition zone without injury to the periprostatic structures. The authors suggested that optimal treatment parameters and monitoring techniques were likely to improve as more experience was gained.

Madersbacher et al. also reported their experience with HIFU in 1994, with an updated report in 1997 and again in 2000 (24–26). The 1994 report included phase I and phase II clinical trials. The phase I trial consisted of HIFU treatment in 22 patients before surgical removal for other disease (suprapubic prostatectomy, 4; radical prostatectomy, 12; cystoprostatectomy, 6) at various intervals after HIFU treatment (30 min to 10 d). Whole mount sections were used to assess histologic changes. Well-demarcated coagulative necrosis was identified. Accurate targeting was also confirmed, as the posterior prostate capsule remained intact and proctoscopy immediately posttreatment was unremarkable. The phase II trial was updated in 1997 after 54 prostates were assessed. The conclusions were similar to those of the earlier report.

The initial clinical data presented in 1994 included 50 men with symptomatic BPH (24). The inclusion criteria were Qmax ≤15 mL/s, AUA symptom score ≥18, prostate volume ≤75 mL, PSA ≤ 10.0 ng/mL, and sterile urine. Standard exclusion parameters were used. Of note was the exclusion of a large intravesicle median lobe. Transrectal HIFU using a 4-MHz transducer with the acoustic energy at the focal site adjusted to 1680 Wcm2. A fixed focal length of 3.0 or 3.5 cm was used. Most were treated using general anesthesia. A 4-s energy-on cycle followed by a 12-s energy-off interval was used.

The trial lasted 1 year, with interim reporting on 44 patients at 3 mo, and only 20 patients reported at 12 mo. Improvements in symptoms, urinary flow rates, and residual urine volumes were noted (Table 2). Four patients crossed over to transurethral resection.

Transient urinary retention was noted in 92% (46/50) of patients. Erectile function was not altered, but one patient had retrograde ejaculation. Other side effects were minor, except for one patient who had a

Table 2
Clinical Outcomes for High-Intensity Focused Ultrasound

Author	Study design	Baseline N	Follow-up (months)	AUA Symptom Scores			Mean Qmax (cc/sec)			Comments
				N	Baseline	Follow-up	N	Baseline	Follow-up	
Madersbacher 1994 (24)	Prospective	50	3	44	24.5	13.3	44	8.9	12.7	TURP 8% (4/50)
Madersbacher 1997 (25)	Prospective	102	12	56	24.5	13.2	56	9.1	13.3	TURP 15%
Madersbacher 2000 (26)	Prospective	80	41	45	19.6	8.5	45	9.1	10.2	TURP 44%
Sanghvi 1999 (22)	Multicenter, Prospective	22	12	22	23.5	10.7	23	8.7	12.6	TURP 8% (2/24) US Pilot Study
Sanghvi 1999 (22)	Prospective	24	14	14	22.6	6.5	11	9.1	13.9	Male Health Centre, Canada
Mulligan 1997 (21)	Prospective	13	24	NR	23	7	NR	9.9	10.6	TURP 15% (2/13)
Sullivan 1997 (19)	Prospective	20	3	20	20.2	9.5	20	9.2	13.7	

perforation of the descending colon. This was not a thermal injury but related to rectal balloon overfilling. This problem subsequently led to a redesign of the filling mechanism.

Madersbacher et al. updated the clinical series in 1997, reporting on 102 patients treated for BPH *(25)*. Similar clinical results were seen with respect to the outcome parameters, however, the failure rate as measured by the need for TURP increased from 8 to 15%. A second severe complication was reported. This was a thermal injury to the rectum caused by inappropriately high power intensity, which was subsequently adjusted.

A trial update by Madersbacher et al. was reported in 2000 *(26)*. They reported on 80 patients, followed for a mean of 32.5 mo. Of the 80 patients, 35 (44%) eventually required TURP because of treatment failure. The authors concluded that the long-term efficacy of HIFU was limited in spite of the early favorable results because of the high rate of TURP with longer follow-up. Possible explanations for failure were considered. These included the learning curve (as with any new technology), inadequate treatment volume, or inadequate treatment at the bladder neck.

Sanghvi et al. summarized the results of seven centers that had treated 92 patients using the SB-100 HIFU device (Focus Surgery Inc., Indianapolis, IN) *(22)*. Three different protocols were reviewed. These included the United States Pilot Study (*n* = 25), the Male Health Centre Study in Canada (*n* = 14), and The Kitasato University Study (*n* = 22). The significant differences in these protocols relate to the treatment parameters and reflect attempts to optimize the outcomes. The United States Pilot Study used the least-aggressive tissue ablation protocol consisting of a minimum focal intensity of 1640 Wcm2 and made nine lesions in the transverse plane from the bladder neck to the verumontanum after the alignment catheter was removed. The other two studies used the same focal intensity but left the catheter in place during treatment and used almost twice as many thermal lesions (17). In addition, in the Kitasato study, two or more focal length probes were used in an effort to more effectively treat the anterior prostate tissue. Leaving the catheter in place during treatment is significant because the increased acoustic impedance leads to higher tissue temperature and more tissue treated. The less-aggressive treatment regimen is referred to as HIFU1 and the more-aggressive treatment protocol as HIFU2.

In reviewing the various outcome parameters, more aggressive treatment has the most significant impact in improving urinary flow rates, but has no corresponding additional reduction in symptom scores or quality of life measures over less-aggressive HIFU1 therapy. This comparison of treatment strategies was reported by Uchida and co-workers *(27)*. In this report, 35 patients were treated with HIFU1 and 22 were treated with HIFU2 (Sonoblate 200). Both systems provided improvement in symptom scores and quality of life measures. Compared with HIFU1, HIFU2 showed greater improvements in urinary flow rates (8.9 to 15 mL/s) and reduction in prostate volume (32.2 to 22.8 mL). Cavity formation within the prostate was noted in 83% of patients treated with HIFU2 (10/12 patients) compared with 40% of patients treated with HIFU1 (6/15). Urinary retention occurred more frequently after HIFU2 therapy (64 vs 31%), and TURP rates within 3 yr also decreased (5 vs 31%). No additional complications were noted with HIFU2 treatment.

Summary

HIFU therapy represents an intriguing ablative therapy because of its ability to target tissue without direct contact. Accurately targeting the transition zone or more aggressive ablation for prostate cancer with unquestionable tissue ablation has been achieved. The initial clinical outcomes are quite similar to those of other minimally invasive techniques for BPH. The widespread use of HIFU has not occurred for several reasons. The technology is expensive, and treatment times are rather long. Although treatment of the median lobe was generally not performed in the initial trials, it would seem that given the imaging and targeting capabilities of HIFU that a median lobe treatment protocol could eventually be developed. The high TURP rates reported after long-term follow-up would seem to reflect the conservative ablation protocols during the initial experience. In principle, this device would seem to be very attractive if treatment times could be shortened, costs reduced, and clinical outcomes improved. Competing technologies that are less expensive, have shorter treatment times, are easy to use, and are reimbursed already exist.

REFERENCES

1. Gormley GJ, Stoner E, Bruskewitz RC, et al. The effect of finasteride in men with benign prostatic hyperplasia. N Engl J Med 1992;327:1185–1191.
2. Lepor H, Auerbach S, Puras-Baez A, et al. A randomized, placebo-controlled multicenter study of the efficacy and safety of terazosin in the treatment of benign prostatic hyperplasia. J Urol 1992;148:1467–1474.
3. Issa MM, Ritenour C, Greenberg M, Hollabaugh R Jr, Steiner M. The prostate anesthetic block for outpatient prostate surgery: World J Urol 1998;16: 378–383.
4. Issa MM, Townsend M, Jiminez KV, Miller LL, Anastasia K. A new technique of intraprostatic fiber placement to minimize thermal injury to prostatic

urothelium during indigo interstitial laser thermal therapy. Urology 1998; 51:105–110.

5. Cohen MS, Steiner MS, et al. Local anesthesia techniques. World J Urol 2000;18:S18–S21.

6. Cohen MS. Considerations for office-based ILC. World J Urol 2000;18: S16–S17.

7. Muschter R, Hofstetter A. Interstitial laser therapy outcomes in benign prostatic hyperplasia. J Endourol 1995;9:129.

8. Mueller-Lisse UG, Heuck AF, Schneede P, et al. Postoperative MRI in patients undergoing interstitial laser coagulation thermotherapy of benign prostatic hyperplasia. J Comput Assist Tomogr 1996;20:273–278.

9. Muschter R, De La Rosette JJMCH, Pellerin JP, et al. Initial human clinical experience with diode laser interstitial treatment of benign prostatic hyperplasia. Urology 1996;48:223–228.

10. William JC. Interstitial laser coagulation of the prostate: introduction of a volume-based treatment formula with 12-month follow up. World J Urol 1998;16:392–395.

11. Greenberger M, Steiner MS. The University of Tennessee experience with the indigo 830e laser device for the minimally invasive treatment of benign prostatic hyperplasia interim analysis. World J Urol 1998;16:386–391.

12. Martenson AC, de la Rosette JJMCH. Interstitial laser coagulation in the treatment of benign prostatic hyperplasia using a diode laser system: results of an evolving technology. Prostate Cancer Prostatic Dis 1999;2:148–154.

13. Mebust WK, Holtgrewe HL, Cockett ATK, Peters PC, and Writing Committee. Transurethral prostatectomy: immediate and postoperative complications. A cooperative study of 13 participating institutions evaluating 3,885 patients. J Urol 1989;141:243–247.

14. Muschter R, Whitfield H. Interstitial laser therapy of benign prostatic hyperplasia. Eur Urol 1999;35:147–154.

15. de la Rosette JJMCH. Lasers in the treatment of benign prostatic obstruction: past, present, and future. Eur Urol 1996;30:1–10.

16. Steiner MS, Cohen MS, Conn RL, et al. Physician's Dialogue 1999;1:16–31.

17. ter Haar G. High intensity ultrasound. Semin Laparosc Surg 2001;8:77.

18. Foster RS, Bihrle R, Sanghvi N, et al. Production of prostatic lesions in canines using transrectally administered high-intensity focused ultrasound. Eur Urol 1999;23:330.

19. Sullivan LD, McLoughlin MG, Goldenberg LG, Gleave ME, Marich KW. Early experience with high-intensity focused ultrasound for the treatment of benign prostatic hyperplasia. Br J Urol 1997;79:172.

20. Hegarty NJ, Fitzpatrick JM. High intensity focused ultrasound in benign prostatic hyperplasia. Eur J Ultrasound 1999;9:55.

21. Mulligan ED, Lynch TH, Mulvin D, et al. High-intensity focused ultrasound in the treatment of benign prostatic hyperplasia. Br J Urol 1997;79:177.

22. Sanghvi NT, Foster RS, Bihrle R, et al. Noninvasive surgery of prostate tissue by high intensity focused ultrasound: an updated report. Eur J Ultrasound 1999;9:19.

23. Bihrle R, Foster RS, Sanghvi NT, Donohue JP, Hood PJ. High intensity focused ultrasound for the treatment of benign prostatic hyperplasia: early United States clinical experience. J Urol 1994;151:1271.

24. Madersbacher S, Kratzik C, Susani M, Marberger M. Tissue ablation in benign prostatic hyperplasia with high intensity focused ultrasound. J Urol 1994; 152:1956.

25. Madersbacher S, Kratzik C, Marberger M. Prostatic tissue ablation by transrectal high intensity focused ultrasound: histological impact and clinical application. Ultrasonics Sonochem 1997;4:175.
26. Madersbacher S, Schatzl G, Djavan B, Stulnig T, Marberger M. Long-term outcome of transrectal high-intensity focused ultrasound therapy for benign prostatic hyperplasia. Eur Urol 2000;37:687.
27. Uchida T, Muramoto M, Kyunou H, et al. Clinical outcome of high-intensity focused ultrasound for treating benign prostatic hyperplasia: preliminary report. Urology 1998;52:66.
28. Van Leenders GJLH, Beerlage HP, Ruijter ETh, de la Rosette JJMCH, van de Kaa CA. Histopathological changes associated with high intensity focused ultrasound (HIFU) treatment for localized adenocarcinoma of the prostate. J Clin Pathol 2000;53:391.
29. Beerlage HP, Thuroff S, Debruyne MJ, Chaussy C, de la Rosette JJMCH. Transrectal high-intensity focused ultrasound using the ablatherm device in the treatment of localized prostate carcinoma. Urology 1999;54:273.
30. Chaussy C, Thuroff S. Results and side effects of high-intensity focused ultrasound in localized prostate cancer. J Endourol 2001;15:437.
31. Beerlage HP, van Leenders GJLH, Ossterhof GON, et al. High-intensity focused ultrasound (HIFU) followed after one to two weeks by radical retropubic prostatectomy: results of a prospective study. Prostate 1999;39:41.
32. Gelet A, Chapelon JY, Bouvier R, et al. Transrectal high-intensity focused ultrasound: minimally invasive therapy of localized prostate cancer. J Endourol 2000;14:519.
33. Gelet A, Chapelon JY, Bouvier R, Pangaud C, Lasne Y. Local control of prostate cancer by transrectal high intensity focused ultrasound therapy: preliminary results. J Urol 1999;161:156.
34. Chaussy C, Thuroff S. High-intensity focused ultrasound in prostate cancer: results after 3 years. Mol Urol 2000;4:179.
35. Kiel H-J, Wieland W-F, Rossler W. Local control of prostate cancer by transrectal HIFU-therapy. Arch Ital Urol Androl 2000,4:314.
36. Chaussy CG, Thuroff S. High-intensity focused ultrasound in localized prostate cancer. J Endourol 2000;14:293.
37. Sedelaar JPM, Aarnick RG, van Leenders GJLH, et al. The application of three-dimensional contrast-enhanced ultrasound to measure volume of affected tissue after HIFU treatment for localized prostate cancer. Eur Urol 2000;37:559.
38. Wu F, Chen W, Bai J, et al. Pathological changes in human malignant carcinoma treated with high-intensity focused ultrasound. Ultrasound Med Biol 2001;27:1099.

11 Transurethral Resection of the Prostate

Harris E. Foster, Jr., MD
and Micah Jacobs, BA

Contents

Introduction
Indications for TURP
Anesthesia
Technique
Complications of TURP
Outcome Studies
Conclusions
References

INTRODUCTION

Benign prostatic hyperplasia (BPH) causes a multitude of urinary symptoms as a result of obstruction of the bladder outlet. There are many phytotherapeutic and pharmacologic agents to treat BPH. BPH is more likely to be managed initially by primary care physicians and internists (49% of cases) than by urologists (37%) *(1)*. Furthermore, minimally invasive techniques such as transurethral microwave hyperthermia (TUMT), transurethral needle ablation (TUNA), water-induced thermotherapy (WIT), and interstitial laser therapy have expanded the treatment options for BPH. Nevertheless, transurethral resection of the prostate (TURP) continues to be the mainstay of therapy and the gold standard surgical technique. In the United States, approx 25% of men are treated for BPH by the age of 80 yr, and more than 300,000 surgical procedures are performed annually for BPH. TURP is

From: *Management of Benign Prostatic Hypertrophy*
Edited by: K. T. McVary © Humana Press Inc., Totowa, NJ

the second most commonly performed surgical procedure, at a cost estimated to be $2 billion *(2)*. Despite the availability of pharmaco- therapy and minimally invasive options, TURP remains a popular treat- ment for BPH because of its familiarity among urologists and superiority in treating the symptoms of prostatism, particularly urinary retention.

INDICATIONS FOR TURP

Patients selected for TURP should have clinical symptoms and signs caused by bladder outlet obstruction from BPH, because this procedure is thought to work by removal of obstructing prostate tissue. Most patients (90%) who undergo TURP do so because of the bothersome irritative and obstructive symptoms associated with BPH, termed pros- tatism, or more recently, lower urinary tract symptoms (LUTS) *(3)*. Other patients, however, are treated for increased postvoid residual urine, urinary retention, urinary tract infection, hematuria, renal insuf- ficiency, and vesical calculi.

Conditions with symptoms that mimic those of BPH must be elimi- nated during the preoperative assessment. The medical history should search for clues that suggest neurologic, infectious, and other causes that can result in lower urinary tract dysfunction and similar symptoms. Although the symptoms of BPH are not specific for the disorder, deter- mining the severity of these symptoms is quite helpful when evaluating a patient for possible TURP. A useful tool is the American Urological Association (AUA) Symptom Index, which has been found to be both valid and reliable *(4)*. It cannot be used alone to diagnose BPH, how- ever, because the symptoms measured are not specific for the disease.

Physical examination, at minimum, should include palpation of the lower abdomen for evidence of bladder distention and digital rectal examination of the prostate. The latter should assess for prostate consis- tency, symmetry, and size. An estimate of prostate size, albeit inaccu- rate by digital examination, is important because there is a limitation to the amount of tissue that can be safely resected transurethrally. Bladder outlet obstruction caused by very large prostates (>75 g) is generally better treated with an open prostatectomy (suprapubic or retropubic) *(5)*. Decreased or absent anal sphincter tone, perineal sensation, or bulb- ocavernosus reflex suggests a neurologic process and should be studied further to determine the correct diagnosis. Urinalysis is necessary to detect the presence of urinary tract infection and can also reveal hema- turia, which may suggest the presence of urinary tract calculi or neopla- sia. Patients with hematuria but no infection should undergo upper tract imaging (intravenous pyelogram, computed tomography [CT] scan, or

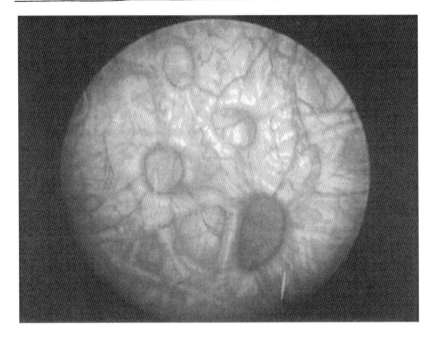

Fig. 1. Bladder trabeculation and cellules seen on cystoscopy in a patient with bladder outlet obstruction caused by BPH.

renal ultrasound), urine cytology, and cystoscopy. When performed, cystoscopy may reveal the secondary effects of obstruction on the bladder such as the presence of trabeculation, cellules, and diverticuli (Fig. 1). Bladder calculi, which form as a result of incomplete emptying associated with obstruction, may also be detected. Cystoscopy findings, in particular occlusion of the urethra by the prostatic lobes, cannot reliably predict bladder outlet obstruction from BPH and should not be used alone to justify proceeding with a TURP (Fig. 2).

Whether urodynamic studies are necessary in the evaluation of patients with LUTS caused by bladder outlet obstruction is controversial. Simple studies such as postvoid residual urine measurement and noninvasive uroflowmetry are generally well accepted. Nevertheless, their ability to predict obstruction and successful surgical outcome has not been established. A postvoid residual urine measurement can be helpful because an elevated residual level implies a problem with either detrusor contractility or outlet resistance. Elevated residual urine by itself, however, does not necessarily indicate obstruction. Basic cystometry can provide useful information about bladder compliance, capacity, and contractility, but it is not recommended as a necessary

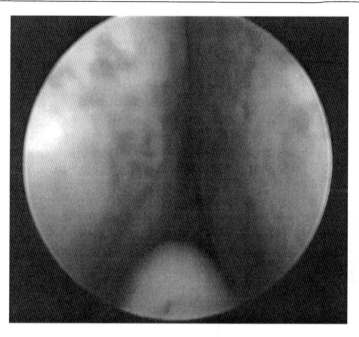

Fig. 2. Cystoscopic appearance of prostatic urethra in a man with LUTS. This is insufficient evidence for obstruction.

preoperative study. The gold standard test is the pressure-flow study, in which detrusor contractility and urinary flow are measured simultaneously. Elevated detrusor pressure in conjunction with low urinary flow rate is evidence of bladder outlet obstruction. This diagnosis is further supported by the findings of external sphincter relaxation and poor posterior urethral opening on electromyography and fluoroscopy, respectively. Those who favor the use of urodynamic studies believe that unequivocal bladder outlet obstruction should be demonstrated before a procedure that is designed to eliminate it is performed. On the other hand, those in opposing camps believe that the expense and invasiveness of urodynamics, and knowledge that most patients do well after TURP despite urodynamic findings, argue against performing this procedure routinely. Although the usefulness of preoperative urodynamic studies in the average patient can be debated, if there is clinical evidence that suggests a potential underlying neurologic cause for voiding dysfunction (i.e., diabetes mellitus, Parkinson's disease, multiple sclerosis), urodynamic studies must be performed before considering TURP.

The Agency for Health Care Policy and Research published guidelines for the evaluation of men with symptoms caused by BPH *(2)*.

Recommended evaluations include a medical history, physical examination, urinalysis, and serum creatinine level. In addition, it is recommended that the AUA Symptom Index be administered initially and used as a measure of a treatment efficacy at follow-up. Studies felt to be optional include noninvasive uroflowmetry, postvoid residual urine measurement, pressure-flow urodynamics, and urethrocystoscopy. The latter is recommended for consideration only when invasive treatment is being planned or when there is evidence of hematuria, urethral stricture (or its risk factors), bladder cancer, or prior lower urinary tract surgery (particularly TURP). Filling cystometry, initial evaluation with urethrocystoscopy, and upper tract imaging studies were not felt to be necessary for the evaluation of the typical patient with BPH.

ANESTHESIA

The use of a regional or a general anesthetic is usually required for TURP. The choice of anesthesia should be tailored to the patient's needs and the surgeon's preference. Although the use of local anesthesia for TURP has been reported, this technique is infrequently used (6–8). The use of regional anesthesia such as a subarachnoid or an epidural block offers the advantage of allowing close interaction with the patient during the procedure. Changes in mental status, particularly those that occur with hyponatremia, may be detected earlier when the patient is awake. Furthermore, a patient who is awake can report to the anesthesiologist other symptoms of excess fluid absorption such as shortness of breath. If the level of anesthesia is T10 or below, the presence of shoulder and/or abdominal pain or abdominal distention could suggest bladder perforation (9). Additional advantages of regional anesthesia are thought to include a more stable anesthetic during the procedure and smoother patient recovery. Subarachnoid block is preferred to epidural anesthesia because TURP is usually of short duration. Spinal block is believed to be the most common type of anesthesia used for patients undergoing TURP (3).

Complications following spinal anesthesia typically include intraoperative hypotension, an occipital headache caused by leakage of cerebrospinal fluid at the dural puncture site, and postoperative paresthesias.

Patients often prefer general anesthesia because they fear the technique used to administer the regional block, although that fear is unwarranted. This type of anesthesia, however, precludes the detection of mental status changes and respiratory difficulties. Considering the relatively low incidence of hyponatremia and fluid overload during TURP, this is generally overlooked as a shortcoming of general anesthesia.

In addition, in patients with contraindications to regional anesthesia, general anesthesia provides a safe and similarly effective alternative. Concerns about general anesthesia include variability in the depth of anesthesia resulting in inadvertent patient movement during the procedure and postoperative nausea and vomiting as a result of the residual effects of the systemic drugs administered.

Comparisons have been made between the use of regional and general anesthesia during TURP and have generally revealed no significant differences. Nielsen et al. found no significant difference in blood loss based on the type of anesthesia (10). Theoretically, increased blood flow to the extremities as a result of sympathetic blockade with regional anesthesia may decrease the incidence of deep venous thrombosis in patients undergoing prostatectomy; however, the risk of deep vein thrombosis is extraordinarily low in patients undergoing TURP. Furthermore, multiple studies have revealed that the risks of a variety of complications such as myocardial infarction, pulmonary embolus, cerebrovascular accident, renal or hepatic insufficiency, and the need for prolonged ventilation are no different between the two modes of anesthesia (9). Although there may be theoretical advantages to regional anesthesia, at this point there are not enough data to support favoring this technique over general anesthesia in the average patient.

TECHNIQUE

Patient Population

Routine assessment of the complete blood cell count, serum electrolytes, and coagulation parameters is typically performed. Patients should stop taking pharmacologic agents that prolong bleeding time by inhibition of platelet function or by impairment of coagulation parameters at least a few days before undergoing TURP unless clinically contraindicated. In the latter case, anticoagulant therapy can be converted to one with a short half-life (i.e., heparin) that can be stopped a few hours before the procedure. Systemic abnormalities in coagulation parameters should be addressed before performing TURP. In cases where anticoagulation cannot be discontinued or when there is a coagulopathy that cannot safely be corrected, other options for treating the bladder outlet obstruction must be considered, such as intermittent catheterization or one of the minimally invasive procedures (i.e., TUMT, WIT, noncontact laser prostatectomy, prostatic urethral stents).

The need for perioperative antibiotics is controversial. Urinary tract infection is a potential complication of TURP, and it can progress to bacteremia and subsequently septicemia. Urinary tract infection has been reported to occur in 6–60% of patients undergoing TURP *(11)*. Risk factors include preoperative bacteriuria and the presence of an indwelling catheter *(12)*. It is generally accepted that the use of perioperative antibiotics is indicated in patients at high risk for postoperative urinary tract infection, such as those indicated above. Consensus has not been reached, however, regarding the utility of this regimen in patients with sterile urine and low risk factors. Although Gibbons et al. reported that the use of prophylactic antibiotics did not prevent postoperative urinary tract infections, many other studies have come to the opposite conclusion *(13)*. Recently, Berry and Barratt performed a meta-analysis on 32 randomized controlled trials, examining the incidence of postoperative bacteriuria and septicemia in patients with sterile urine undergoing TURP *(14)*. Following preoperative treatment with antibiotics, the incidence of bacteriuria decreased from 26 to 9.1%, a 65% reduction, and septicemia was reduced 77%, from 4.4 to 0.7%. A variety of treatment regimens were found to be effective, although short-term protocols were more effective than those in which only a single dose was administered. Useful antibiotics included quinolones, cephalosporins, co-trimoxazole, and aminoglycosides. In light of these data and those from other studies, prophylactic antibiotics should be administered before TURP, even in the absence of bacteriuria.

Surgical Procedure

TURP is generally performed in the dorsal lithotomy position via the urethral meatus. In certain situations where the dorsal lithotomy position is not possible or the urethral caliber is insufficient for easy, safe passage of the resectoscope, TURP can be performed by means of a perineal urethrostomy without much difficulty. Cystoscopy should typically precede TURP in the operating room so that disease in the bladder, urethra, and prostate (i.e., transitional cell carcinoma, urolithiasis, urethral stricture) can be detected. This may not be necessary preoperatively unless there is reason to do so, including the presence of hematuria or a high suspicion for other disorders (i.e., bladder cancer) that may mimic the symptoms of BPH. Periodically, the urethra is too narrow for passage of the resectoscope or there is a urethral stricture. In this situation, the urethra can be gently dilated with urethral sounds to allow easy passage of the scope. Some have advocated the use of an Otis urethrotome to achieve this outcome *(15)*. If a urethral stricture is encountered when performing cystoscopy before TURP, it must be considered as a possible cause of the urinary symptoms. In this situation, the urethral stricture should be treated by visual urethrotomy. The surgeon should then strongly entertain the possibility of canceling the TURP and assessing the patient's response to the urethrotomy. Because many patients who are scheduled for TURP have elevated postvoid residual urine volume levels, they are also at increased risk for the development of vesical calculi. Often these calculi are not apparent on preoperative evaluation since cystoscopy has ceased to be a routine study. Consequently, vesical calculi are often diagnosed initially at the time of TURP. Removal of the calculi following fragmentation using the surgeon's technique of choice (i.e., electrohydraulic, laser, or mechanical lithotripsy) should precede TURP. Some have advocated the performance of a small cystolithotomy before TURP *(16)*.

Instruments

INSTRUMENTS

A variety of instruments are available to perform TURP. The basic requirements are a standard cystoscopy lens (usually 30°), a bridge that accommodates a resection loop, and a cystoscopy sheath specifically designed for resection (Fig. 3A,B). This entire setup is typically called a resectoscope. Each one of the segments of a resectoscope can be altered to fit the needs and preferences of the surgeon. A major improvement in the sheath element has been the development of the ability for continuous irrigation. This required creating an inner sheath that provides inflow with an outer sheath that has fenestrations and is connected to suction for aspiration of the irrigation fluid. In addition, a continuous flow pump is necessary to help evacuate the fluid and dispose of it. There are two common types of bridges, the Stern-McCarthy and the Iglesias (Fig. 4). The latter is probably used more frequently because it allows the surgeon to move the resection loop through the tissue predominately with the thumb. Other options for the resectoscope include the type of loop used for resection and/or cauterization (Fig. 5). The thin-wired loop has been in use the longest and is still the most popular. Advantages include the ability to cut through the prostate tissue easily and the ability to accurately cauterize bleeding vessels. More recently, surgeons have used one of the many types of loops in which the cutting element is wider, often with serrated edges. A theoretical advantage is the ability to reduce the amount of bleeding during the resection because the wider loop allows for some cauterization even in the cut mode. The thickness of these types of loops and the goal of trying to cauterize as one cuts reduce the speed with which it can be pulled through the prostate tissue, a distinctive disadvantage. Loops with rollerballs are also available, and although not generally used to ablate tissue, can be helpful in obtaining hemostasis because of the wider surface area in contact with the tissue.

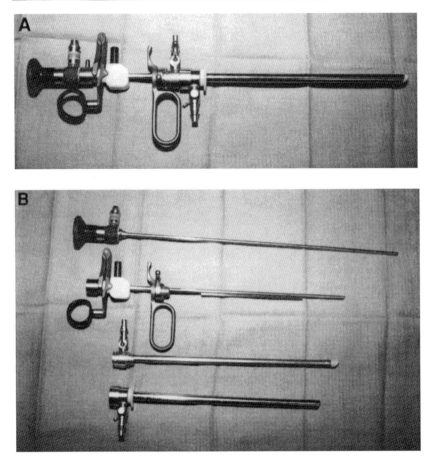

Fig. 3. (A) Compete resectoscope. (B) Components of resectoscope (from top to bottom): lens, Iglesias bridge, inner and outer portion of continuous flow sheath.

Various devices are available to assist with recovery of the prostate chips. One of the most common is the Ellik evacuator, consisting of dual connected glass chambers, oriented vertically, and attached to a suction bulb (Fig. 6). The upper chamber is connected to the suction bulb and allows the surgeon to irrigate the bladder in and out. The lower chamber collects the prostatic chips as they fall by gravity from the upper chamber. Other devices of similar design (albeit with different composition) and piston-like devices are also available for prostatic chip evacuation, and are used at the discretion of the surgeon. Finally, the use of fiberoptic technology to transmit the image from the cystoscope lens to a television monitor has greatly improved the surgeon's ability to perform the

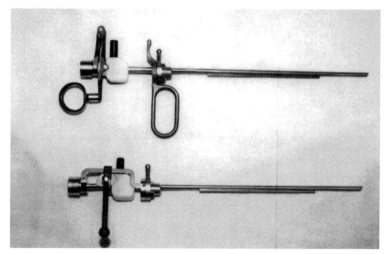

Fig. 4. Resectoscope bridges. Top, Iglesias; bottom, Stern-McCarthy.

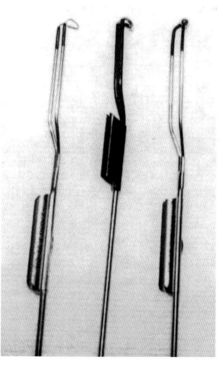

Fig. 5. Resection loops. From left to right: standard, thick loop, rollerball.

172

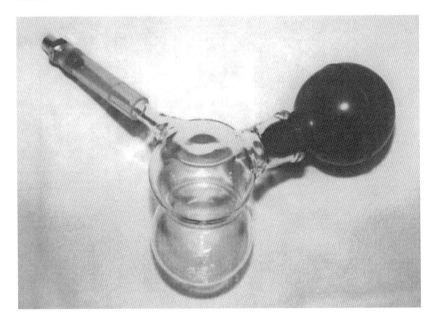

Fig. 6. Ellik evacuator.

procedure, reduced exposure to the blood-contaminated irrigant, and enhanced resident learning (Fig. 7 A,B).

IRRIGATION FLUID

Irrigation is required for visualization during TURP because bleeding begins once the prostate tissue is incised. Sterile water was initially used for the irrigant during TURP until it was recognized that absorption of large volumes could result in complications, particularly hemolysis and hyponatremia *(17–19)*. Although sterile water can still be effective as an irrigant when used appropriately, the use of more isotonic solutions has become practically universal. These relatively isotonic and nonionizing irrigants typically are made by adding glucose, mannitol, and/or glycine to sterile water, increasing the osmolality. Common solutions include 1.5% glycine, Cytal (a combination of sorbitol and mannitol), 2.5% glucose, mannitol, and 3% sorbitol. It should be recognized, however, that even though the likelihood of hemolysis is dramatically reduced, use of these irrigants might still result in dilutional hyponatremia when they are absorbed in high volumes.

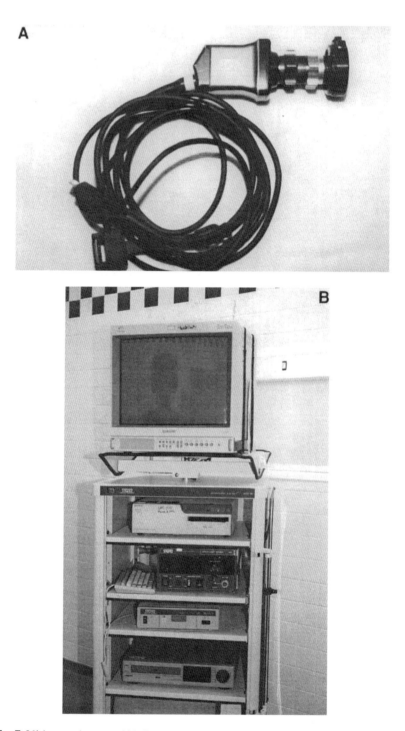

Fig. 7. Video equipment. (**A**) Camera. (**B**) Tower (monitor, printer, light source, video conduit for camera, video recorder).

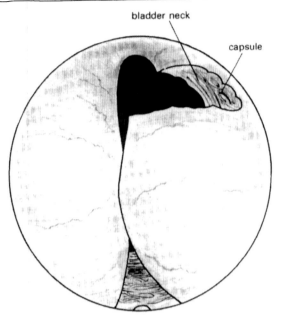

bladder neck

capsule

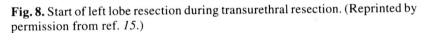

Fig. 8. Start of left lobe resection during transurethral resection. (Reprinted by permission from ref. *15*.)

RESECTION TECHNIQUE

There are many techniques for performing TURP, all of which have advantages and disadvantages. In each, the technique involves resection of transition zone prostate tissue from the bladder neck to the verumontanum. Differences in the various techniques revolve primarily around the initial stages of the resection. Most advocate resection of the anterior and lateral portions of the prostate first, allowing the tissue on each side to fall to the floor. This tissue is then subsequently resected, followed by the apex. Others believe that initial resection of the bladder neck and median lobe, when present, allows better flow of irrigation into the bladder, thereby facilitating easier resection of the remaining tissue. Nevertheless, most of the other aspects of the resection remain the same, and the choice of technique should be based on the individual surgeon's experiences, preferences, and judgment based on patient anatomy.

When performing the first technique, the resection should start at either the 12 o'clock position or slightly lateral to this position, at the level of the bladder neck. Typically, there is a paucity of hyperplastic tissue in this area, which primarily encompasses the anterior fibromuscular zone of the prostate (Fig. 8). To facilitate resection down to the appropriate depth throughout the entirety of the procedure, early identification of the surgical capsule is desirable. Although distinct from the true fibrous capsule of the prostate, and furthermore not an anatomic capsule in the traditional sense, this important landmark identifies the ideal depth of resection. It is formed by the compression of normal, nontransition zone prostate tissue by the expanding transition zone that enlarges as a result of the hyperplastic process. Resection deep to this level often results in perforation of intraprostatic and periprostatic venous sinuses, causing excessive bleeding and impairing visualization during the procedure. In addition, prolonged irrigation with relatively hypo-osmolar fluid increases the risk for the development of absorptive hyponatremia, fluid overload, and other manifestations of the transurethral resection syndrome (TUR). Very deep resection may also reveal perivesical or periprostatic fat.

Resection should then proceed from the 12 o'clock position approximately down to the 4 and 8 o'clock positions, extending distally to a point just proximal to the verumontanum (Fig. 9A,B). Throughout this phase, care must be taken to maintain the appropriate depth of resection as described above. This maneuver effectively causes the lateral tissue of the prostate to fall to the floor. The remaining portions of the lateral lobe on each side are then resected (Fig. 10). The arterial supply to the prostate and vesical neck generally enters at the 5 and 7 o'clock positions. Brisk bleeding should be expected from this area and should be rapidly controlled with electrocautery. At this point, the floor of the prostate is resected, including the median lobe if it is present. The latter should be resected completely down to the circular fibers of the bladder neck; however, the resection should be distal enough to avoid injury to the ureteral orifices.

A fair amount of apical tissue often remains at this point, and resection of this area requires extra care. Sacrifice of the internal urethral sphincter (bladder neck) is an accepted consequence of TURP. Consequently, preservation of the external urethral sphincter complex, particularly the intrinsic rhabdosphincter, which projects into the distal prostatic urethra, is paramount in maintaining continence with increasing intraabdominal pressure. This remaining tissue should be resected carefully, with particular attention to the location of the verumontanum, as this represents the proximal extent of the external sphincter complex. This tissue can often be better visualized by elevating it with a gloved finger placed in the rectum (Fig. 11A,B). Once this has been done, an open prostatic urethra should be seen when the cystoscope is positioned at the level of the verumontanum (Fig. 12A,B).

Resection of the prostate using the second technique begins with removal of the median lobe/median bar and some of the bladder neck

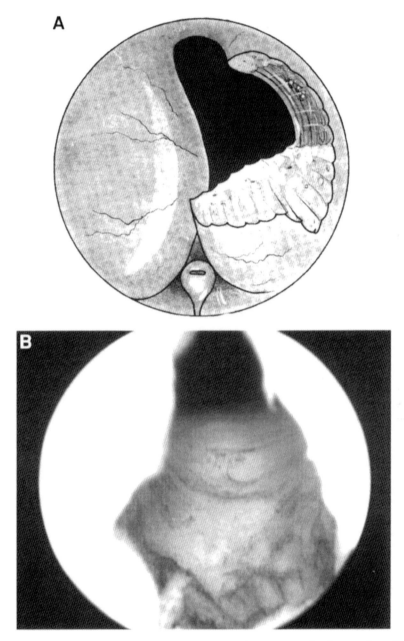

Fig. 9. (A) Drawing of left lobe resection during transurethral resection. **(B)** Intraoperative photo of left lobe resection. (Reprinted by permission of ref. *15.*)

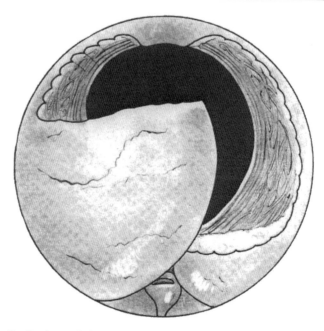

Fig. 10. Beginning of right lobe resection during transurethral resection. (Reprinted by permission of ref. *15.*)

from approximately the 4 o'clock to 8 o'clock positions. Resection is carried down to the circular fibers of the bladder neck. In theory, removal of this tissue early in the procedure allows better flow of irrigation fluid from the prostatic fossa into the bladder, thereby optimizing visualization. The rest of the resection proceeds similarly to the former technique by starting anteriorly and resecting the lateral lobes, followed by the apex.

After completion of the resection portion of the procedure, all prostatic chips should be evacuated. As mentioned above, the Ellik evacuator and similar devices allow this to be done efficiently. It is imperative that prostatic chips be removed because those that go undetected may occlude the urethral catheter postoperatively and interfere with bladder irrigation, possibly necessitating reexploration. Following complete evacuation, all prostate tissue should be collected and sent to the pathologist for histologic evaluation to rule out the presence of occult prostate cancer.

Finally, once the prostate tissue has been completely evacuated from the bladder, hemostasis should be achieved. The level of hemostasis obtained before completion of the procedure will vary among individual surgeons and individual patients. In general, smaller prostates tend to

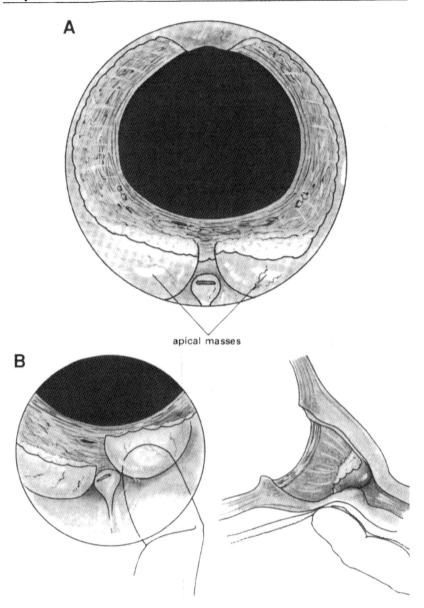

A

apical masses

B

Fig. 11. (A) Residual apical tissue. **(B)** Elevation of apical tissue by finger in rectum. (Reprinted by permission of ref. *15.*)

bleed less and larger prostates more. Some surgeons are more comfortable than others with greater amounts of bleeding. In all situations, however, arterial bleeding must be stopped because catheter placement

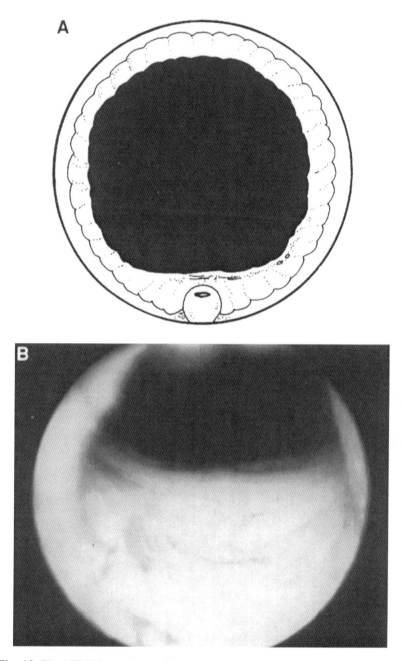

Fig. 12. Final TURP result. (**A**) Open prostatic urethra. (Reprinted by permission of ref. *15*.) (**B**) Intraoperative photo.

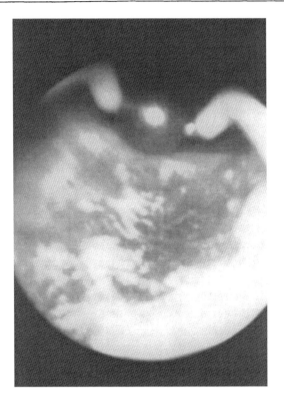

Fig. 13. Intraoperative photo demonstrating rollerball coagulation of prostatic fossa.

and drainage will generally not provide satisfactory hemostasis. The prostatic fossa should be examined carefully, and bleeding sites should be cauterized with either the resection loop or rollerball electrode (Fig. 13). Ideally, cessation of the irrigation should allow reasonable visualization of the prostatic fossa. If any bleeding persists, further cauterization should occur, recognizing that bleeding from venous sinuses deep to the surgical capsule may be difficult or even impossible to stop. When hemostasis is thought to be sufficient, the resectoscope should be removed and a three-way urethral catheter should be inserted. Occasionally, because of an undermining of the bladder neck, this is difficult. In these situations, a catheter guide should be used to ensure that the balloon is not inadvertently inflated in the prostatic fossa. Following inflation of the balloon, irrigation of the catheter should reveal at most a pink-tinged effluent. If bright red blood is obtained on irrigation, the catheter should be removed and the prostatic fossa reexamined with the resectoscope for additional sites of bleeding, particularly arterial sites.

Once adequate hemostasis has been obtained, with confirmation by placement of the urethral catheter and drainage as indicated above, the three-way urethral catheter should be connected to continuous irrigation, if necessary. Gentle traction on the catheter, maintained by attaching it to the leg with tape or other specifically designed devices, can prevent entrance of prostatic fossa blood into the bladder and allow for slower irrigation rates. The patient is then transported to the post-anesthesia recovery unit.

If used, continuous bladder irrigation should be performed until the effluent is essentially clear. Time on catheter traction should be minimized because it may promote ischemia of the bladder neck and subsequent contracture formation. Furthermore, it could also mask significant bleeding in the prostatic fossa. Therefore, traction should be released before determining whether or not continuous irrigation can be discontinued. When the urine is clear without traction and continuous irrigation, the catheter is removed, the patient is given a trial of void, and if successful, is discharged home. Most patients require at least 1 to 2 d of hospitalization; however, some patients can be discharged following 23 h or less. Occasionally, patients are unable to void following catheter removal. This can be a result of persistent obstruction, edema of the prostatic urethra, retained prostatic tissue, or unrecognized detrusor dysfunction as a cause for urinary retention. If a retained prostatic chip is suspected, evacuation with cystoscopy if often required. On the other hand, the remaining causes of postoperative urinary retention are usually managed by re-inserting the urethral catheter or instituting clean intermittent catheterization. In the former case, the catheter can be removed at a later date and another trial of void performed. In the latter case, the patient can be discharged with instructions to carry out clean intermittent catheterization and is told to continue this procedure until postvoid residual urine measurements decrease to an acceptable level.

COMPLICATIONS OF TURP

There are several complications of TURP that are unique to the procedure. These can generally be divided into three categories: intraoperative, perioperative, and long-term morbidity. Although the overall rate of complications is similar between the time periods (about 20%), the nature of the complications differs. In the 1960s, a large percentage of complications involved systemic infections caused by pneumonia and pyelonephritis, whereas in the 1980s and 1990s, urinary retention and urinary tract infection accounted for most complications (3,20,21).

Intraoperative Complications

There are many potential intraoperative complications that can occur during TURP. These include significant bleeding (at times requiring transfusion), perforation of the prostatic capsule, perforation of the bladder, injury to the rectum, and development of TUR syndrome resulting from overabsorption of hypotonic fluid and its resultant dilutional hyponatremia. The most significant improvement in TURP complications over the last 10 years has been in the number of intraoperative complications. In the 1990s, bleeding requiring transfusion was the most common intraoperative complication associated with TURP, affecting more than 2% of patients who underwent the operation. This was followed closely by TUR syndrome (2%) and myocardial arrythmia (just over 1%) *(3)*. After the development of more sophisticated equipment, shorter operative time, and better irrigant solutions, transfusion requirements and TUR syndrome now affect less than 1% of patients *(21)*. Interestingly, in the last 10 years, myocardial arrhythmia, occurring in just over 1% of patients, has been more prevalent *(3)*. Timely and meticulous performance of TURP, with careful attention to detail, can help prevent many of these complications.

BLEEDING

Excessive bleeding can occur for a variety of reasons. A frequent cause is failure to control early bleeding, particularly from arteries, which subsequently impairs visualization to the extent that identification of bleeding vessels becomes increasingly difficult. Perforation of the surgical capsule, especially early in the procedure, is another common culprit. Although generally venous and not arterial, this type of bleeding can be particularly difficult to control with cauterization because of the size of the vessels. When this occurs early, especially in large prostates, some surgeons advocate completing the resection on the side of the perforation and aborting the rest of the procedure. If necessary, TURP can be completed at a later date. Late perforation of the capsule generally allows completion of the procedure; however, this complication must be recognized, thereby prompting the surgeon to finish the procedure expeditiously. In all situations, aggressive attempts at hemostasis should occur before stopping the procedure and inserting the urethral catheter. Persistent bright red blood in the urethral catheter after irrigation suggests the presence of an uncontrolled artery, mandating removal of the catheter with repeat cystoscopic examination and fulguration. Weighted averages of the risk for blood transfusion associated with TURP approx 12%; however, recent reviews of the literature suggest that the rate has decreased to less than 1% *(2,21)*.

PERFORATIONS

Perforations of the surgical prostatic capsule and bladder are not uncommon during TURP. Perforation of the surgical capsule generally results in the unroofing of periprostatic venous channels, causing bleeding that can be difficult to control. Similar results (i.e., excessive bleeding) can also be obtained by perforating or undermining the bladder neck. In contrast to the periprostatic veins, this bleeding is often arterial and amenable to cauterization using the resectoscope loop. Perforation of the bladder is generally the result of poor visualization from excessive bleeding and bladder overdistention. When this problem is recognized, the procedure should be terminated as soon as possible. Because perforation is almost always extraperitoneal, management with urethral catheterization is sufficient. In the rare instance of intraperitoneal extravasation, open surgical repair is necessary. If a rectal injury occurs during TURP, initial treatment with prolonged urinary diversion by means of a urethral or suprapubic catheter is reasonable. On the other hand, if there is persistent drainage of feculent material into the urinary tract, fecal diversion with a colostomy is the treatment of choice.

TUR SYNDROME

As mentioned earlier, resection deep to the surgical capsule can uncover large prostatic venous sinuses. When this occurs, irrigation (continuous or not) can result in the absorption of large volumes of relatively hypo-osmolar fluid. When sterile water was used as the irrigant, hemolysis was a potential complication that could eventuate in hemoglobinuria and acute tubular necrosis. With the advent of more isotonic solutions, the incidence of hemolysis has been dramatically reduced. Nevertheless, unopposed large infusions of these substances can still produce life-threatening dilutional hyponatremia. The constellation of symptoms associated with these occurrences is the TUR syndrome, which occurs in less than 1% of patients undergoing TURP *(21)*. Typical symptoms and signs include mental confusion, nausea, vomiting, hypertension, bradycardia, and other arrhythmias. The neurologic symptoms are thought to be the result of cerebral edema caused by a relative hypoproteinemia. The latter decreases serum osmolality, predisposing the patient to a fluid shift into the brain. Patients typically do not become symptomatic until the serum sodium is less than 125 meq/mL. Mebust et al. also found that the risk of this complication increased with prostate size, particularly if >45 g *(3)*. In addition, duration of surgery also correlated with development of TUR syndrome, especially when this exceeded 90 min. Another suggested cause of this syndrome is ammonia toxicity because glycine is metabolized into glycolic acid and ammonia. Although this is plausible, that the syndrome occurs even when other irrigation fluids are used would support the more accepted cause of hyponatremia.

Most patients with normal renal function are able to withstand large increases in intravascular volume by diuresis. This ability is reduced in patients with renal insufficiency (even mild) and in those with myocardial dysfunction. When excessive fluid absorption occurs, even patients with normal renal function are unable to increase diuresis enough to prevent dilutional hyponatremia. When recognized during TURP, TUR syndrome should prompt a rapid conclusion of the procedure, even if additional tissue needs to be resected. This, of course, must be preceded by establishment of an acceptable level of hemostasis. Initial treatment with intravenous diuretics (i.e., furosemide) is reasonable; however, if there is not a rapid amelioration of the symptoms of hyponatremia, 3% hypertonic saline should be administered slowly over 3–6 hr.

Perioperative Complications

Perioperative complications primarily include bleeding, urinary tract infection, and urinary retention. These occur in approx 7% of patients, sometimes extending the hospital stay by a few days or requiring discharge with an indwelling catheter (3,21).

BLEEDING

It is imperative that optimal hemostasis be achieved before TURP is concluded and the patient is transported from the operating room. Methods to manage mild-to-moderate persistent bleeding, such as catheter traction and continuous bladder irrigation, have been described earlier. Despite these maneuvers, persistent or recurrent bleeding can complicate postoperative management, potentially causing obstruction of the urethral catheter and clot retention. Initial management should include aggressive hand irrigation of the bladder to remove clots and changing the catheter to a larger caliber with more eyes, as necessary. If the clots can be completely evacuated, another attempt at traction and continuous bladder irrigation is not unreasonable. Patients with continuous bleeding after TURP that cannot be abated by these techniques should be returned to the operating room for clot evacuation and fulguration of bleeding vessels. Recurrent bleeding can also occur after discharge from the hospital. Often it is transient, obviating the need for medical intervention. On occasion, however, catheterization, irrigation, and cystoscopy with fulguration may be necessary.

Urinary Tract Infection and Urinary Retention

Recently studies have shown that urinary tract infections occur in approx 2% of patients during the postoperative period, although it had been reported to occur in as many as 60% of patients (11,21). As stated above, the use of prophylactic antibiotics during TURP is unquestioned when the patient is managed with continuous or intermittent catheterization because bacteriuria can be expected to occur in these situations. Recently, it has been established that all patients undergoing TURP will likely benefit from the use of prophylactic antibiotics administered preoperatively and perioperatively (14). Urinary retention has been reported to occur in approx 7% of patients after TURP (21). This can usually be managed with continuous or intermittent catheterization. The latter is generally preferable because it allows the patient an opportunity to spontaneously void. Nevertheless, most patients eventually regain the ability to void unless there is underlying detrusor dysfunction.

Mortality

Mortality associated with TURP is generally low according to most studies. Over the last several decades, the mortality rates have dropped significantly from over 2% in the 1960s to well below 1% more recently (3,20). Roos et al. compared the mortality rate between open prostatectomy and TURP, finding that it was higher in the TURP group, approx 3% (22). A potential explanation for this difference may be that patients undergoing TURP in this study were more likely to have significant comorbidities. Other studies have found that mortality rates following TURP are no different from those of age-matched controls (23,24). These data suggest that TURP is a safe treatment for the treatment of BPH.

Long-Term Complications

Long-term complications following TURP primarily include urinary tract infection, obstruction, incontinence, and erectile dysfunction, although there is debate about whether the latter is truly associated with the procedure. Interestingly, despite the use of prophylactic and perioperative antibiotics, delayed genitourinary infection is still a significant problem after TURP, accounting for nearly half of long-term complications (4%) (21). This is probably not a result of persistent bacteriuria from the procedure but is more likely the result of some of the complications discussed below, including obstruction and incontinence.

Bladder Neck Contracture/Urethral Stricture

Recurrent obstruction can occur at the level of the bladder neck and urethra following TURP. In either case, patients return with symptoms similar to their original ones, in particular the obstructive symptoms such as retention, hesitancy, and weak stream. Bladder neck contracture (BNC) has been reported to occur in approx 2% of patients *(21)*. Methods thought to help prevent this complication include avoiding aggressive resection of the bladder neck, limiting cauterization at this site, and decreasing the duration of catheter traction in the postoperative period. BNC can be treated using a variety of techniques. Although not generally successful in the long term, soft dilation can sometimes be effective. More often, however, some type of incision or resection of the fibrous tissue is necessary to achieve a durable response. Bladder neck incision with either electrocautery or the laser is thought to be preferable because it theoretically reduces the likelihood of recurrence as the result of less tissue being damaged by the procedure. Urethral strictures following TURP are relatively uncommon (1%), however, they can be problematic when they develop *(21)*. Often they occur in the bulbous urethra and fossa navicularis. Preventative strategies include adequate calibration and lubrication of the urethra during TURP. Similar to BNC, the occurrence of urethral strictures following TURP can be treated with urethral dilation, but they generally require visual urethrotomy. In situations where these treatments are unsuccessful and recurrence is frequent, open urethroplasty may be required, although insertion of urethral stents represents another possibility.

BLEEDING

Bleeding requiring return to the hospital occurs in 1.4% of patients *(21)*. This can usually be avoided by controlling the initial bleeding during hospitalization as described above and discharging the patient only when the urine is essentially clear. Patients are counseled to restrict heavy lifting for 4–6 wk and to avoid constipation by maintaining adequate fluid intake and taking stool softeners. However, the inherent increase in activity with departure from the hospital inevitably puts patients at risk for recurrent hematuria. When hematuria does recur, it generally can be managed conservatively by restricting activity and increasing fluid intake. If hematuria is more significant, clot formation can occur, with a strong potential for obstruction and urinary retention. In this situation, all clots should be removed with a large irrigating catheter, after which continued bleeding can be managed with continuous bladder irrigation and catheter traction. Continued bleeding usually requires repeat transurethral fulguration, although the use of clot-promoting drugs such as aminocaproic acid can be considered. Recurrent hematuria not requiring surgical intervention can sometimes be successfully managed with 5α-reductase inhibitors *(25)*.

INCONTINENCE

Because TURP includes the removal of tissue at the bladder neck that encompasses smooth muscle of the internal sphincter, stress urinary incontinence can result if care is not taken to protect the external urethral sphincter complex. As described earlier, critical in avoiding injury to this sphincteric complex is the identification of the verumontanum and the resection of prostate tissue only proximal to this landmark. Stress urinary incontinence should be uncommon after TURP when the procedure is performed correctly, with an incidence well below 1%. Risk factors for postoperative stress incontinence include prostatic scarring from prior prostate surgery, radiation, and prostate cancer, all of which have the potential to obscure the verumontanum, making resection more difficult and increasing the likelihood of injury to the external sphincter. In fact, patients with a history of advanced prostate cancer who require TURP for relief of obstructive symptoms have an approx 20% risk for the development of postprostatectomy stress incontinence (26). Management of this complication generally requires insertion of an artificial urinary sphincter, although newer techniques such as the male sling procedure may provide a suitable alternative. Transurethral injection therapy with collagen and other agents has not demonstrated similar efficacy or durability. Finally, when addressing the issue of incontinence after TURP, it is important to recognize that detrusor abnormalities (i.e., detrusor instability and/or poor compliance) related to the original bladder outlet obstruction may be the cause. For this reason, urodynamic studies should play an important role in the evaluation of postoperative incontinence in these patients, certainly before any surgical intervention.

SEXUAL DYSFUNCTION

Sexual dysfunction, in particular erectile and ejaculatory disturbances, has been reported with varying incidences after TURP, occurring in approx 13% and 75% of patients, respectively, according to recent systematic reviews (2,27). The risk of retrograde ejaculation is substantial because the muscle of the bladder neck/internal sphincter is frequently disrupted, allowing entrance of ejaculate into the bladder, thereby interfering with emission. The cavernous nerves run in the neurovascular bundles at approximately the 4 and 8 o'clock positions posterior to the prostate. These nerves are potentially susceptible to injury from the electrocautery current during the resection. Therefore, it has been suggested that maintaining an appropriate depth of resection is important, particularly posteriorly, to prevent this complication. Men with relatively small prostates have in some instances been shown to be at greater risk for perforation of the capsule and thus may be more susceptible to problems with erection (28). Rates of new-onset erectile dysfunction are debatable, ranging from 5 to 33% depending on the study and risk factors of the patient (28,29). Wasson et al. found no differences in the incidence between men with BPH managed with either watchful waiting or with TURP (30). Interestingly, a most recent study found that erectile function actually worsened with conservative management in men with LUTS and improved in men who underwent TURP (31). Furthermore, following TURP, pain and discomfort on ejaculation improved compared with baseline. Clearly, there are conflicting data regarding the incidence of erectile dysfunction after TURP; however, if it does occur, it is probably uncommon.

OUTCOME STUDIES

TURP has been in practice since the early 20th century, and there is a fair amount of outcome data available for analysis. The results of this procedure have been scrutinized over the years, largely by patient feedback and surgeon reporting, and in the latter half of the last century by uroflowmetry and urodynamic parameters as well. These studies are useful in measuring the efficacy of TURP, particularly when comparing it to pharmacotherapy and the use of minimally invasive procedures.

Assessment of the symptoms of BPH has been greatly improved by the development of the various symptom questionnaires such as the AUA Symptom Index. These questionnaires have allowed for objective characterization of subjective symptoms. The symptom score can be obtained before and after treatment, ultimately providing reliable and accurate information on changes in response to intervention. Although the patient's assessment of symptoms (i.e., by means of symptom indices) is paramount in determining the success of the procedure, using this parameter as an indicator of treatment success has some shortcomings. The symptoms of BPH are not specific for the disease, and therefore, symptom scores can be confounded by concomitant disorders. As a result, later in the course of follow-up, it can be difficult to determine whether symptom severity is increasing because of BPH or because of another disease process. When urinary symptoms recur, it is useful to compare the severity of symptoms with those present preoperatively. In addition, several clinical tools provide additional information to corroborate with the qualitative patient symptom score. These include postvoid residual urine measurements and urodynamic studies. Some of the most effective analyses on outcome of TURP have been urodynamic studies, either simple uroflow (primarily maximum flow rate) or pressure/flow studies.

Multiple studies have demonstrated the superiority of TURP in improving symptoms associated with BPH. Data from randomized clinical trials are very convincing. When compared to watchful waiting over 3 yr, TURP resulted in more men improving (90% vs 39%), as indicated by a reduced bother of difficulty from urinary symptoms *(30)*. During the course of the study, 24% of men in the watchful waiting arm underwent TURP. Further follow-up of these patients for 5 yr was reported by Flanigan et al., demonstrating treatment failure rates of 10 and 21% for patients managed by TURP and watchful waiting, respectively *(32)*. In addition, 36% of men in the watchful waiting arm eventually crossed over to invasive therapy. Treatment failure was defined as death, acute urinary retention, high residual urine volume, renal azotemia, vesical calculi, persistent urinary incontinence, or a high symptom score. The major categories of treatment failure reduced by TURP were acute urinary retention, large bladder residual (>350 mL), and severe deterioration in urinary symptoms.

Several studies have attempted to clarify the usefulness of minimally invasive procedures compared with TURP. In addition to assessing the effectiveness of the procedures, these studies also provide useful information on the outcome of TURP. When compared with transurethral incision of the prostate in the largest trial to date, with almost 3 yr of follow-up, outcomes were similar for both treatments *(33)*. This was further confirmed in a meta-analysis of studies comparing the two procedures by Yang and co-workers *(34)*. Although improvements in symptom score were equivalent between the treatments, maximum urinary flow rate was higher in the TURP group. The authors correctly noted, however, that long-term information (i.e., 5–10 yr) on the effectiveness of both procedures is lacking. Recently, one group looked at a large number of patients in the ClasP study to determine the benefits of laser therapy. Donovan and colleagues randomized over 300 patients to receive laser therapy, TURP, or conservative therapy *(35)*. Using maximum urinary flow as the basis for evaluation, the study showed that laser therapy was effective in 67% of patients and TURP was successful in 81%. Conservative therapy was effective in 15% of patients. In addition, the two other papers containing data from the CLasP study showed significantly better prostate symptom scores and significantly fewer treatment failures with TURP than with laser therapy *(36,37)*.

CONCLUSIONS

In summary, TURP should clearly be considered the gold standard treatment for BPH. The effectiveness of the procedure has withstood the test of time, despite advances in pharmacotherapy and the development of minimally invasive techniques. When performed correctly, the incidence of intraoperative, perioperative, and late complication is low. When compared with other treatments, TURP is clearly superior and should remain the mainstay of surgical treatment of BPH until data from well-performed prospective studies suggest otherwise.

REFERENCES

1. Bruskewitz R. Medical management of BPH in the US. Eur Urol 1999; 36(suppl 3):7–13.
2. McConnell JD, Barry MJ, Bruskewitz RC, et al. Benign Prostatic Hyperplasia: Diagnosis and Treatment; Clinical Practice Guideline Number 8. U.S. Department of Health and Human Services, Public Health Service, Agency for Health Care Policy and Research, Rockville, Maryland, 1994.
3. Mebust WK, Holtgrewe HL, Cockett ATK, Peters PC, and Writing Committee. Transurethral prostatectomy immediate and postoperative complications: a cooperative study of 13 participating institutions evaluating 3,885 patients. J Urol 1989;141:243–247.
4. Barry MJ, Fowler FJ, O'Leary MP, et al. The American Urological Association's symptom index for benign prostatic hyperplasia. J Urol 1992;148:1549–1557.
5. Oesterling JE. Retropubic and suprapubic prostatectomy. In: Walsh PC, Retik AB, Vaughan ED Jr, Wein AJ, eds., Campbell's Urology, ed. 7, vol 2, Philadelphia: WB Saunders, 1998, p. 1529.
6. Sinha B, Haikel G, Lange PH, Moon TD, Narayan P. Transurethral resection of the prostate with local anesthesia in 100 patients. J Urol 1986:135:719–721.
7. Birch BR, Gelister JS, Parker CJ, Chave H, Miller RA. Transurethral resection of prostate under sedation and local anesthesia (sedoanalgesia). Experience in 100 patients. Urology 1991;38:113–118.
8. Chander J, Gupta U, Mehra R, Ramteke VK. Safety and efficacy of transurethral resection of the prostate under sedoanalgesia. BJU Int 2000;86:220–222.
9. Malhotra V. Transurethral resection of the prostate. Anesth Clin N Am 2000;18:883–897.
10. Neilsen KK, Andersen K, Asbjorn J, Vork F, Ohr-Nissen A. Blood loss during transurethral prostatectomy: epidural versus general anesthesia. Int Urol Nephrol 1987;19:287–292.
11. Madsen P, Larsen E, Dorflinger T. The role of antibacterial prophylaxis in urological surgery. Urology 1985;26:38–42.
12. McEntee GP, McPhail S, Mulvin D, Thomson RW. Single dose antibiotic prophylaxis in high risk patients undergoing transurethral prostatectomy. Br J Surg 1987;74:192–194.
13. Gibbons RP, Stark RA, Correa RJ, Cummings KB, Mason JT. The prophylactic use–or misuse–of antibiotics in transurethral prostatectomy. J Urol 1978; 119:381–383.
14. Berry A, Barratt A. Prophylactic antibiotic use in transurethral prostatic resection: a meta-analysis. J Urol 2002;167:571–577.
15. Blandy JP, Notley RG. Transurethral Resection of the Prostate, 3rd ed, Oxford, UK: Butterworth-Heinemann, 1993, p. 52–104.

16. Richter S, Ringel A, Sluzker D. Combined cystolithotomy and transurethral resection of prostate: best management of infravesical obstruction and massive or multiple bladder stones. Urology 2002;59:688–691.

17. Creevy CD. Hemolytic reactions during transurethral prostatic resection. J Urol 1947;58:125–131.

18. Creevy CD, Webb EA. A fatal hemolytic reaction following transurethral resection of the prostate gland: a discussion of its prevention and treatment. Surgery 1947;21:56–66.

19. Beirne GJ, Madsen PO, Burns RO. Serum electrolyte and osmolality changes following transurethral resection of the prostate. J Urol 1954;93:83–86.

20. Holtgrewe H, Valk W. Factors influencing the mortality and morbidity of transurethral prostatectomy: a study of 2,015 cases. J Urol 1962;87:450–459.

21. Borboroglu PG, Prodromos G, Kane C, et al. Immediate and postoperative complications of transurethral prostatectomy in the 1990s. J Urol 1999; 162:1307–1310.

22. Roos NP, Wennberg JE, Malenka DJ, et al. Mortality and reoperation after open and transurethral resection of the prostate for benign prostatic hyperplasia. N Engl J Med 1989;320:1120–1124.

23. Chute CG, Stephenson WP, Guess HA, Lieber M. Benign prostatic hyperplasia: a population based study. Eur Urol 1991;20(suppl 1):11–17.

24. Fuglsig S, Aagaard K, Jonler M, Olesen S, Norgaard JP. Survival after transurethral resection of the prostate: a 10-year follow-up. J Urol 1994;151:637–639.

25. Kearney MC, Bingham JB, Bergland R, Meade-D'Alisera P, Puchner PJ. Clinical predictors in the use of finasteride for control of gross hematuria due to benign prostatic hyperplasia. J Urol 2002;167:2489–2491.

26. Hirshberg E, Klotz L. Post transurethral resection of prostate incontinence in previously radiated prostate cancer patients. Can J Urol 1998;5(2):560–563.

27. Soderdahl DW, Knight RW, Hansberry KL. Erectile dysfunction following transurethral resection of the prostate. J Urol 1996;156:1354–1356.

28. Bieri S, Iselin C, Rohner S. Capsular perforation localization and adenoma size as prognostic indicators of erectile dysfunction after transurethral prostatectomy. Scand J Urol Nephrol 1997;31:545–548.

29. Perera N, Hill J. Erectile and ejaculatory failure after transurethral prostatectomy. Ceylon Med J 1998;43:74–77.

30. Wasson JH, Reda DJ, Bruskewitz RC, et al. A comparison of transurethral surgery with watchful waiting for moderate symptoms of benign prostatic hyperplasia. The Veterans Affairs Cooperative Study Group on transurethral resection of the prostate. N Engl J Med 1995;332:75–79.

31. Brookes ST, Donovan JL, Peters TJ, Abrams P, Neal DE. Sexual dysfunction in men after treatment for lower urinary tract symptoms: evidence from randomized controlled trial. BMJ 2002;324:1059–1061.

32. Flanigan RC, Reda DC, Wasson JH, et al. Five year outcome of surgical resection and watchful waiting for men with moderately symptomatic benign prostatic hyperplasia: a Department of Veterans' Affairs cooperative study. J Urol 1998;160:12–16.

33. Riehmann M, Knes JM, Heisey D, Madsen PO, Bruskewitz RC. Transurethral resection versus incision of the prostate: a randomized, prospective study. Urology 1995;45:76–775.

34. Yang Q, Peter TJ, Donovan JL, Wilt TJ, Abrams P. Transurethral incision compared with transurethral resection of the prostate for bladder outlet obstruction:

a systematic review and meta-analysis of randomized controlled trials. J Urol 2001;165:1526–1532.

35. Donovan JL, Peters TJ, Neal DE, et al. A randomized trial comparing transurethral resection of the prostate, laser therapy and conservative treatment of men with symptoms associated with benign prostatic enlargement: the CLasP study. J Urol 2000;164:65–70.

36. Gujral S, Abrams P, Donovan JL, et al. A prospective randomized trial comparing transurethral resection of the prostate and laser therapy in men with chronic urinary retention: the CLasP study. J Urol 2000;164:59–64.

37. Chacko KN, Donovan JL, Abrams P, et al. Transurethral prostatic resection or laser therapy for men with acute urinary retention: the ClasP randomized trial. J Urol 2000;164:166–170.

12 Transurethral Vaporization of the Prostate

Joe O. Littlejohn, MD, Young M. Kang, MD, and Steven A. Kaplan, MD

CONTENTS

INTRODUCTION
HISTORIC BACKGROUND
INDICATION/CONTRAINDICATIONS
EQUIPMENT/POWER SETTINGS
TECHNIQUE
OUTCOME
DISCUSSION
REFERENCES
FURTHER READING

INTRODUCTION

There are numerous abbreviations used to signify transurethral vaporization of the prostate: TVP, TUVP, TUEVP, and TUVRP. Regardless of which acronym is used, transurethral vaporization of the prostate entails the simultaneous vaporization, desiccation, and coagulation of prostatic tissue, using a rollerball or thick loop. TUVRP, which stands for transurethral vapor resection of the prostate specifically refers to the use of the thick-loop electrode and adds resection to the vaporization, desiccation, and coagulation accomplished with other electrodes. Otherwise the equipment is identical to that used for transurethral resection of the prostate (TURP). The generator must be capable of producing 25–45% higher wattage *(2,4)*. The indications for TUVP are the same as those for TURP. This chapter will demonstrate that this modality is a modification of TURP.

From: *Management of Benign Prostatic Hypertrophy*
Edited by: K. T. McVary © Humana Press Inc., Totowa, NJ

There are numerous transurethral modalities available for the treatment of benign prostatic hyperplasia (BPH). The final common pathway of each of these methods is heat. The differences occur in whether one uses microwave, radio frequency, laser, or high-intensity focused ultrasound, and how the energy form of choice is converted to heat, which yields the desired effect in the prostatic tissue. Vaporization is the effect of a specific range of temperature exerted on tissue, resulting in cellular lysis and evaporation of the intracellular fluid. This technology is a modification of TURP; however, vaporization is quite distinct from standard electrosurgical resection. This distinction can be easily overlooked when working with familiar equipment and using a familiar technique; however, there are subtle but critical technical nuances.

The efficacy of transurethral vaporization and vapor resection is comparable to that of TURP. However, there are differences in operative time, length of catheterization, blood loss, and fluid absorption. TUVP using the roller electrodes and TUVRP using the thick loop are not assumed to be equivalent, and outcome data from each will be presented separately.

HISTORIC BACKGROUND

TURP has been the gold standard for the surgical treatment of BPH for prostates <80 g. This established technique is based on the use of high-frequency electrical current to cut and fulgurate tissue and obtain hemostasis. Furthermore, standard TURP uses a thin-wire resectoscope loop and removes prostatic tissue by resection of chips, with minimal tissue vaporization and no desiccation.

However, well-recognized morbidities associated with TURP (bleeding, hospital stay, electrolyte disturbances, and anesthetic requirement) have led many urologists to seek other alternatives. One of the earliest modifications of TURP was transurethral electrovaporization of the prostate (TUVP, TVP, TUEVP, EVAP), which entered mainstream urology in 1995 after successful pilot studies in 1994 and 1995 (1–3).

Transurethral electrovaporization stems from the concept of ablating the tissue by means of simultaneous vaporization and desiccation, allowing for better visualization and minimal blood loss. TUVP requires the use of a slower loop resection speed; a lack of tissue specimens; use of new, more powerful generators; and use of an electrode with a grooved, fluted, or rollerbar design. The procedure was well received by urologists because of its technical similarities to TURP.

Technological advancements have resulted in modification of the vaporizing electrode, creating an electrode that enables simultaneous vaporization and resection. Various names have been given to this new technique, including vaporizing-resection, transurethral vaporization-resection of the prostate (TVRP, TUVRP), vapor-cut, electrovaporization-resection, and thick-loop TURP. This electrode features a thin leading edge to aid in resection and a thick trailing edge for vaporization and desiccation.

INDICATION/CONTRAINDICATIONS

Indications for TUVP are same as those for TURP. Primarily, they include moderate-to-severe symptoms on the International Prostate Symptom Score (I-PSS) or the American Urologic Association Symptom Index (AUA SI), and/or prostatism refractory to medical therapy. Other absolute indications for surgery are acute refractory urinary retention, recurrent infection, recurrent hematuria, cystolithiasis, and postrenal azotemia.

There are no absolute size requirements. The literature generally recommends TUIP for prostatic glands <30 g without a median lobe because of reported low morbidity. For the same reason, an open prostatectomy is recommended for glands >80 g. The median lobe is not a contraindication for TUVP, unlike for some of the other new minimally invasive procedures.

Contraindications for the procedure are same as for any other surgery and include active infection and coagulopathy. Preoperative laboratory testing is routinely done to identify these contraindications. Of note, patients with pacemakers will need careful monitoring during the perioperative period.

Although studies have shown mixed outcome results for post-TURP infection rates, the administration of prophylactic first-generation cephalosporin (unless other antibiotics are indicated) is used (e.g., mitral valve prolapse) (5).

Although there have been reports of performing transurethral surgery of prostate with the patient under local anesthesia, we generally recommend using a general or spinal anesthesia. There are no differences in blood loss, postoperative morbidity, or mortality between using a spinal anesthesia and a general anesthesia, according to the literature (5).

EQUIPMENT/POWER SETTINGS

To perform TUVP or TURVP, minor additional equipment is needed beyond the standard TURP set. This includes different resectoscope electrodes and impedance-free electrosurgical generators. This section will cover various power generators and their respective effective power settings and electrode designs in depth.

Electrosurgical Generators

Generator power plays a crucial role in vaporization. Intuitively, an insufficiently powered generator will not provide adequate power for vaporization. Although many generators may provide sufficient power wattage at low impedance levels, some of the older generators are not efficient at delivering the same power at increased resistances. In electrovaporization, prostatic tissue is desiccated after the initial swipe. The desiccated, vaporized tissue raises the tissue impedance. Thus, the next swipe is going to meet higher resistance and require greater power to achieve the same desired current or effect.

For example, conventional TURP power generators, including the Valley-Labs Force 2 and Force 4 (Valley-Labs, Boulder, CO) are not as efficient in delivering consistent power over a wide range of impedances as Force 40 (6,7). Power/resistance curves should be available for every generator. Moreover, newer generators, such as the Valley-Labs Force 300, FX, or ERBE ICC 350 (Erbe, Tubingen, Germany) contain microprocessors that adjust for changing tissue impedance (6). Hence, for maximal vaporization to occur, an impedance independent electrosurgical unit should be used. If inadequate power current is used, excessive fulguration will result in coagulation necrosis and subsequent irritative voiding symptoms.

Electrovaporization is best performed with a cutting current set at 25–75% higher power than standard TURP (6). Van Swol et al. reported that minimum power of 150 watts to tissue is needed to achieve vaporization (7). For a Force 40 unit, a power setting of 240–250 watts (pure cut) is recommended; for a Force 300, 150 watts is required. For a Force FX or ERBE units, 130–150 watts is suggested (6).

For vaporizing-resection, different investigators have used various power settings. Kaplan used an ERBE ICC 350 unit set at 200 watts (pure cut), whereas Perlmutter used 120–150 watts (pure cut) with the same unit for vaporization-resection (6). Kupeli et al. used a Valley-Lab Force 40 unit set at 250–300 watts (pure cut), whereas Talic et al. used an Eschmann TD411-RS unit set at 250 watts (8,9). Additionally, the different technique used for resection and the unique electrode must be taken into account when considering power settings during vaporizing-resection.

Electrodes

Electrode design is also important in achieving desired electrosurgical effects on tissue. An electrode with a broad surface area of contact and multiple ridges or grooves produces more vaporization than a smooth

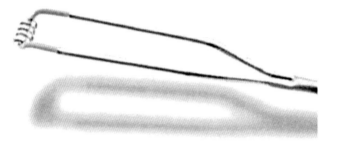

Roller Electrode

Fig. 1. Roller electrode for TUVP (Karl Storz, Tuttlingen, Germany).

electrode with a thin loop configuration. Optimum tissue-electrode contact must be maintained for maximal vaporization.

Figure 1 shows a roller electrode comparable to the VaporTrode electrode (Circon, Santa Barbara, CA), which is essentially a 3-mm (diameter) × 3-mm (width) grooved cylinder, composed of nickel silver with Teflon insulation. The large surface area of this electrode and its ability to roll, permit delivery of high-density current to broad areas of tissue at its leading edge. Most studies have been conducted using the VaporTrode. Other manufacturers have produced similar products, including the EVAP Multi-Ridge Barrel Electrode or Screw Design Electrode (Richard Wolf, Germany).

Figure 2 shows the Vaporcut electrode, which is comparable to the VaporTome (Circon), which consists of a thick loop with grooves, a thin leading edge for vaporization, and a thick trailing edge for coagulation and desiccation. The Wedge by Microvasive (Natick, MA) is another vaporizing-resection electrode that uses the differential loop thickness concept. The Wing EVAP electrode (Richard Wolf) is a semicircular designed, gold-plated wire loop that is wider and thicker than a standard TURP loop.

Bipolar electrovaporization technology (Gyrus Plasmakinetic Electrosurgical System, Buckinghamshire, UK) is the latest technology that has entered the electrovaporization market. This system allows for use of isotonic saline as the irrigating solution, which essentially elimi-

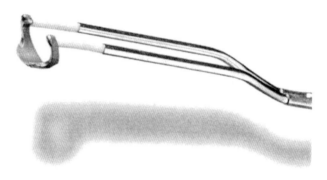

Vaporcut® Electrode

Fig. 2. Thick loop electrode for TUVRP (Karl Storz, Tuttlingen, Germany).

nates the risk of hyponatremia and allows longer operative time. There is also no need for a monopolar return pad, which removes the risk of patient burns. The Gyrus Endourology system can be used with common existing cystoscopic equipment but needs a specific electrosurgical generator and electrode.

TECHNIQUE

The technique for TUVRP (thick-loop) and that for TUVP (roller electrode) will be described separately. The techniques described represent the methods of the author, and modification to the individual surgeon's preference is not only acceptable but advised.

TUVRP Technique

The technique for performing TUVRP of the prostate should be very familiar to the urologist. It is essentially the same as that of the standard TURP. The major difference is that the speed of resection is decreased to allow coagulation, desiccation, and vaporization to occur. A rapid motion during an individual swipe will result in resection without substantial coagulation of blood vessels, and hemostasis and visualization will suffer. Another difference of note is that a substantial increase in bubbles will be produced in the vaporization process. This may initially be a minor nuisance, but will later barely be even noticed.

A 28-Fr continuous irrigation sheath is inserted into the bladder under direct vision. An Otis urethrotome is used as indicated to allow meatal entry. A 30°-angle lens is used initially to inspect the bladder and to identify the ureteral orifices. The 30°-angle lens is then replaced with the Iglesias element containing a 12°-angle lens and a thick band loop (e.g., Vaportome). The verumontanum is localized, and the sheath is held fixed just proximal to it. The scope is pointed upward and resection of the left lateral lobe is begun at the 1 o'clock position. The appropriate depth of resection is determined, and a trench is developed in a linear fashion from the bladder neck to the fixed location proximal to the verumontanum. The left lateral lobe is systematically resected in a stepwise fashion from the 1 o'clock to the 5 o'clock position. As with TURP, it is necessary to torque the resectoscope midswipe to achieve the appropriate depth of resection in this curvilinear gland. The right lateral lobe is approached in the identical fashion. The bladder is emptied and manually irrigated as necessary. Hemostasis is achieved as necessary with the thick loop in coagulation mode. However, if a bleeding vessel is encountered within a portion of tissue that requires further resection, it is often beneficial to resect the tissue to the appropriate depth before coagulating the bleeding vessel. More often than not the bleeding vessel will have been coagulated in the course of resection; if not, better localization of the vessel will have been achieved.

The median lobe is usually approached last so that one does not have to contend with lateral tissue falling in during this part of the resection. The protrusion of lateral tissue into the field can be disorienting and thus hinder what can be a rapid, straightforward debulking process. The resection proceeds from the bladder neck to just proximal to the verumontanum. The resection begins on either side, moving systematically to the contralateral side. Finally, short excursions of the resectoscope are used to carefully clear any remaining apical tissue that is thought to be of significance.

Regardless of the sequence of resection, there are two key points that should be followed. Use a systematic approach to resection and use slow individual swipes through the tissue. The slower motion, which is required to achieve optimal vaporization, desiccation, and coagulation of prostatic tissue, takes its toll on the operative time. However, some time may be saved as a result of having clearer visualization if a deliberate systematic course of vapor-resection is taken.

Most urologists place a 20–24-Fr, three-way, 30-mL balloon Foley catheter on traction, with continuous bladder irrigation overnight. Traction and irrigation are removed in the morning, as is the Foley catheter if the urine remains sufficiently clear.

Postoperatively, we measure serum complete blood count and electrolytes. The patient is given parenteral antibiotics before the procedure, which are continued for 24 h or to the time of discharge, for those discharged, prior to 24 h, the patient is given oral antibiotics to take at home.

TUVP Technique

Standard resectoscope equipment is introduced into the patient's bladder, and the procedure is performed with continuous glycine irrigation. A roller electrode element is used instead of a loop element. The electrical current generator is set between 120 and 300 watts for cutting and 60 and 75 watts for coagulation. The vaporization proceeds in much the same way as described above. The roller element should not be dragged through tissue as the loop is; instead it is rolled over the prostatic tissue, with moderate pressure exerted toward the tissue. The motion of vaporizing with the roller element is slower than the motion of resection in the standard TURP; however, it cannot be too slow or a zone of char will form, rendering that tissue virtually impossible to vaporize. Because the tissue is being vaporized, there will be no specimen for pathology. If tissue is needed for evaluation, the element can be switched to a standard loop for the purpose of tissue acquisition.

OUTCOME

Efficacy

The gold standard of transurethral surgical intervention for BPH is TURP. The available literature suggests that vaporization techniques are comparable in improvement by both subjective and objective measures. To assess how effective a treatment is, it is necessary to have standardized reproducible parameters with which to measure the treatment. Surgical intervention for BPH uses both subjective and objective parameters to measure success. The subjective parameters are most commonly assessed using one of two validated questionnaires, the I-PSS or the AUA SI. The objective measures used in most studies include the peak flow rate (PFR) and the postvoid residual (PVR).

TUVRP EFFICACY

The subjective and objective outcomes of TUVRP have been the topic of several studies since its inception. This hybrid between roller vaporization and TURP is proving to be popular in surgical BPH therapy.

In 1999, Talic et al. reported on 31 patients treated with TUVRP over a 2-yr period (10). Of these, 19 patients had urinary retention, and the remainder had lower urinary tract symptoms (LUTS). Baseline I-PSS

Table 1
Comparison of Postoperative Outcomes: TURP vs Vapor Resection

	Gotoh et al. (11)			Talic et al. (9)	
	IPSS	PFR (mL/sec)	PVR (mL)	IPSS	PFR (mL/sec)
TUVRP	3.7 ± 2.4	23.6 ± 13.9	8.1 ± 12.9	4.0 ± 3.4	19.0 ± 6.5
TURP	3.8 ± 2.3	21.2 ± 9.4	9.3 ± 22.1	5.6 ± 3.1	15.2 ± 10.0
	(NS)	(NS)	(NS)	(p = 0.03)	(p = 0.01)

NS, not significant.

was obtained for those with LUTS. The average initial I-PSS was
24.3 ± 8.3. Three months after TUVRP, the average I-PSS had declined
to 4.1 ± 4.9 ($p < 0.001$). The 3-mo postoperative I-PSS for patients with
urinary retention was 3.9 ± 3.1. Baseline PFR was obtained for those
with LUTS. The average initial PFR was 5.2 ± 4.5. Three months
after TUVRP, the average PFR had increased to 16 ± 7.5 ($p < 0.001$).
The 3-mo postoperative PFR in patients with urinary retention was
21.3 ± 10.2.

TUVRP vs TURP

The above referenced study showed that patients derived statistically
significant subjective and objective improvement following
TUVRP. However, it does not give one a direct comparison with TURP.
Two head-to-head comparisons between TUVRP and TURP have been
reported (Table 1) (9,11).

The conclusion of the Gotoh et al. study was that TUVRP was as
effective, both subjectively and objectively, as TURP, but offered no
advantages (11). The conclusion of the Talic et al. study was that TURVP
was as efficacious as TURP and offered some advantages, which will be
discussed in sections to follow (9).

TUVP EFFICACY

The roller vaporization technology has been used longer and thus has
been the subject of numerous studies. Four studies from 1995 to 2000
illustrate the efficacy data regarding TUVP (2,4,12,13).

Subjective Efficacy

The AUA symptoms score decreased from a baseline of 17.8 to 4.2
($p < 0.01$) at the 3-mo follow-up visit after TUVP in a study of 25 men
with mild-to-moderate LUTS (2). Narayan et al. reported a decrease in
I-PSS from a baseline of 24 to 7.8 ($p < 0.0001$) 6 mo after TUVP (12).

Table 2
Comparison of Postoperative Outcomes: TURP vs Vaporization

	Symptom Score	Peak Urinary Flow (mL/sec)	PVR (mL)
TUVP (Baseline)	19.4 ± 3.9	7.2 ± 3.1	77.8 ± 20.3
TUVP Follow-up			
12 mo (30/32 pt)	6.6 ± 2.4	16.9 ± 4.1	43.6 ± 22.4
TURP (Baseline)	18.3 ± 3.9	8.3 ± 3.1	66.9 ± 15.7
TURP Follow-up			
12 mo (31/32 pt)	6.1 ± 1.9	19.6 ± 4.9	34.2 ± 19.6

In the study by Narayan et al., both PFR and PVR improved significantly. In the study by Kaplan et al., the PFR increased from a baseline of 7.4 ± 2.6 mL/s to 17.3 ± 2.7 mL/s ($p < 0.02$) at 3 mo (4). PVR improved from a baseline of 57.56 ± 17.7 mL to 43.78 ± 21.47 at 3 mo in the same study, but the difference was not significant.

TUVP vs TURP

Kaplan et al. used a blinded, prospective, comparative technique to study 32 consecutive men with LUTS treated with TUVP and a cohort of 32 men treated with TURP (4). This study concluded that both modalities improved the subjective and objective parameters of efficacy, but TURP did so to a greater extent (Table 2).

A study by Enkengren et al. compared TURPV and TUVP in 54 men using a randomized, prospective technique (13). These men were scheduled for surgery to relieve urinary outlet obstruction and were randomized to TUVP or TURP. The efficacy outcomes used by this study were I-PSS, quality of life score, prostate-specific antigen, PVR, and PFR as measured at 1 yr after surgery. These authors concluded that there was no statistically significant difference between the two procedures.

Safety

When a new modality or a modification of the standard is being compared with the gold standard, it is not enough to measure it against the efficacy of the standard. Complications and the associated adverse effects of the new treatment must also be compared to those of the gold standard. The complications of these procedures are stratified into three groups: intraoperative, early postoperative, and long-term.

Safety information about TURP was described in a landmark article published in 1989 by Mebust et al. that evaluated data from 3885 patients

Table 3
Outcome Comparison: Kaplan et al.

	Operating Room Time (min)	Change in Na+ (meq/L)	Blood Loss (change in Hgb)
TUVP	47.6 ± 17.6	1.4 ± 0.4	2.8 ± 0.7
TURP	34.6 ± 11.2	3.9 ± 1.9	5.6 ± 3.1
	(p < 0.003)	(p < 0.003)	(p < 0.05)

Table 4
Outcome Comparison: Enkengren et al.

	Operating Room Time (min)	Fluid absorption (mL)	Blood loss (mL/min)*
TUVP	30	125	2.5
TURP	33	154	4.9

*$p < 0.001$.

(14). From this work it was learned that the average resection time was 57 min and that resection times greater than 90 min correlated with a significant increase in intraoperative bleeding. TUR syndrome occurred in 2% of cases, of which 2.5% required intraoperative transfusions and 3.7% required postoperative transfusions. Of those with TUR syndrome, 82% had catheter removal by postoperative day 3; and 78% were discharged from the hospital by postoperative day 5. Refinements in technique, technology, patient monitoring, and preoperative assessment have changed since that time, but these values can be used to orient the reader. Some contemporary TURP data are compared with data from vaporization technique studies below.

TUVP Safety

INTRAOPERATIVE

The most common intraoperative issues are operative time, fluid absorption, and blood loss. These complications were compared with the same complications during TURP in studies by Kaplan et al. and by Enkengren and co-workers *(4,13)*. In the 1998 study by Kaplan et al., operative times were longer with TUVP, but there was less fluid absorption as determined by change in serum sodium levels, and blood loss was less (Table 3). Enkengren et al. reported no difference in operative time or fluid absorption as determined by ethanol-laced irrigation. There was, however, significantly less blood loss with TUVP (Table 4).

Table 5
Complications of TUVP and TURP

	TUVP	TURP
Hematuria	53%	60%
Clot Retention	9%	6%
Blood Transfusion	0	3%
Transurethral Resection Syndrome	0	3%
Bladder-Neck Contracture	0	0
Urethral Stricture	3%	3%
Urinary Tract Infection	16%	13%
Incontinence	0	0

EARLY POSTOPERATIVE

Catheterization time, length of hospital stay, and days lost from work are important considerations of the early postoperative period. Kaplan et al. addressed these issues and found that TUVP yielded more favorable outcomes for all three of these factors (4). Catheters were removed on average at 12.9 ± 4.6 h in patients undergoing TUVP, as opposed to 67.4 ± 13.6 h with TURP. Length of hospital stay was 1.3 ± 0.5 d compared with 2.6 ± 0.9 d with TURP. Days lost from work were 6.7 ± 2.1 d vs 18.4 ± 7.6 d with TURP.

No patient undergoing TUVP later had TUR syndrome, and none required blood transfusion. Clot retention occurred in 3%, and 5% reported urinary tract infection (Table 5).

LONG-TERM

The more common long-term complications of transurethral prostatic procedures include retrograde ejaculation, urethral strictures, bladder neck contractures, incontinence, and late re-operation. There were no significant differences in any of these factors between TUVP and TURP in either the Kaplan et al. or the Enkengren et al. study. However, the total number of complications after TUVP was greater in the Enkengren et al. study ($p < 0.02$).

TUVRP Safety

INTRAOPERATIVE

In the study by Gotoh et al., there were no differences in change in serum sodium levels, blood loss, or operative times between TUVRP and TURP (11).

Talic et al. noted a significant difference in each of those parameters (9). Talic et al. found that operative time was significantly longer for the

Table 6
Blood Test Results Before, During, and 24 Hours Postoperatively

	TUVRP	TURP	p Value
Hemoglobin (g/dL)			
Preoperative	13.6 ± 1.1	13.2 ± 1.4	NS
1 hour after treatment	13.1 ± 1.1	12.5 ± 1.5	0.03
1 day after treatment	12.8 ± 1.1	12.2 ± 1.6	0.03
Hematocrit (mL/dL)			
Preoperative	40.4 ± 3.1	39.3 ± 4.0	NS
1 hour after treatment	38.6 ± 3.0	37.0 ± 4.2	0.03
1 day after treatment	37.8 ± 3.2	35.8 ± 5.1	0.05
Serum sodium (mEq/L)			
Preoperative	140.5 ± 3.5	140.4 ± 2.6	NS
1 hour after treatment	140.5 ± 3.4	139.2 ± 2.5	0.01
1 day after treatment	138.6 ± 3.0	137.3 ± 3.2	0.04

Adapted from ref. 9.
NS, not significant.
Data presented as the mean ± SD.

TUVRP group when compared with the TURP group. However, blood loss and change in serum sodium were significantly lower (Table 6).

EARLY POSTOPERATIVE

Gotoh et al. showed no difference in catheterization time between the groups (11). No data were available regarding length of hospital stay or days lost from work. Talic et al. showed a significant decrease in the catheterization time, with 94% of patients catheter-free at 24 h after TUVRP compared with 60% in the TURP group (9). The mean catheter times were 23.1 ± 10.3 h and 36 ± 17.3 h for the TUVRP and TURP groups, respectively ($p < 0.0001$). Neither length of stay nor days lost from work data were available.

Gotoh et al. reported no TUR syndrome, blood transfusion, or clot retention in either group. In the Talic et al. study, there were no cases of TUR syndrome, and no blood transfusions in either group, but one patient in each group did experience delayed hemorrhage with clot retention.

LONG-TERM

There was no significant difference in long-term complication between TUVRP and TURP in either study. Gotoh et al. found no urethral strictures, bladder neck contractures, urinary tract infection, or incontinence in either group at 3 mo. Talic et al. reported three patients with urethral strictures in each group and one patient in the TURP group who had meatal stenosis. This latter study also mentions that no new cases of erectile dysfunction were encountered. No data on retrograde ejaculation were reported in either study.

DISCUSSION

The vaporization techniques appear to be just as efficacious with somewhat fewer complications than the standard TURP. It is imperative that the surgeon performing vaporization use slower excursion with the resectoscope. This is suggested by a report in which there was no difference in safety parameters between TUVRP and TURP, no difference in operative times, and no difference in the resected tissue weight. In the single study that did show a difference in the safety parameters between TUVRP and TURP, operative times for TUVRP were significantly longer. This implies that slower excursions were taken by the surgeons performing TUVRP. Whether this technology may someday prove to be superior to TURP will require the performance of multicentered, well-designed, properly executed studies. TUVRP appears to have the advantages of decreased blood loss, catheter time, and hospital stay. This modification allows the surgeon to approach larger glands with less trepidation because there is less fluid absorption, and an equivalent amount of tissue is being both vaporized and resected. Surgeons are already accustomed to this familiar form of transurethral prostatectomy, and conversion to this technology is a relatively low-cost endeavor. As further modifications take place with this technology, continued changes in these procedures are expected.

REFERENCES

1. Perlmutter AP, Muschter R, Razvi HA. Electrosurgical vaporization of the prostate in the canine model. Urology 1995; 46:518–523.
2. Kaplan SA, Te AE. Transurethral electrovaporization of the prostate (TVP): a novel method for treating men with benign prostatic hyperplasia. Urology 1995; 45:566–573.
3. Stewart S, Benjamin D, Ruckle HC, et al. Electrovaporization of the prostate: new technique for the treatment of symptomatic benign hyperplasia. J Endourol 1995;9:413–416.
4. Kaplan SA, Laor E, Fatal M, Te AE. Transurethral resection of the prostate versus transurethral electrovaporization of the prostate. A blinded, comparative study with 1-year follow-up. J Urol 1998;159(2):454–458.
5. Mebust WK. Transurethral surgery. In: Walsh PC, Retik AB, Vaughn ED Jr, Wein AJ, eds., Campbell's Urology, ed 7, Philadelphia: WB Saunders Co, 1998, pp. 1511–1528.
6. Cabelin MA, Te AE, Kaplan SA. Transurethral vaporization of the prostate: current techniques. Curr Urol Rep 2000;1:116–123.
7. Van Swol CFP, van Vliet RJ, Verdaaskonk RM, et al. Electrovaporization as a treatment modality for transurethral resection of the prostate: influence of generator type. Urology 1999;53:317–321.

8. Kupeli S, Soygur T, Yilmaz E, et al. Combined transurethral resection and vaporization of the prostate using newly designed electrode: a promising treatment alternative for benign prostatic hyperplasia. J Endourol 1999;13:225–228.
9. Talic RF, El Tiraifi A, El Faqih SR, et al. Prospective randomized study of transurethral vaporization resection of the prostate using the thick loop and standard transurethral prostatectomy. Urology 2000;55(6):886–890.
10. Talic RF. Transurethral electrovaporization-resection of the prostate using the "Wing" cutting electrode: preliminary results of safety and efficacy in the treatment of men with prostatic outflow obstruction. Urology 1999;53:106–110.
11. Gotoh M, Okamura K, Hattori R, Nishiyama N, et al. A randomized comparative study of the bandloop versus the standard loop for transurethral resection of the prostate. J Urol 1999;162:1645–1647.
12. Narayan P, Tewari A, Crocker B, et al. Factors affecting size and configuration of electrovaporization lesions in the prostate. Urology 1996;47:679–688.
13. Ekengren J, Haendler L, Hahn RG. Clinical outcome 1 year after transurethral vaporization and resection of the prostate. Urology 2000;55:231–235.
14. Mebust WK, Holtgrewe HL, Cockett ATK, et al. Transurethral prostatectomy: immediate and postoperative complications. Cooperative study of 13 participating institutions evaluating 3,885 patients. J Urol 1989;141:243–247.

FURTHER READING

Source material not specifically referenced in the text.

Bush IM, Malters E, Bush J. Transurethral vaporization of the prostate (TVP): new horizons [abstract]. Society for Minimally Invasive Therapy 1993; 2(suppl):98.

Chen SS, Chiu AW, Lin AT, et al. Clinical outcomes at 3 months after transurethral vaporization of prostate for benign prostatic hyperplasia. Urology 1997;50:235–238.

Desautel MG, Burney TL, Diaz PA, et al. Outcome of VaporTrode transurethral vaporization of the prostate using pressure-flow urodynamic criteria. Urology 1998;51:1013–1017.

Dineen MK, Brown BT, Cantwell AL, et al. Outpatient transurethral resection of the prostate with vaporization assistance: a two year experience in a free standing ambulatory surgery center. J Urol 1997;157(suppl):314.

Gallucci M, Puppo P, Perachino M, et al. Transurethral electrovaporization of the prostate vs. transurethral resection. Eur Urol 1998;33:359–364.

Hamawy KJ, Siroky MB, Krane RJ, et al. Transurethral vaporization of the prostate (TUVP): an electrosurgical alternative for BPH. J Endourol 1995; 9(suppl 1):S124.

Hammadeh M, Sanjeev M, Singh M, et al. Transurethral electro-vaporization of the prostate, a possible alternative to standard TURP: three years follow up of a prospective randomized trial. J Urol 1999;161(suppl 4):1516A.

Kaplan SA, Te AE. A comparative study of transurethral resection of the prostate using a modified electro-vaporizing loop and transurethral laser vaporization of the prostate. J Urol 1995;154:1785–1790.

Larsen TR, Religo EM, Collins JM, et al. Detailed prostatic interstitial thermal mapping during transurethral grooved rollerball electrovaporization and loop electrosurgery for benign prostatic hyperplasia. Urology 1996;48:501–507.

Lim LM, Patel A, Ryan TP, et al. Quantitative assessment of variables that influence soft-tissue electrovaporization in a fluid environment. Urology 1997;49:851–856.

Meade WM, Mcloughlin MG. Endoscopic rollerball electrovaporization of the prostate-the sandwich technique: evaluation of the initial efficacy and morbidity in the treatment of benign prostatic obstruction. Br J Urol 1996;77:696–700.

Narayan P, Fournier G, Indudhara R, et al. Transurethral evaporization of the prostate (TUEP) with Nd:YAG laser using a contact free beam technique: results in 61 patients with benign prostatic hyperplasia. Urology 1994;43:813–820.

Narayan P, Tewari A, Aboseif S, et al. A randomized study comparing visual laser ablation and transurethral evaporization of prostate in the management of benign prostatic hyperplasia. J Urol 1995;154:2083–2088.

Narayan P, Tewari A, Garzotto M, et al. Transurethral vaportrode electrovaporization of the prostate: Physical principles, technique, and results. Urology 1996;47(4):505–510

Okada T, Terai A, Terachi T, et al. Transurethral electrovaporization of the prostate: preliminary clinical results with pressure-flow analysis. Int J Urol 1998;5:55–59.

Patel A, Fuchs GJ, Gutierrez-Aceves J, et al. Prostate heating patterns comparing electrosurgical transurethral resection and vaporization: a prospective randomized study. J Urol 1997;157:169–172.

Patel A, Fuchs GJ, Gutierrez-Aceves J, et al. Transurethral electrovaporization and vapour-resection of the prostate: an appraisal of possible electrosurgical alternatives to regular loop resection. BJU Int 2000;85:202–210.

Perlmutter AP, Schulsinger DA. The "Wedge" resection device for electrosurgical transurethral prostatectomy. J Endourol 1998;12:75–79.

Perlmutter AP, Vallancien G. Thick loop transurethral resection of the prostate. Eur Urol 1999;35:161–165.

Reis RB, Cologna AJ, Suaid HJ, et al. Electrovaporization of the prostate (VAP): an electrosurgical alternative for BPH [abstract]. J Urol 1996;155:406A.

Reis RB, Cologna AJ, Suaid HJ, et al. Interstitial thermotherapy in men undergoing electrovaporization: is it safe? J Urol 1996;155(suppl):707A.

Te AE, Kaplan SA. Electrovaporization of the prostate. Curr Opin Urol 1996;6:2–9.

Te AE, Kaplan SA. Transurethral electrovaporization of the prostate: the year in review. Curr Opin Urol 1997;7:25–36.

13 Treatment of Benign Prostatic Hyperplasia with Ethanol Injections, Water-Induced Thermotherapy, and Prostatic Urethral Luminal Stents

Jay Y. Gillenwater, MD

Contents

ETHANOL INJECTION
TRANSURETHRAL WATER-INDUCED THERMOTHERAPY (WIT)
  OF THE PROSTATE
PROSTATIC STENTS FOR TREATMENT OF BPH
SUMMARY
REFERENCES

ETHANOL INJECTION

Injection of sclerosing solutions into the prostate for the treatment of benign prostatic hyperplasia (BPH) was reported early in the 20th century. Sclerosing solutions including phenol, glacial acetic acid, and glycerin were injected transperineally and were successful in four of nine patients reported by Broughton and Smith *(1)*. However, this therapy was discontinued because of perineal pain occurring within minutes and lasting up to 24 hr in five of the nine patients. Broughton and Smith found extravasation of contrast medium in the region of the apex of the prostate in a patient who had undergone transperineal prostate injection. Transperineal injection of sclerosing solutions was associated with extraprostatic leakage and caused sphincter necrosis in three of seven canines in an animal study *(2)*.

From: *Management of Benign Prostatic Hypertrophy*
Edited by: K. T. McVary © Humana Press Inc., Totowa, NJ

Two groups have subsequently reported success with transurethral prostatic injections of dehydrated ethanol, avoiding some of the earlier complications *(3,4)*. Goya and associates used an endoscopic injection set through a cystoscope to inject 0.5–2.0 mL of dehydrated ethanol per site in four to eight sites in each lateral lobe in 10 patients *(3)*. The median lobe was also injected if present. A urethral catheter was left for 1 wk. No ethanol could be measured in the patient's blood. The treatment was successful in 8 of 10 patients, as evidenced by patient satisfaction and improvement in symptom scores, peak flow rates (PFR), and residual urine volume. Ditrolio and associates recently reported 1-yr success in 13 patients using an INJEC Tx endoscopic device to inject absolute ethanol transurethrally into the prostate *(4)*. In this study, patients with prostate cancer, urinary retention, or prostatic volumes >100 g were excluded. The INJECT Tx is a new device with a 20-G needle with multiport infusion designed to give homogenous diffusion throughout the prostate gland. The volume of alcohol injected ranged from 2 to 5 mL per injection site. If a median lobe was present, it was also injected. In their studies in animals and humans, the alcohol solution remained confined to the prostatic parenchyma. Plasma ethanol levels were not detectable 60 min after the injection. Postoperative catheter drainage averaged 3.6 d. Gross hematuria was present for the first two to three postoperative days, but there was no clot retention. At 1 yr after surgery, these patients had relief of their symptoms (73% reduction), improved flow rates (200% improvement), and reduced prostate volume (55% of the preoperative volume). In one patient, subsequent transurethral resection of the prostate (TURP) had to be done because of lack of relief of the patient's symptoms after the ethanol injection.

The mechanism of action of ethanol injection is hemorrhagic coagulation necrosis and thrombotic closure of local arterioles and venules. Two human studies of transurethral prostatic ethanol injection show that it can effect relief of lower urinary tract symptoms (LUTS) associated with BPH with no apparent morbidity *(3,4)*. Both of these studies are small, and therefore some caution is warranted until larger series with longer follow-ups are available.

TRANSURETHRAL WATER-INDUCED THERMOTHERAPY (WIT) OF THE PROSTATE

A variety of techniques have been introduced over the last 15 years using heat to destroy prostate tissue to relieve obstruction and other symptoms of BPH. The latest of these is transurethral WIT (ArgoMed Inc., Cary NC). This technique was conceived, designed, and a company (ArgoMed) was formed to produce the catheter. After initial testing, the WIT treatment was investigated in a multiinstitutional Food and Drug Administration-approved study reported by Muschter and associates *(5)*.

The mechanism of action of WIT is coagulation necrosis, which does not occur below 45°C. The correlation of time and temperature is not fully known and may vary; however, it may take up to an hour at 45.5°C and only minutes at 60°C. Between 60° and 100°C, coagulation is nearly instantaneous. Temperatures over 100°C may vaporize tissue *(6)*.

WIT is performed using the Thermoflex (ArgoMed Inc, Cary NC) system. The system consists of a console that heats and pumps the water into a treatment balloon inflated to 50 Fr within the prostatic fossa, which receives 60°C water for 45 min. There is also a balloon inflated with 16 mL of air located in the bladder. The catheter is insulated except for the balloon in the prostatic urethra. Treatment balloons are available in lengths of 20–60 mm in 5-mm increments, allowing balloon length to be matched to prostate length. The treatment is not effective for median lobe prostatic hypertrophy.

Topical urethral anesthesia is given with 2% lidocaine gel. We have not found it necessary to use other analgesia. The treatment 18 Fr catheter is passed; if there is a problem, the catheter can be passed over a wire placed in the bladder with a flexible cystoscope. All patients are discharged home the day of treatment with a Foley catheter to manage prostatic swelling. Half of the patients need the catheter for only a week. An additional 30% are catheter-free at 2 wk, but some patients require a catheter for 3–5 wk.

The depth of necrosis from WIT therapy was around 10 mm in prostate specimens studied by Corica and co-workers *(7)*. In the European multiinstitutional study, at 2 yr, peak flow was increased by 96%, International Prostate Symptom Score (I-PSS) decreased 52%, and quality of life scales decreased by 41% *(5)*.

We have treated 40 patients at our institution. Of these, 25 had chronic urinary retention with catheter drainage or had residual urine levels >600 mL. All of these patients were in poor health and averaged 79.6 yr of age; many were in nursing homes. Treatment was done on an outpatient basis without sedation or analgesics. One patient had a thalamic stroke 1 mo later and was not given a voiding trial because he could not stand or ambulate. One passed his voiding trial but died of bladder cancer 13 mo later. Voiding trials have failed in five; one is on intermittent catheterization; four had a subsequent TURP. In two, the pathology report revealed prostatic cancer. Two had a median lobe that was not recognized on flexible cystoscopy. Interestingly, one had a concave hollowing out of the middle lobe from the heat therapy. On cystogram, only one patient had a hollowed-out prostatic fossa. In the 19 patients who can void, the postvoid residual volume (PVR) averaged 38.7 mL, time-to-removal of the catheter was 4.8 wk, flow rates were 6–10 mL/s, and urodynamic studies showed mild obstruction of 2–4/6 (1 is normal and 6 is obstructed).

PROSTATIC STENTS FOR TREATMENT OF BPH

During my training, I was taught that splints were used externally, for instance to stabilize fractures, whereas stents were for internal use. A recent biographic paper on Dr. Charles Stent, a dentist who invented stents around 1856 in England said that it was invented to get dental impressions, originally called Stent's mass (8). This formulation was also used as a tissue expander for neck and knee surgery and later to hold tubes open and in facial reconstruction during the WWI. The ancestry of the stent would appear to be by way of dentistry and plastic surgery.

Prostatic stents are divided into three categories: prostate springs, which include Urospiral, Prostacath, Prostacoil stents; self-expandable stents such as the Urolume; and balloon-expandable stents such as the Titan and the newer Memotherm, including intraurethral catheters and the new biodegradable ones. The available literature concerning the various types of stents consist of small series with short follow-up and no controls. There are, however, excellent recent reviews (9,10).

The use of ureteral stents began in the 1960s with the use of Silastic tubing to keep obstructed ureters open. It was used more as an indwelling catheter than as a stent to hold scarred ureters open. The tubing was passed from below. In 1969, stents were placed in peripheral arteries to prevent re-stenosis after balloon angioplasty in the peripheral vascular system (11). Since that time, stents have been adapted for use in every vessel, duct, and tube in the body.

The first described use of intraprostatic stents in the treatment of prostatic obstruction dates to 1980 when Fabian described placing a temporary stent through the prostate for high-risk patients (the urospiral) (12,13). The urospiral reportedly had problems with migration, encrustation, and recurrent infections, and did not allow cystoscopy.

The second permanent prostatic stent system was reported by Chapple et al. in 1990 (14). This group had previous experience with stents for managing strictures in the male urethra and thought it was a logical extension of the procedure to use it in prostate obstruction. The stent was made of wire mesh that became epithelialized in 6–8 mo. Most of the patients had urinary retention from BPH and were poor operative candidates. Patients with atonic neurogenic bladders were excluded. The stent was successful in 11 of 12 patients. One patient was unhappy with the procedure because of persistent frequency of urination and was found to have severe detrusor instability. In two patients, encrustations of the proximal end of the stent developed, which were dislodged and removed endoscopically. The same group's expanded experience of 54 patients was reported in 1993 (15). In this group, 93% were able to void, and 74% had no to minimal voiding symptoms. Encrustations developed in 26% and 6 of 54 required subsequent removal.

Expandable Stents

Favorable experiences have been reported with the Urolume wallstent endoprosthesis in the treatment of BPH. The wallstent is a woven tubular mesh of corrosion-resistant superalloy wire compressed and elongated inside the delivery system. A large multicenter trial of 126 patients was reported by Oesterling and associates (16). In this study, 95 of the patients had moderate or severe prostatism, and 31 had urinary retention. For those without retention, the symptom score decreased from 14.3 to 5.4 at 24 mo, peak urine flow increased from 9.1 to 13.4 mL/s, and PVR decreased from 86 to 48 mL. In the group with retention, the symptom score at 24 months was 4.1, peak urinary flow averaged 11.4 mL/s, and PVR was 46 mL. There was a 13% removal rate. At 12 mo, most stents were covered by epithelium.

Guazzoni et al. reported on 30 patients who were poor operative risks who had bladder outlet obstruction resulting from BPH (17). Twelve could void spontaneously and 18 had retention. One of 30 could not void after insertion of the Urolume wallstent. At 1 yr, flow rates in those without retention were increased from 8 to 15.8 mL/s and residual urine decreased from 127 to 38 mL. In the group with retention, PFR were 13.2 mL/s and residual urine was 32 mL. The one patient who could not void did successfully void after the stent was repositioned. The Urolume wallstent has been shown to provide relief for patients with urinary retention caused by advanced prostate cancer and in patients with bladder outlet obstruction after prostate brachytherapy (18,19).

The results of the intraprostatic spiral (Prostakath device) in 150 patients were reported by Nordling and associates (20). Eighty patients had urinary retention and 70 had severe prostate obstruction. By 4 mo, 75 patients had the stents removed (17 to do a prostatectomy, 16 for urinary retention, 10 for incontinence, 7 for local discomfort, because of no improvement in 13, and other causes such as stroke in 7). Migration occurred 55 times, but only led to coil removal in five patients. Voiding symptoms improved in the majority of patients. There were no or few symptoms in two of three patients and 10% had severe prostatism. The reported success rate was 66%.

Braf et al. reported on their use of Prostakath (coated with 24-karat gold) in 65 patients and of the Urospiral (made entirely of stainless steel) in 45 patients *(21)*. The complications reported at 1 yr with the Prostakath were migration in one patient, incontinence in one patient, encrustation in one patient, clinical infection in two patients, failure to void in four patients, and stent removal in 16%. Complications at 1 yr with the Urospiral were migration in four patients, incontinence in one patient, encrustation in two patients, clinical infection in three patients, failure to void in one patient, and stent removal in 16%. A bad complication of late strictures at the postsphincteric end of the device occurred once in each group. Open prostatectomy with retrieval resulted in death in one patient in each group.

Self-Expandable Stent: ProstaCoil and Gianturco-Z

The ProstaCoil is 17 Fr before insertion and expands to 24–30 Fr. Yachia and associates reported on their experience in 65 patients *(22)*. Of these, 37 had their stents removed at the time of prostatectomy. Complications were urinary tract infections in 32 patients, repositioning in 5 patients, and dysuria or perineal pain in 14 patients.

The Gianturco-Z stent, a zigzag arrangement of stainless steel wires that expands to 36 Fr, was initially used within the biliary system. Morgentaler and DeWolf reported on the use of this stent in 21 patients *(23)*. Spontaneous voiding resumed in 95%, with long-term success in 76%. Two patients had failure as a result of stent migration within 1 mo.

Balloon-Expandable Stent: Titan Intraprostatic Stent

Kaplan et al. reported a multicenter study of the Titan intraprostatic stent in 68 patients *(24)*. This stent is made of titanium and has a tubular mesh appearance. It is expanded under direct vision in the prostatic urethra. All patients in this series were able to void spontaneously within 36 hr of stent insertion. At 18 mo, peak PFR increased from 3.9 to 14.4 mL/s and PVR volumes decreased from 74.4 to 40.2 mL. Of the initial 68 patients, 5 died of underlying problems but had satisfactory voiding, and 17 underwent uneventful stent removal (10 for technical failure and 7 for treatment failure). Technical failures were caused by inaccurate positioning or improper stent sizing.

Thermosensitive Nitinol Stent

The thermosensitive nitinol stent (an alloy of nickel and titanium) can expand to its maximal diameter of 42 Fr at body temperatures. After expansion, the stent loses its compressibility but keeps its flexibility so

that it can adjust to the course of the prostatic urethra. Nitinol is biologically inert. The nitinol stent becomes soft and pliable again if it is cooled,
and it can then be pulled out like a string. A nitinol stent (Memotherm)
was reported by Gesenberg and Sintermann to be successful in 95% of
123 patients, of whom 37% had urinary retention (25). The maximum
PFR increased from 7.4 to 16.1 mL/s and PVR decreased to 26 mL.
Early stent dislocation was experienced by 8.9%, which could be
corrected.

Marks et al. tested another nitinol prostatic stent (Horizon) in
10 patients (26). Insertion was easily done after the patients received
anesthesia. Removal was easily accomplished by unraveling after the
stent was cooled with iced saline. One patient required stent removal
because of dysuria. Residual urine volume decreased from 189 mL to
50 mL, and PFR improved from 6.6 to 10.8 mL/s.

Temporary Nonbioresorbable Prostate
and Posterior Urethral Stents

Two publications describe a new type of temporary stent that is placed
in the prostatic urethra and attached by a suture going through the sphincter to a short stent in the bulbous urethra. Djavan and associates reported
on the prostatic bridge catheter in 54 patients, which is used after transurethral microwave therapy for 1 mo to prevent urinary retention (27).
Extraction is by an attached string. The prostatic bridge catheter
remained indwelling in 48 of 54 patients (88.9%), and while in place,
significant improvements were observed in mean PFR (59%), I-PSS
(33%), and quality of life score (24%) compared with baseline. Early
prostatic bridge catheter removal was required in three patients (5.6%)
because of urinary retention and in three (5.6%) because of catheter
migration.

Similar success was reported in 42 patients by Devonec and
Dahlstrand (28). The same temporary prostatic stent (Trestle, Boston
Scientific Microvasive) was also reported by Traxer and associates (29).
In this study, the stents were inserted in 20 patients with BPH patients
and urinary retention in whom surgery was contraindicated. The stents
remained in place for an average of 3.5 mo. Two migrations were
reported. The maximum PFR was 13.7 mL/s, and the mean PVR volume
was 110 mL. The stents were easily removed by the protruding attached
suture. Little encrustation was observed.

Temporary Bioresorbable Prostatic Stents

In the early 1980s, high-strength, self-reinforced, biodegradable
polymeric composites were developed for tissue management. They

were polymers of organic acids with a molecular weight of up to 1,000,000 D. The properties of these polymers depend on the basic molecules and the degree of polymerization. The degradation depends on the structure and strength of the individual materials. The use of these polymers in temporary bioresorbable prostatic stents in 11 men was reported by Isotalo and associates (30). They used a temporary bioresorbable self-reinforced poly-L-lactic acid prostatic urethral stent plus finasteride. The strength of the stent is retained for 35 wk in vitro and the total degradation time is 1 yr. The stent expands 45% to hold itself in place. All patients were able to void spontaneously, and their bladders emptied properly. In this trial, there were three cases of incorrect positioning of the stent and three urinary tract infections. The stents held the prostatic urethra open until finasteride could shrink the prostate.

Laaksovirta and associates reported their results in 39 men treated with a self-reinforced lactic and glycolic acid copolymer prostatic spiral stent after interstitial laser coagulation of the prostate (31). This stent expands 100%, locking it into the prostatic urethra. All but one patient voided on postoperative day 1, and when the stent was properly relocated, this patient was also able to void. At 4 mo, the stent was degraded into small pieces. Three patients had asymptomatic urinary tract infections. The authors felt the combination of interstitial laser therapy with a temporary stent was successful.

SUMMARY

Prostatic stents have a future role in managing patients with bladder neck obstruction. An ideal stent needs to be easily inserted and large enough in diameter to work, and it must be biologically inert and easy to remove. There is a definite need for temporary stents after the various forms of heat therapy now used for BPH and after brachytherapy for prostate cancer because of the temporary swelling of the prostate. The ideal temporary prostatic stent has yet to be reported; currently available temporary stents break down into spicules that stick in the urethra.

The various forms of heat therapy offer an attractive alternative to clean intermittent catheterization or chronic urethral catheterization. An alternative therapy would be the use of long-term prostatic stents. Anjum and associates (32) reported improvements in urine flow that have been maintained for as long as 5 yr. Long-term stents have not had adverse effects on sexual activity. There are favorable reports about resecting epithelial overgrowth into the lumen of the stents. The problems reported with long-term stents are migration, encrustations, misplacements, recurrent infections, and lack of efficacy with large median lobes.

REFERENCES

1. Broughton AC, Smith PH. The significance of perineal pain after injection of the prostate. Br J Urol 1970;42:73–75.
2. Littrup PJ, Lee F, Borlaza GS, et al. Percutaneous ablation of the canine prostate using transrectal ultrasound guidance, absolute alcohol and Nd:YAG laser. Invest Radiol 1988;23:734–739.
3. Goya N, Ishikawa N, Ito F, et al. Ethanol injection therapy of the prostate for benign prostate hyperplasia: preliminary report on the application of a new therapy. J Urol 1999;162:383–386.
4. Ditrolio J, Patel P, Watson RA, Irwin RJ. Chemo-ablation of the prostate with dehydrated alcohol in the treatment of prostatic obstruction. J Urol 2002;2100–2104.
5. Muschter R, et al. Transurethral water-induced thermotherapy for the treatment of benign prostatic hyperplasia: a prospective multicenter clinical trial. J Urol 2000;164:1565–1569.
6. Perlmutter AP. The new invasive therapies for benign prostatic obstruction. In: Walsh PC, Retik AB, Vaughan ED Jr, Wein AJ, eds., Campbell's Urology Update 24, Philadelphia: W. B. Saunders, 1997, p. 1.
7. Corica FA, et al. Transurethral hot-water balloon thermoablation for benign prostatic hyperplasia: patient tolerance and pathologic findings. Urology 2000;56:76–80.
8. Ring ME. How a dentist's name became a synonym for a life-saving device: the story of Dr. Charles Stent. J Hist Dent 2001;49:77–80.
9. Lam JS, Volpe MA, Kaplan SA. Use of prostatic stents for the treatment of benign prostatic hyperplasia in high risk patients. Curr Urol Rep 2001;2:277–284.
10. Kapoor R, Liatsikos EN, Badlani G. Endoprostatic stents for management of benign prostatic hyperplasia. Curr Opinion Urol 2000;10:19–22.
11. Dotter CT. Transluminally-placed coilspring endoarterial tube grafts: long-term patency in canine popliteal artery. Invest Radiol 1969;4:329–332.
12. Fabian KM. Der intraprostatische "partielle katheter" (urologische spirale). Urologe A 1980;19:236–238.
13. Fabian KM. Der intraprostatische "partielle katheter" (urologische spirale). II. Urologe A 1980;23:229–233.
14. Chapple CR, Milroy EJ, Rickards D. Permanently implanted urethral stent for prostatic obstruction in the unfit patient. Preliminary report. Br J Urol 1990;66:58–65.
15. Milroy E, Chapple CR. The Urolume stent in the management of benign prostatic hyperplasia. J Urol 1993;150:1630–1635.
16. Oesterling JE, Defalco AJ, Kaplan SA, et al. The North American experience with the Urolume endoprosthesis as a treatment for benign prostatic hyerplasia: long-term results. Urology 1994;44:353–362.
17. Guazzoni G, Bergamaschi F, Montorsi F, et al. Prostatic Urolume wallstent for benign prostatic hyperplasia patients at poor operative risk: clinical, uroflowmetric and ultrasonographic patterns. J Urol 1993;150:1641–1646.
18. Guazzoni G, Montorsi F, Bergamaschi F, Consonni P, Rigatti P. Prostatic Urolume wallstent for urinary retention due to advanced prostate cancer: a 1-year followup study. J Urol 1994;152:1530–1532.
19. Konety BR, Phelan MW, O'Donnell WF, Antiles L, Chancellor MB. Urolume stent placement for the treatment of postbrachytherapy bladder outlet obstruction. Urology 2000;55:721–724.

20. Nordling J, Ovesen H, Poulsen AL. The intraprostatic spiral: clinical results in 150 consecutive patients. J Urol 1992;147:645–647.

21. Braf Z, Chen J, Sofer M, Matzkin H. Intraprostatic metal stents (Prostakath® and Urospiral®): more than 6 years' experience with 110 patients. J Endourol 1996;10:555–558.

22. Yachia D, Beyar M, Anidogan IA. A new large caliber, self expanding and self retaining temporary intraprostatic stent (ProstaCoil) in the treatment of prostatic obstruction. Br J Urol 1994;74:47–49.

23. Morgentaler A, DeWolf WC. A self-expanding prostatic stent for bladder outlet obstruction in high risk patients. J Urol 1993;150:1636–1640.

24. Kaplan SA, Merrill DC, Mosely WG, et al. The titanium intraprostatic stent: the United States experience. J Urol 1993;150:1624–1629.

25. Gesenberg A, Sintermann R. Management of benign prostatic hyperplasia in high-risk patients: long-term experience with the Memotherm stent. J Urol 1998;160:72–76.

26. Marks LS, Ettekal B, Cohen MS, Macairan ML, Vidal J. Use of a shape-memory alloy (nitinol) in a removable prostatic stent. Tech Urol 1999;5:226–230.

27. Djavan B, Fakhari M, Shariat S, Ghawidel K, Marberger M. A novel intraurethral prostatic bridge catheter for prevention of temporary prostatic obstruction following high energy transurethral microwave thermotherapy in patients with benign prostatic hyperplasia. J Urol 1999;161:144–151.

28. Devonec M, Dahlstrand C. Temporary urethral stenting after high energy transurethral microwave thermotherapy of the prostate. World J Urol 1998;16:120–123.

29. Traxer O, Anidjar M, Gaudez F, et al. A new prostatic stent for the treatment of benign prostatic hyperplasia in high risk patients. Eur Urol 2000;38:272–280.

30. Isotalo T, Talja M, Hellstrom P, et al. A double-blind, randomized, placebo-controlled pilot study to investigate the effects of finasteride combined with a biodegradable self-reinforced poly L-lactic acid spiral stent in patients with urinary retention caused by bladder outlet obstruction from benign prostatic hyperplasia. BJU Int 2001;88:30–34.

31. Laaksovirta S, Talja M, Valimaa T, et al. Expansion and bioabsorption of the self-reinforced lactic and glycolic acid copolymer prostatic spiral stent. J Urol 2001;166:919–922.

32. Anjum MI, Chari R, Shetty A, Keen M, Palmer JH. Long-term clinical results and quality of life after insertion of a self-expanding flexible endourethral prosthesis. Br J Urol 1997;80:885–888.

14 Suprapubic Transvesical Prostatectomy and Simple Perineal Prostatectomy for the Treatment of Benign Prostatic Hyperplasia

James M. Kozlowski, MD, FACS,
Norm D. Smith, MD,
and John T. Grayhack, MD

Contents

Introduction
Indications for Open Prostatectomy
Preoperative Considerations
Anesthetic Considerations
Surgical Technique
Complications of Open Prostatectomy
Operative Results and Retreatment Rates
Conclusions
References

INTRODUCTION

There are a variety of well-defined goals associated with the surgical management of benign prostatic hyperplasia (BPH) voiding dysfunction. It is imperative that the operative approach selected adequately correct all of the significant pathophysiologic effects of bladder neck obstruction, including the following: (1) recurrent urinary tract infections; (2) the development of bladder stones; (3) episodes of gross hematuria unresponsive to finasteride; (4) urinary retention unresponsive to α-blocker therapy; (5) the development of large bladder diverticula with narrow necks and associated urinary stasis; (6) postrenal

From: *Management of Benign Prostatic Hypertrophy*
Edited by: K. T. McVary © Humana Press Inc., Totowa, NJ

azotemia; and (7) chronically elevated postvoid residual levels (PVR) with or without overflow incontinence *(1)*.

Ideally, surgical treatment should also improve the quality of the patient's life by allowing him to void to near completion at normal intervals with an adequate urinary stream and maintain good urinary control and unaltered sexual function. The therapeutic approach that best accomplishes these goals with the least morbidity and disability should be selected. Logical issues that impact decision-making include the patient's general medical status, the size and configuration of the obstructing prostatic tissue, the functional status of the bladder, the surgeon's skill, and realistic patient preferences.

Open prostatectomy (suprapubic, retropubic, perineal) has become an infrequently performed procedure and currently comprises about 5% of all surgical prostatectomies *(2)*. Undoubtedly, this infrequency reflects the favorable impact of medical management strategies, the availability of minimally invasive approaches, and continuing refinements of transurethral resection of the prostate (TURP).

This chapter will address the techniques of transvesical and perineal prostatectomy. For obvious reasons, the suprapubic approach will be emphasized. Retropubic prostatectomy for the management of BPH is addressed elsewhere in the text.

INDICATIONS FOR OPEN PROSTATECTOMY

There are a number of factors that should prompt the serious consideration of suprapubic transvesical prostatectomy. These include the following: (1) adenomas > 75 g; (2) transition zone hyperplasia associated with a large, prominent subtrigonal component; (3) presence of a physiologically relevant diverticulum; (4) multiple large bladder calculi; (5) confounding orthopedic problems such as severe spinal stenosis and fusion/ankylosis of the hip joints; (6) large scrotal hernia or massive hydrocele; (7) rigid or semirigid penile prosthesis; (8) multiple urethral strictures; (9) trigonal distortion resulting from trauma or previous surgery that places the ureteral orifices in close proximity to the bladder neck; (10) expectations/prejudices of the patient; and (11) skill/experience of the surgeon *(1)*.

Ideally, simple perineal prostatectomy warrants consideration in those patients with large, low-lying prostates who are capable of withstanding prolonged exaggerated lithotomy. Preferably, patients selected for posterior capsulotomy by means of perineal exposure should be free of significant perineal or anorectal disease and never have had surgery in that area. Achieving perineal access is also attractive in those patients with large glands who have undergone previous pelvic surgery. This approach is also attractive because it allows exposure of the prostate at its most superficial location, allows exposure of the prostate beneath the pelvic venous plexus and peritoneal reflection, minimizes the risk of bleeding from periprostatic veins and significant ileus, provides the most direct and dependent route for drainage of extravasated urine and blood, and allows a postoperative course associated with minimal pain and reduced analgesic requirements (3).

There are two major reasons for the infrequent use of simple perineal prostatectomy for the management of BPH. First, there is a general attrition of perineal surgical skills. Second, this approach has been historically associated with a 15% risk of impotence and is therefore unattractive to potent patients. The well-appreciated anatomy of the cavernous nerves and their relationship to the dorsolateral prostatic capsule permits the successful preservation of these neurovascular bundles in skilled hands (3).

PREOPERATIVE CONSIDERATIONS

It is important to emphasize that prostatectomy represents an elective procedure. For that reason, it is imperative to optimize the patient's condition before surgery. Even in those individuals with the most severe degree of bladder neck obstruction and its adverse sequelae, the obstruction can be relieved and the associated problems reversed or optimized by catheter drainage. Improving the patient's condition before surgery helps to achieve a good outcome by optimizing renal function in patients with postrenal azotemia; normalizing platelet function, which can be adversely affected in patients with renal failure; resolving any attendant postobstructive diuresis; correcting any concomitant fluid, electrolyte, and acid-base abnormalities; and eradicating superimposed bacterial infection (1).

General Assessment of Comorbid Status

The elderly patient with BPH requiring open surgery often has associated cardiovascular, pulmonary, neurologic, or other significant medical comorbidities that may impact on the preoperative surgical evaluation and on the choice of anesthetic management. It is important that the urologic surgeon personally perform a thorough physical examination and get a complete medical history. In addition, a standard preoperative database must be accumulated. The input of the primary care physician and other relevant medical specialists is essential to optimize the patient's medical status.

For example, patients with underlying chronic obstructive pulmonary disease may benefit from pulmonary function testing and arterial blood gas sampling to determine whether they require the initiation or modification of bronchodilator therapy. Similarly, evaluation of cardiac risk using exercise-based (i.e., stress echocardiogram) or pharmacologic (dobutamine echocardiography) stress testing may provide strategically important preoperative insight.

Hematologic Issues

Clotting abnormalities are best identified by questioning the patient about familial or personal episodes of unusual bleeding. Indeed, recognized risk factors in clinical screening include bleeding or clotting problems during previous surgery, a family history of bleeding, and the use of medications that interfere with clotting (anticoagulants, nonsteroidal anti-inflammatory drugs, and herbal preparations containing gingko biloba). Supportive findings on physical examination might include petechiae, purpura, or splenomegaly. Studies have suggested that even if there is no clinical evidence of a bleeding tendency, there is still an 0.008% probability that a clotting disorder will be present during surgery [4]. Therefore, the use of routine clotting profile studies (prothrombin time, partial thromboplastin time, platelet, and platelet function testing) is probably limited. However, these tests should be done for any patient with possible hematologic concerns. In addition, significant persistent azotemia predisposes to platelet dysfunction and bleeding that is often at least partially reversible by presurgical dialysis and the administration of the antidiuretic hormone analog L-desamino-8-D-arginine vasopressin [1].

The incidence of significant bleeding that requires transfusion after open prostatectomy has been reported to range from 1.7 to 35.5% [2]. Indeed, the lowest rates, 0.8 and 1.7%, respectively, were reported by Meier and associates in 1995 [5]. The latter rate represents one of the more recent reviews of open prostatectomy and probably reflects currently anticipated outcomes. Obviously, the anticipated blood loss after simple perineal prostatectomy should fall in the low end of this range. We always submit blood for typing and screening. We do not, as a matter of routine, submit blood for typing and cross-matching, nor do we routinely encourage the donation of autologous units. However, patients with hemoglobin levels less than 13 g/dL who are scheduled to undergo prostatectomy and who are anxious or who are religiously opposed to allogeneic blood use may benefit from the preoperative administration of epoetin-alfa (recombinant human erythropoietin). The rational for its administration is to increase the rate of red blood cell production in the bone marrow with the resultant increase in red cell volume. Two doses of 600 IU/kg epoetin-alfa administered 14 and 7 d before surgery significantly increases red blood cell mass and decreases the need for allogeneic blood transfusion *(6)*. When used in this manner, erythropoietin-induced complications (hypertension, cerebrovascular accident, influenza-like symptoms, and an increase in thromboembolic events) are infrequently encountered.

Finasteride (Proscar) used preoperatively has further reduced the need for transfusion in patients undergoing surgery for BPH. Current evidence suggests that gross hematuria in patients with BPH is associated with increased microvessel density in the suburethral portion of the prostate *(7)*. Hoschberg et al. demonstrated that finasteride significantly decreased suburethral prostatic microvessel density in patients with BPH *(8)*. This finding may explain the why 5α-reductase inhibitor is useful to limit bleeding related to BPH and BPH surgery. Therefore, patients not already taking finasteride as a component of long-term drug therapy should be given the drug (5 mg every day) 2–4 wk before anticipated surgery.

Infection Risk and Preoperative Antimicrobial Therapy

As stated previously, documented preoperative urinary tract infection must be eradicated with appropriate antimicrobial therapy. This is very important given the observation that bacteremia occurs postoperatively in 10–32% of patients without recognized preoperative bacteriuria and occurs much more frequently in patients with infected urine *(9,10)*. Prophylactic antibiotic administration to reduce immediate and long-term infection-related risks in patients without preoperatively documented infection has a limited effect on perioperative infections or fever, although a reduced incidence of postoperative bacteremia has been noted *(9)*. Gorelick and associates documented demonstrable bacteria in as many as 20% of prostatectomy tissue specimens *(11)*. As a result, antibiotics used for prophylaxis should eradicate bactericidal tissue as well as reduce levels in urine. In low-risk patients with negative preoperative urine cultures, we commonly initiate coverage about 1 h before surgery using intravenous levofloxacin or cefazolin. Patients with increased risk factors for infection such as azotemia, upper tract calculi, a history of an elevated PVR, debility, diabetes mellitus, and those who are immunocompromised are given a longer course of preoperative oral antimicrobial prophylaxis. All patients currently receive empiric intravenous antimicrobial therapy for 24–48 h after surgery. Before catheter removal, urine is again submitted for culture and sensitivity testing. If infection is documented, appropriate targeted antimicrobial therapy is provided. If the cultures are negative, patients are given a 3-d course of nitrofurantin or a fluoroquinolone to begin on the day of catheter removal.

The American Heart Association recommends endocarditis prophylaxis at the time of prostatic surgery for those with the following conditions: (1) a prosthetic cardiac valve; (2) congenital cardiac malformation; (3) surgically constructed systemic-pulmonary shunts; (4) rheumatic and other acquired valvular dysfunction; (5) idiopathic hypertrophic cardiomyopathy; (6) history of baterial endorcarditis; (7) mitral valve prolapse with regurgitation or thickened leaflets; or (8) cardiac surgery within the preceding 6 mo. Enterococci bacteria are the most common cause of endocarditis after gastrointestinal and genitourinary procedures. For genitourinary surgery and instrumentation, a standard parenteral antibiotic regimen would include 2.0 g ampicillin (50 mg/kg) intramuscularly or intravenously plus 1.5 mg/kg gentamicin (maximum 120 mg) administered within 30 min of beginning surgery. Oral ampicillin (1 g intramuscularly or intravenously) or 1 g of oral amoxicillin should be administered 6 hr later for high-risk patients. Moderate-risk patients can be treated with 2 g of amoxicillin orally 1 hr before or 2 g of ampicillin intramuscularly or intravenously within 30 min of the planned procedure. Vancomycin (1 g intravenously infused slowly over 1 h, beginning 1 h before surgery) is used in penicillin-allergic patients. High-risk patients include those individuals with prosthetic heart valves, a history of endocarditis, and those patients taking continuous oral penicillin for rheumatic fever prophylaxis (1).

Prevention of Venous Thromboembolism

Urologic patients are at increased risk for the development of postoperative deep vein thrombosis (DVT) and pulmonary emboli. Benizri et al. found that 10% of patients not given prophylactic medication had DVT after TURP (12). Generic risk factors for postoperative phlebothrombosis and pulmonary embolism include hypercoagulability (antithrombin III deficiency, circulating lupus anticoagulant estrogen use, malignancy); stasis cause by obstructed venous outflow, congestive heart failure, or immobility; and vascular endothelial injury as a result of previous surgery or trauma. A particularly high-risk group includes those patients with a history of previous thromboembolism resulting from atrial fibrillation. In those patients with standard risk factors, we prefer conservative measures such as the use of anti-embolic stockings, pneumatic sequential compression boots, adequate hydration, and early ambulation. Consultation should be obtained for patients perceived to be at intermediate or high hematologic risk because those patients will probably require pharmacologic management with a low-molecular-weight heparin preparation or may even require formal anticoagulation. The risk of fatal pulmonary embolism or stroke must be balanced in these patients with the markedly increased risk of postoperative bleeding that could result in clot retention, wound hematomas, or hemodynamically significant pelvic or retroperitoneal bleeding (1).

Preoperative Genitourinary Evaluation

Before surgery, it is our practice to obtain an updated American Urological Association symptom score, assess PVR (if feasible), and perform pressure/flow urodynamic tests (if not already done), cystoscopy, and imaging studies. The availability of this data preoperatively permits a more objective assessment of treatment efficacy after surgery and adequate postoperative recovery.

Bowel Preparation

Finally, before transvesical prostatectomy or a perineal prostatectomy, patients are placed on a liquid diet 24 h before surgery. A gentle mechanical bowel preparation consisting of either oral Fleets phosphosoda or enemas is also used. For patients destined to undergo perineal surgery, a neomycin enema on the morning of surgery is used as an adjunct.

ANESTHETIC CONSIDERATIONS

Suprapubic prostatectomy can be comfortably performed with the patient under a general or regional anesthetic. With respect to the latter, options include a continuous spinal or epidural anesthetic. Regional anesthesia is advantageous because it is an excellent skeletal and smooth muscle relaxation, airway-related complications (unexpected coughing, gagging, or bucking) can be mostly avoided, and postoperative hemostasis is enhanced in because the patient is more comfortable and tranquil patient (1). Potential disadvantages include a history of documented central or peripheral neurologic deficits after the use of regional anesthetic, potential bleeding tendencies associated with this method, documented chronic low back pain after receiving regional anesthetic, spinal stenosis and/or severe degenerative disk disease after regional anesthetic, and associated osseous metastasis (6). In addition, patient acceptance is low. Given the need for prolonged exaggerated lithotomy necessary to conduct simple perineal prostatectomy, most patients are best served by general endotracheal anesthesia with full muscle relaxation.

SURGICAL TECHNIQUE

Suprapubic Transvesical Prostatectomy

Following the induction of satisfactory general or regional anesthesia, the operating table should be gently flexed in the modified Trendelenburg position. Care must be taken to avoid injudicious flexion that might induce a sacral stretch injury. When properly performed, this simple position change facilitates exposure within the narrow male pelvis and permits more facile mobilization of the peritoneal reflection. At this point, thigh-high anti-embolism stockings should be placed along with pneumatic sequential compression boots and heel protectors. The patient is comfortably secured to the table once these preliminary steps have been completed. The abdomen and genitalia are shaved and then prepped and draped in sterile standard fashion. It is our preference to prepare the penis and genitalia into the sterile operative field. Once this has been established, a 22-Fr Foley catheter is inserted and the balloon is inflated to 30 mL. Using a piston-tipped syringe, the bladder is then filled to approx 200 to 300 mL. The catheter is then clamped to maintain bladder distension. It is useful for the operating surgeon and/or the assistant to wear a fiberoptic headlight, which facilitates visualization of the prostatic fossa after enucleation.

A sterile marking pen is then used to delineate the line of intended incision. With respect to the latter, a transverse (Pfannenstiel) or lower midline incision may be used depending on the need for adjunctive procedures (i.e., diverticulectomy, concomitant inguinal hernia repair), the patient's body habitus, and the presence of previous surgical scars. If a transverse approach is chosen, the incision should be placed approximately two finger-breadths above the pubic symphysis in a suitable skin crease. Care must be taken to avoid extending the transverse incision too far laterally to decrease the risk of postoperative hernia. Awareness of potential injury to the underlying inferior epigastric vessels is important. We prefer the transverse approach whenever feasible given the superior cosmetic quality of the healed incision. The remainder of this discourse will be predicated on that operative approach.

After creation of the skin incision, the subcutaneous tissues are incised with electrocautery. Larger bleeding vessels that may be encountered with the transverse approach are delineated with blunt dissection, clamped, severed, and tied with 3-O or 4-O Vicryl sutures. The anterior fascia is then further delineated with sharp and blunt dissection. At this point the surgeon has the option of securing wound towels to the subcutaneous tissues using 3-O silk sutures. The approach to the fascia can be facilitated using small self-retaining retractors. A fresh scalpel is used to score the fascia in the midline aspect of the established wound. The fascial incisions are generally extended to the lateral border of each rectus abdominis muscle. At this point, it is necessary to raise the superior and inferior fascial flaps. This is done easily using three Kocher clamps applied equidistantly at each edge. The assistant provides gentle uplift, and the surgeon provides counter traction on the underlying rectus muscles. Using the Bovie, the superior flap is raised to a point halfway to the umbilicus. The inferior flap is raised to the pubic symphysis. The exposed rectus abdominis muscles are then separated one from the other in the midline aspect. Careful sharp and blunt dissection permits mobilization of the rectus muscle bellies and good exposure to the underlying umbilicoprevesical fascia. The latter is gently uplifted and incised. At this point, the peritoneal reflection is identified and gently reflected from the dome of the nicely distended bladder. Obtaining good exposure of the bladder in the space of Retzius is important, along with optimal identification of the bladder neck and prostate. However, injudicious dissection over the vesicle neck is unnecessary. Further exposure is provided by the use of a Balfour retractor. The padded blades are placed gently alongside and under each rectus muscle belly. Additional exposure of the bladder, bladder neck, and anterior prostatic surface can be facilitated by the careful placement of small-medium malleable retractors.

In general, it is our preference to establish a transverse incision approx 2 to 3 cm above the bladder neck. The placement of stay sutures of 2-O chromic catgut above and below the line of intended incision is helpful. This approach to the bladder is quite useful in that it optimizes exposure of the prostatic fossa and causes minimum disruption of the bladder neck and prostatic capsule. In theory, the latter developments are somewhat more likely if a vertical incision is chosen. The initial stay sutures are uplifted, and the bladder muscle is incised using electrocautery. The underlying mucosa is then easily identified and entered. The instilled fluid is then evacuated. The transverse incision can be extended with a careful spreading maneuver or with electrocautery. In any event, appropriately spaced 2-O chromic catgut sutures are placed in equidistant fashion along the superior and inferior bladder flaps. We tag the true midline sutures and the lateral sutures with straight clamps for identification purposes. If necessary, these sutures can be placed in figure-eight fashion and tied for additional hemostasis. A padded malleable or Deaver retractor is then placed in the bladder dome to optimize exposure. Indigo carmine is administered intravenously to facilitate exposure of the ureteral orifices. Baby malleable retractors can be used to optimize exposure within the bladder. At this point, it should be emphasized that

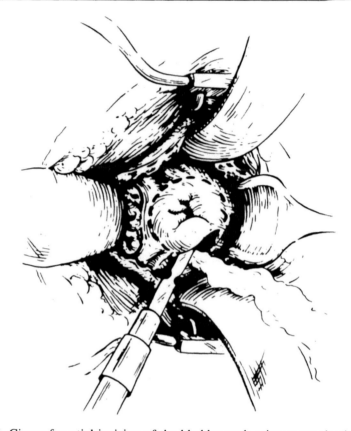

Fig. 1. Circumferential incision of the bladder neck prior to enucleation of prostatic adenoma. Exposure is facilitated by placement of a medium malleable or Deaver retractor in the superior aspect of the bladder. Additionally, the use of small malleable or Deaver retractors adjacent to the bladder neck greatly enhances visualization. Electrocautery is used to initiate the incision through the mucosa overlying the intruding adenoma at the level of the bladder neck. Sharp dissection can be used subsequently to further free the adenoma from the surrounding tissue. Care must be taken to avoid injury to the bladder neck and trigone. (Reprinted with permission from ref. *13.*)

procedures to be done in conjunction with the prostatectomy (removal of bladder stones, diverticulectomy, preperitoneal repair of an inguinal hernia) should be performed before enucleation of the adenoma.

Careful inspection of the bladder, especially with respect to the location of the trigonal complexes and identification of associated bladder disease, is important before initiating enucleation of the obstructing adenoma. Scoring the mucosa circumferentially around the protruding adenoma with electrocautery prevents excessive tearing during enucleation

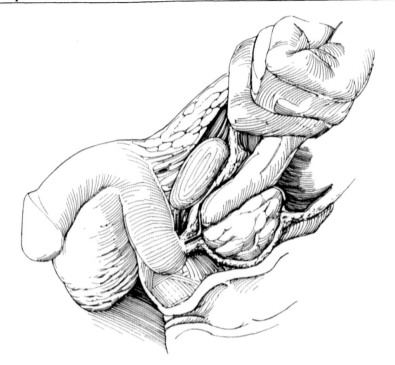

Fig. 2. Finger enucleation of the prostatic adenoma. This maneuver is accomplished by using the index finger inserted into the prostatic urethra. The anterior commissural tissue is then cracked by gentle manipulation using the ip of the index finger. The proper plane is then established between each component of the adenoma and the surgical capsule on the lateral aspects, respectively (Reprinted with permission from ref. *13.*)

of the prostate. The instrument can be used on the fulguration mode and applied repetitively for deeper penetration. At this point, fine scissors can be used to separate the mucosa from the underlying adenoma. Alternatively, careful use of the cutting current can accomplish this goal as well (Fig. 1) *(13)*.

The enucleation should be initiated by inserting the index finger into the prostatic fossa and cracking the anterior commissure using anterolateral pressure against the larger adenoma. Using the fingernail as a wedge is helpful (Figs. 2, 3) *(13,14)*. A sweep and roll maneuver should be used, with the tip of the index finger within the cleavage plane between the surgical capsule and the adenoma. The lateral sweeping maneuvers should be alternated and pressure should be exerted primarily against the adenoma. It is preferable to initiate the enucleation of each lobe before proceeding to definitive detachment of either lobe. Each lobe

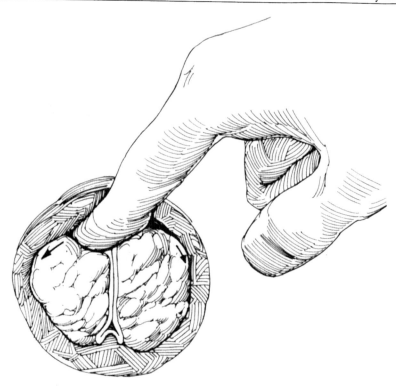

Fig. 3. Depiction of the lateral plane of cleavage the adenoma and surgical capsule. This plane is best developed by using the tip of the index finger to initiate a sweep and roll maneuver. This should be done sequentially on one side and then the on other to establish the optimal plane of cleavage for each component of the adenoma. This should be done thoroughly before any attempt is made to sever the urethra and evacuate the adenoma. (Reprinted with permission from ref. *14*.)

should be freed laterally, then posteriorly across the midline and behind the middle lobe (if present). The mucosa should be pushed distally with the fingernail at the apex and either pinched off between the thumbnail and finger or occasionally divided sharply with scissors hugging the adenoma (Fig. 4) *(14)*. In any event, the apex of the adenoma should be separated from the area adjacent to the external sphincter bilaterally, and both lateral lobes should be free before completing the enucleation. Traction on the distal urethra should be avoided while the capsule is being teased from the apex of the adenoma to avoid sphincter injury. In obese patients, enucleation may be facilitated by placing the fingers of the free hand or an assistant's hand in the rectum to push the prostate

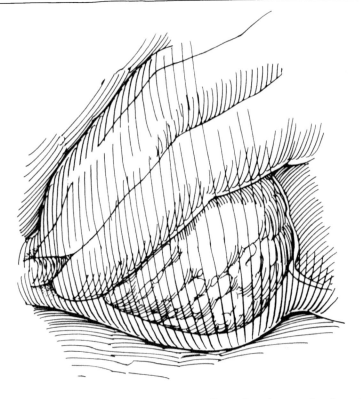

Fig. 4. Transection of the prostatic urethra. Once the adenoma has been thoroughly mobilized, the tether point represents the prostatic urethra. Pinching it off between the thumbnail and index finger is a useful maneuver. If adhesions are encountered and easy transection is not forthcoming, the surgeon can angulate the elbow or try standing with his or her back to the table. (Reprinted with permission from ref. *14*.)

ventrally in a cephalad direction. The potential need for this maneuver should be anticipated preoperatively to permit adequate patient positioning. The adenoma should be separated with care from the bladder neck, especially posteriorly in the area of the ureteral orifices. A thyroid clamp is occasionally useful to grasp the adenoma and facilitate extraction (Fig. 5) *(14)*. The sequence of the enucleation must be varied depending on the configuration of the adenoma and the ease of enucleation. At times, the median or subtrigonal lobe should be worked on first. In a large gland with multiple adenomas, sequential removal is preferable to the traumatic intact removal of the adenomatous growth. Obviously, unusual adherence of the adenoma to the capsule should increase suspicion of carcinoma.

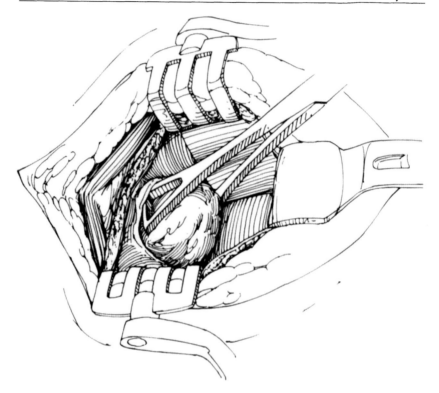

Fig. 5. Use of sponge or lobe forceps to grasp a large adenoma. Once the adenoma has been mobilized to near completion, grasping it with suitable forceps can facilitate extraction. During this process, any adherent mucosa should be trimmed with scissors. Following removal of the adenoma, the prostatic fossa should be inspected and palpated for residual tissue. The latter should be removed with additional blunt and sharp dissection. (Reprinted with permission from ref. *14.*)

Once the adenoma has been enucleated, rapid control of bleeding is a paramount concern. Figure 6 shows the primary and secondary arterial supply to the prostate *(15).* The first and probably most strategic hemostatic maneuver at this point is to tightly pack the evacuated prostate fossa using a vaginal gauze roll or a Kerlex roll. Baby malleable retractors and an empty ring forceps can be used to facilitate this packing maneuver. Once established, compression should be left in place for approx 5 min. The pack can then be removed and, using optimal lighting, the prostatic fossa can be inspected. It may be possible at this point to spot fulgurate discrete bleeding vessels within the fossa. It is our preference to repetitively pack the fossa for 5-min intervals until hemostasis has been optimized and discrete bleeding areas better defined.

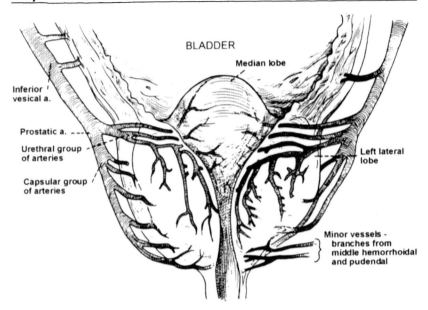

Fig. 6. Primary and secondary arterial supply to the prostate gland. The primary (inferior vesical) and secondary (middle rectal and pudendal) arteries are derived from the anterior division of the hypogastric artery. As depicted here, the urethral branches generally enter the bladder neck at the 5 and 7 o'clock positions, but this relationship is inconstant and variable. (Reprinted with permission from ref. *15*.)

Patience with this particular phase of the procedure can greatly enhance a successful outcome.

Because the primary arterial supply enters at the 5 o'clock and 7 o'clock positions of the bladder neck, purposeful or anticipatory figure-eight 2-O chromic catgut sutures are placed in these positions (Fig. 7) *(13)*. These sutures can also be used to anchor the bladder neck to the surgical capsule posteriorly. Persistent discreet bleeding can be fulgurated or controlled with interrupted figure-eight suture ligatures of 2-O chromic catgut. More diffuse but accessible oozing within the prostatic fossa can be treated with the careful application of the Argon beam photocoagulator. When using this approach, care must be taken to avoid contact with the bladder neck to prevent postoperative contracture. Plication of the capsule (Fig. 8) is a very simple and useful maneuver when bleeding persists even though no artery is obviously exposed *(16)*. Two sutures of 0 chromic catgut on 5/8 curved needles are placed in the prostatic capsule, running from one side of the fossa to the other, to plicate these tissues. This simple approach induces immediate mechani-

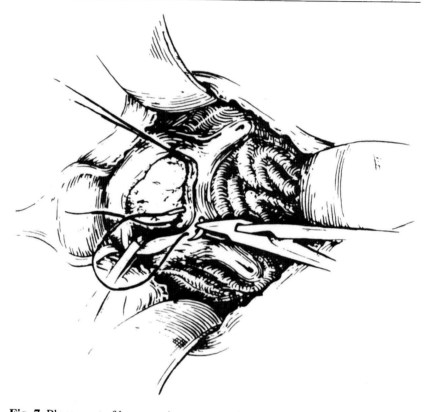

Fig. 7. Placement of hemostatic sutures at the 5 and 7 o'clock positions of the bladder neck. 2-O chromic catgut sutures placed in figure-eight fashion generally control the urethral branches of the prostatovesicular artery, which enters in these locations. This maneuver is facilitated by the use of 5/8 curved genitourinary needles and optimal exposure. Care must be taken to avoid injury to the trigonal complex at this time. (Reprinted with permission from ref. *13*.)

cal contraction of these tissues, which facilitates hemostasis. In most instances, the use of hemostatic agents (oxidized cellulose, thrombin-soaked Gelfoam, fibrin glue) is unnecessary, but their use should be considered (along with prolonged packing) in extraordinary circumstances.

In the very unlikely event of severe persistent bleeding, consideration can be given to the insertion of a resectoscope and directed fulguration of bleeding vessels within the prostatic fossa using a rollerball electrode. Another infrequently needed adjunct is the placement of a Malament purse-string suture. This consists of a double-armed suture of 1-O or 2-O nylon placed through the mucosa and into the muscle and then carried around in both directions to cross in the midline and exit the entire bladder wall (Fig. 9; *14*). Before the purse string is tied, a 24- or

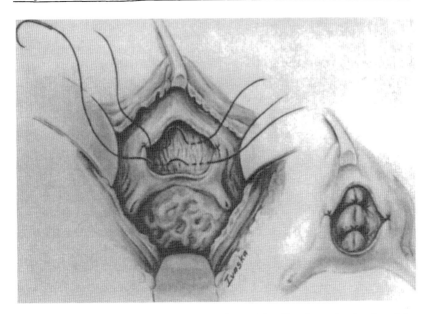

Fig. 8. Hemostatic plication sutures. Persistent bleeding from the depths of the posterior prostatic fossa can be controlled by placing three transverse plication sutures of 0 chromic catgut. The sutures should engage the opposing lateral aspects of the fossa as well as the midzone component. Once tied, they induce an accordion-like affect, which facilitates hemostasis. (Reprinted with permission from ref. *16*.)

26-Fr 30-mL catheter is inserted into the bladder and its balloon inflated. The purse-string sutures are then drawn up close to the neck of the bladder around the catheter (Fig. 10; *14*). Following bladder closure, the needles are cut off at each end of the nylon sutures, which are then threaded on large straight cutting needles, passed out above the symphysis, and tied over a button (or some other anchor) under slight tension. Under ideal circumstances, the Foley catheter would be removed on the second or third postoperative day, and the suprapubic catheter would be removed on the sixth or seventh postoperative day. The nylon purse string would then be removed to complete the process. In general, hemostasis is easy to achieve after simpler surgeries, and this particular maneuver should be required in only the most extreme circumstances.

Anchoring the bladder neck to the posterior aspect of the prostatic fossa facilitates hemostatis and helps prevent the formation of an obstructing membrane. This process of trigonalization of the prostatic fossa is illustrated in Figure 11. This maneuver also facilitates any sub-

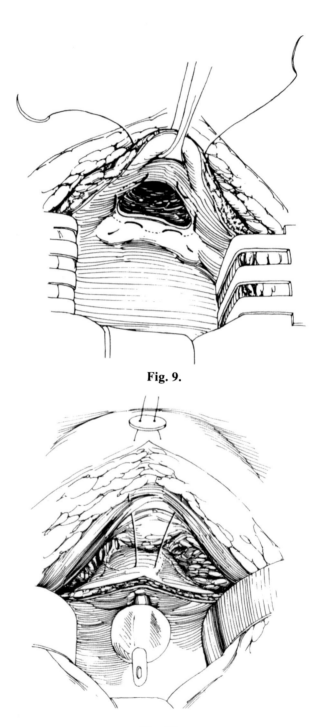

Fig. 9.

Fig. 10.

238

sequent catheter placement. Obviously, before completing this step, it should be determined whether the bladder neck is inordinately tight. If so, a V-shaped wedge can be removed from the 6-o'clock position (Fig. 12) *(1)*. Once completed, the surgeon should proceed with the trigonalization step. Before bladder closure, a 24-Fr catheter is inserted in each urethra. The balloon is inflated to approx 60 to 70 mL, placed on general traction, and temporarily clamped. A separate opening is made in the dome of the bladder for the placement of a 28-Fr Malecot suprapubic catheter. Ultimately, that catheter will traverse the abdominal wall through another opening made in the superior fascial flap. It is helpful to gently anchor the Malecot catheter to the bladder wall using one or two 3-O or 4-O chromic catgut sutures. A two-layer bladder closure is initiated with interrupted figure-eight 2-O chromic catgut sutures, taking care to avoid injury to the hyperinflated Foley balloon (Fig. 13) *(17)*. Once the bladder is closed, the catheter is unclamped and through and through irrigation is initiated to validate catheter patency and adequacy of hemostasis. In addition, it helps to determine the watertight integrity of the closure. Additional interrupted sutures can be placed if necessary. Bladder closure is facilitated by pairing the previously placed suture tags.

Before embarking on closure of the abdominal wall, drains should be placed. Some surgeons favor small-to-medium Penrose drains for this purpose. Others, including our group, prefer the use of closed suction sump drains. Generally, a single 7- or 10-mm flat-type sump drain is adequate for this purpose. We generally place it through an inferior opening. It should be positioned well away from the bladder suture line. It has been reported that inaccurate placement of sump drains may result in a risk for persistent urinary leakage, but this has not been our general experience *(2)*.

Fig. 9. *(previous page)* Placement of the Malament purse-string suture. In rare instances, severe persistent bleeding may prompt additional hemostatic procedure. Depicted here is placement of a purse-string suture around the bladder neck using a doubly armed suture of 1-O or 2-O nylon. The sutures are placed through the mucosa and into muscle and carried around the bladder neck in both directions exiting in the 12 o'clock orient position. (Reprinted with permission from ref. *14*.)

Fig. 10. *(previous page)* Completion of the Malament circumferential purse-string suture. In this figure, a 24- or 26-Fr Foley catheter is inserted into the bladder. Its balloon is hyperinflated (60–70 mL). At that point, the respective ends of the purse-string are delivered through the anterior abdominal wall at the level of the symphysis. The sutures are then snugly tied over a bolster or button. (Reprinted with permission from ref. *14*.)

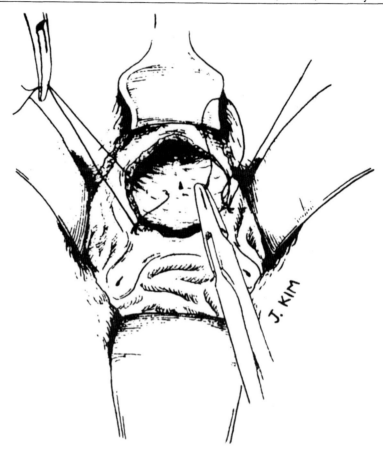

Fig. 11. Trigonalization of the prostatic fossa. This can be accomplished using previously placed hemostatic sutures that are located at the 5 and 7 o'clock positions at the bladder neck. Alternatively, separate suture placement can be used for this maneuver. This simple approach aids in achieving hemostasis, facilitates appropriate healing, and prevents the development of a lip or ridge, which can be an obstructing element, particularly for catheter passage. (Reprinted with permission from ref. *8*.)

The rectus diastasis can be obliterated with loosely tied interrupted figure-eight 2-O or 3-O monofilament absorbable suture. The fascia is reapproximated with 1-O or 2-O monofilament absorbable suture placed in interrupted figure-eight fashion. The subcutaneous tissues are irrigated with an antimicrobial solution and closed with running 3-O monofilament absorbable suture. The skin is generally closed with a running subcuticular suture of 4-0 Maxon. The suprapubic tube should be secured to the skin level with several 2-O silk sutures.

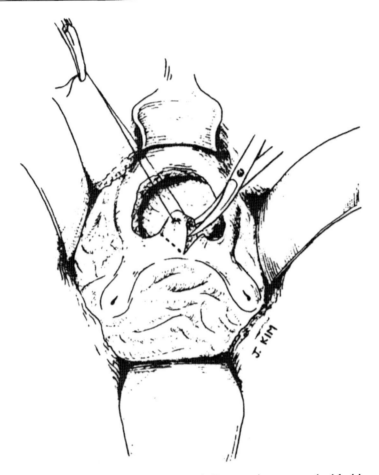

Fig. 12. Wedge resection of bladder neck. In some instances, the bladder neck will appear unduly snug following enucleation of the adenoma. In those cases, a ventrally directed wedge resection can be performed. When necessary, the wedge resection should precede retrigonalizing the posterior aspect of the prostatic fossa. (Reprinted with permission from ref. *1*.)

During the process of abdominal wall closure, periodic reassessment of catheter patency and hemostasis should be done. When the operation is completed, it is our preference to place the Foley catheter on a gentle traction and initiate a rather brisk, continuous irrigation with flow directed through the Foley catheter and out the suprapubic tube. The rate of infusion should be titrated to achieve a color that approaches crystal clear to light pink. In general, the irrigation is stopped on the first post-operative day. The Foley catheter is removed on the second or third

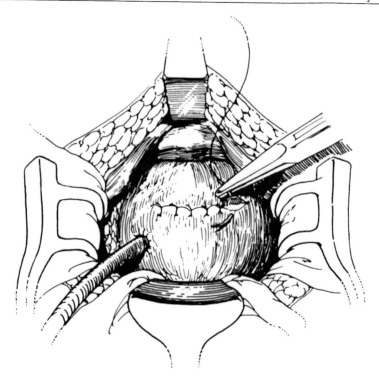

Fig. 13. Bladder closure. Before closing the transverse bladder incision in two layers with interrupted figure-eight sutures of 2-O chromic catgut, two catheters should be placed into the bladder proper. The first is a 24-Fr Foley catheter. Its balloon should be hyperinflated to about 70 mL and initially placed on gentle traction. The second catheter is a 28-Fr Malecot suprapubic tube. It should exit the superior aspect of the bladder. Following bladder closure, through and through irrigation is initiated to validate catheter patency and to assess the degree of hemostasis. That maneuver is performed periodically during the remainder of the closure. (Reprinted with permission from ref. *17.*)

postoperative day. Barring complications, the suprapubic catheter is left indwelling for 7–10 d. In most instances, a cystogram is not required before its removal but should be considered in situations where bladder closure was tenuous. The drain maybe removed when clinically apparent drainage ceases or after removal of the suprapubic catheter. Of note, prolonged suprapubic drainage might be considered prudent in patients whose preoperative pressure-flow studies demonstrated profound detrusor hypocontractility.

If voiding is not resumed and the suprapubic site closed by 48–72 h, re-insertion of a urethral catheter may be necessary. In most instances, short-term catheter drainage will facilitate closure of the suprapubic tract. Persistent suprapubic drainage usually requires endoscopic and, at times, cystographic assessment to evaluate the possible presence of persistent obstructing tissue or foreign body. More remote causes within the context of the rule of fistulas may warrant consideration if suprapubic drainage persists.

It is a good practice to obtain a urine culture one or two days before removing the final catheter. In most instances, the cultures will be negative. When infection is documented, appropriate antimicrobial agents should be provided before catheter removal. Patients with negative cultures are treated with oral antimicrobial therapy (nitrofurantin or fluoroquinolone) on the date of catheter removal and for two additional days.

Simple Perineal Prostatectomy

Currently, adenomectomy for the treatment of BPH is rarely performed by means of the perineal route. Previously, this approach was associated with significantly lower mortality than the abdominal route. However, this latter advantage has disappeared in the modern era as the mortality from all forms of prostatectomy has decreased to exceedingly low levels (18).

Resurgence of interest in the radical perineal prostatectomy has resulted in an increasing number of urologists becoming familiar with the perineal approach. This, in addition to a more precise understanding of anatomic relationships of the prostate (sphincter mechanism, neurovascular bundles), may encourage reevaluation of the perineal approach for the management of BPH in selected cases. In any event, knowledge that a perineal adenomectomy is a feasible procedure that has been performed with satisfactory results is important to maintain (1).

Proper establishment of the exaggerated lithotomy position is critical in establishing optimal perineal exposure and obviating positioning-related morbidity. The desirable flat perineum lying parallel to the floor can be achieved by elevating the buttocks or by marked flexion of the thighs. This requires avoiding pressure on the legs and the shoulders by using proper padding and careful placement of supports. The arms should be kept as close to the body as possible. In many instances, this can be accomplished by simply taping the hands (properly padded) to the knees.

Following the establishment of optimal positioning, the perineum is shaved, prepared, and draped in sterile standard fashion. A curved Lowsley tractor is placed into the bladder and then carefully withdrawn into the prostatic fossa. A semicircular skin incision between the ischial

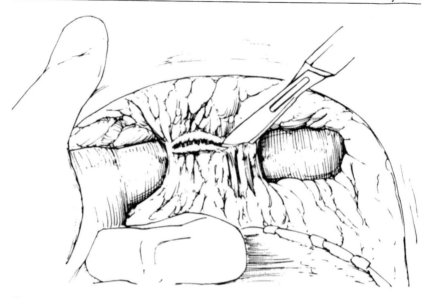

Fig. 14. Transection of the central tendon. Before doing this maneuver, the superficial perineal fascia must be entered and the ischiorectal fossa developed on both sides of the midline. If the central tendon is not easily identified and undermined, the index fingers should be inserted most posteriorly. It is important to stay behind the transverse muscles and the bulbar urethra. (Reprinted with permission from ref. *19*.)

tuberosities is placed just above the mucocutaneous junction. The incised skin and subcutaneous tissues are then anchored with sutures or clips to an inferiorly placed drape or towel. Posteroinferior pressure applied to the Lowsley tractor helps push the prostate toward the perineum. The superficial fascial layers are incised carefully, preserving the central tendon. Each ischiorectal fossa is developed superiorly and posteriorly, with the handle of the knife working on the superior aspect of the inferiorly placed index finger until the posterior aspect of the prostate is felt. The index fingers of each hand should encounter very little resistance as they are then used in a gentle seesaw motion ventral to the rectum and behind the central tendon to isolate this structure. The central tendon is then sharply divided (Fig. 14; *14*).

Following transection of the central tendon, the whitish longitudinal muscle fibers of the rectum should become readily apparent. That structure constitutes an important regional landmark. At this point, it can be helpful to place an extra glove on the nondominant hand. Once done, an index finger can be placed in the rectum to better define that structure. It is also helpful to use a moist 4 × 4 gauze pad under the left thumb to

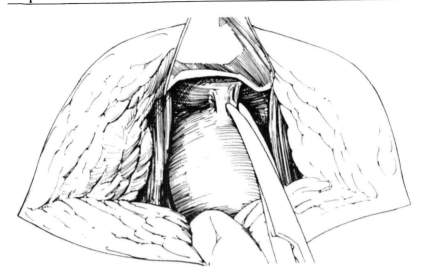

Fig. 15. Incision of the rectourethralis. Once the rectourethralis is identified, gentle but deliberate spreading of the levator ani muscles in this area will often reveal the distinctive white surface covering the prostate on either side near the apex. It is important to recall that the rectum is still tented and can be entered. (Reprinted with permission from ref. *19*.)

draw the rectal wall taut. With the knife handle, the external rectal sphincter can be lifted away from the rectal lamina propria if this approach is desired. At this point it is useful to insert specially designed right-angle (often designated lateral) retractors to help achieve the exposure desired and to use a pediatric or perineal Omni retractor to maintain exposure.

The fibers of the levator ani muscle covering Dnomvilliers' fascia should be readily apparent. These fibers often fuse in the midline, thus constituting the so-called rectourethralis muscle. Once identified, it is helpful to insert a Lowsley or similar tractor into the bladder and open the blades. The assistant can then use the properly positioned tractor to elevate the prostate into the wound for better definition of the prostatic apex. The rectourethralis can then be sharply divided, avoiding the rectal wall (Fig. 15) but keeping in mind the relative safety of a limited misadventure into the surgical capsule of the prostate *(19)*.

The assistant should then raise and tilt the Lowsley tractor to move the prostate into the wound. By doing so, the pubic symphysis acts as a fulcrum. Blunt dissection should now permit definition of the apical portion of the ventral rectal fascia (also referred to as the posterior layer of Dnomvilliers fascia). This is best done with the knife handle.

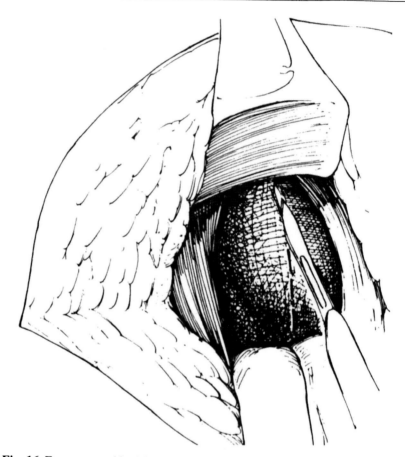

Fig. 16. Exposure and incision into the posterior layer of Denonvilliers fascia. A vertical incision in the posterior lamella protects the cavernous nerves, which are located in a lateral position. This figure also depicts the levator ani muscles standing in relief lateral adjacent to the respective borders of the prostate. (Reprinted with permission from ref. *19*.)

This layer is also designated the pearly white gates of Young. By making a superficial vertical incision in the posterior lamella below the apex, the cavernous nerves (which are located laterally) can be avoided (Fig. 16; *19*). The rectal fascia should then be bluntly dissected laterally over the body of the prostate to preserve the neurovascular bundles (Fig. 17); again, the knife handle is often useful in this maneuver *(19)*.

Following exposure of the prostatic capsule, an inverted U-shaped or V-shaped incision should be made in the surgical capsule of the prostate. The apex of this incision should be slightly proximal to the verumon-

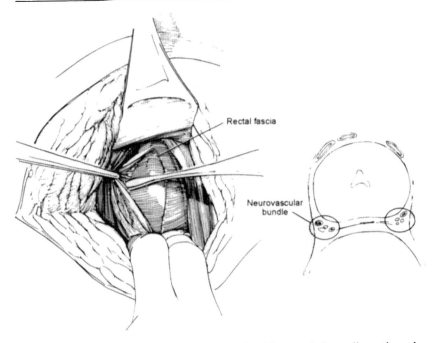

Fig. 17. Dissection of the rectal fascia. Using blunt and sharp dissection, the rectal fascia should be mobilized laterally over the body of the prostate. By doing so, the neurovascular bundles can be preserved. (Reprinted with permission from ref. *19.*)

tanum. The latter is often demonstrable as a soft spot in the capsule. The incision into the surgical capsule should be deep enough to expose the cleavage plain of the adenoma (Fig. 18; *19*). An Allis clamp can be used to grasp the apex of the U-flap and turn it downward (Fig. 19; *19*). Both sharp and blunt dissection should be used to define the lateral border of the adenoma and its interface with the surgical capsule (Fig. 20; *20*). Digital dissection can be used to further mobilize the adenoma in its apical aspect and better outline the urethra. The dorsal wall of the urethra should be divided to free the apical extent of the adenoma. Once accomplished, the remainder of the urethra can be divided at the apex to avoid injudicious tension placed on the sphincters (Fig. 21; *19*). Before completing digital enucleation, it is prudent to remove the long tractor and the lateral and posterior retractors to avoid injury and tearing during the process of enucleation. The digital enucleation should stop when the adenoma has been completely mobilized except for its attachment to the bladder neck. The bladder wall should be grasped with an Allis clamp and the adenomectomy completed with sharp transection of this remain-

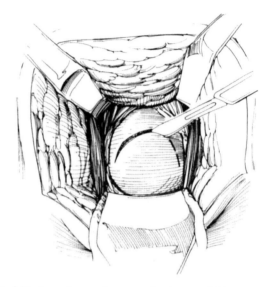

Fig. 18. Inverted U-shaped capsulotomy. An inverted U-shaped or V-shaped incision provides optimal exposure for enucleation of the adenoma. The apex should be slightly proximal to the verumontanum. The incision through the capsule should be deep enough to define the cleavage plain between surgical capsule and adenoma. (Reprinted with permission from ref. *19*.)

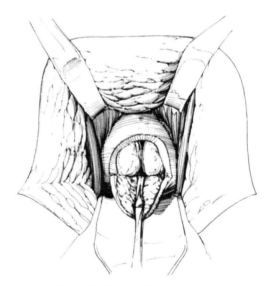

Fig. 19. Development of the U-shaped flap and exposure of the underlying adenoma. This figure depicts optimal retraction of the rectum inferiorly and the levator muscles laterally and superiorly. The U-shaped flap is grasped with an Allis clamp and turned downward. This exposes the underlying adenoma. (Reprinted with permission from ref. *19*.)

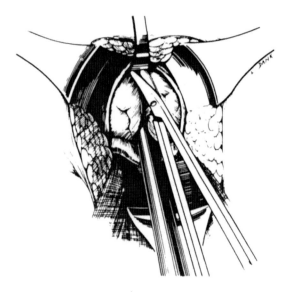

Fig. 20. Separation of the adenoma from the prostatic capsule. In this figure, sharp dissection is used to initiate the plane of cleavage between the adenoma and the surgical capsule. This is facilitated by a Young's tractor that is positioned into the bladder and permits mobilization of the adenoma and ultimately amputation of the urethral apex. (Reprinted with permission from ref. *20*.)

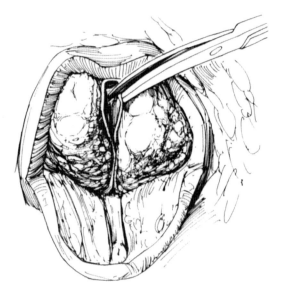

Fig. 21. Division of the prostatic urethra. Before this point, the adenoma has been freed in both lateral aspects. Once transection of the urethral apex occurs, an index finger can be inserted into the cleavage plain and completion of the enucleation can take place. (Reprinted with permission from ref. *19*.)

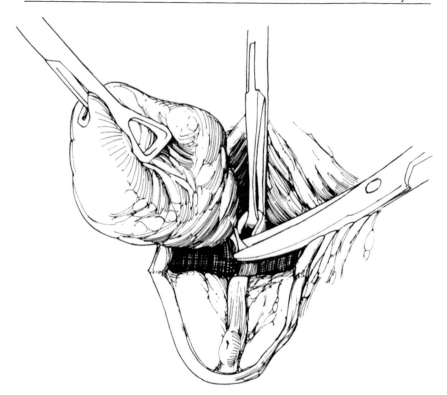

Fig. 22. Detachment of the adenoma. In this figure the adenoma has been grasped with a thyroid clamp. The Allis clamp has engaged the bladder neck. The tether point is being transected to free the adenoma from the bladder neck. (Reprinted with permission from ref. *19*.)

ing tether point (Fig. 22; *19*). As is the case with suprapubic prostatectomy, it is important to remove all significant subtrigonal and subcervical lobes. In the case of a large middle lobe, it may be necessary to dilate the bladder neck digitally and pop this component of the adenoma into the surgical field. Removal of a posteriorly placed V-shaped wedge of tissue will usually allow a fibrotic constricted bladder neck to spring open.

Bleeding can be controlled by spot fulguration or by carefully placed hemostatic mattress sutures of 2-O chromic catgut at the 5 o'clock and 7 o'clock positions. These sutures can also be used to anchor the bladder neck to the prostatic fossa (Fig. 23; *19*). Dead space within the evacuated prostatic fossa can be obliterated (and hemostasis optimized) by leaving the hemostatic figure-eight sutures attached to the bladder neck long, with the ultimate intention of passing them through the

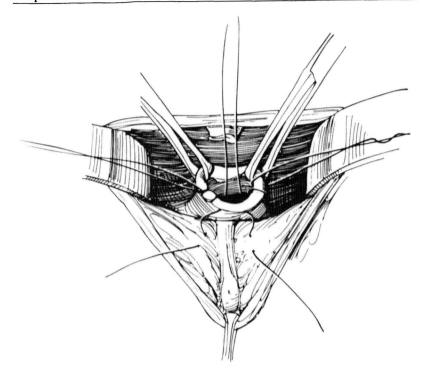

Fig. 23. Reconfiguration of the bladder neck. Allis clamps are used to grasp the 2 and 10 o'clock positions of the bladder neck. Hemostatic figure-eight sutures of 2-O chromic catgut have been placed in the 5 and 7 o'clock positions. Those sutures are intentionally kept long for later use. Posteriorly oriented sutures engage the bladder neck and posterior capsular flap. This maneuver helps to draw the posterior bladder neck into the prostatic fossa. (Reprinted with permission from ref. *19*.)

prostatic capsule and tying them snuggly. A 24-Fr 30-mL balloon catheter should be inserted into the wound and directed into the bladder using a curved clamp. The balloon can be hyperinflated to 60–70 mL if necessary. The catheter should be irrigated to evacuate any clots that may have accumulated and to validate optimal positioning (Fig. 24; *19*). Currently, a perineal drainage tube is almost never placed in the bladder.

The U-shaped flap is closed using interrupted 2-O chromic catgut suture. A Penrose drain is placed in the perineum and brought out through one corner of the perineal wound. The Levator fibers are approximated with interrupted 2-O or 3-O chromic catgut sutures; the subcutaneous tissues are approximated with interrupted 3-O plain catgut; and the skin with a subcuticular closure.

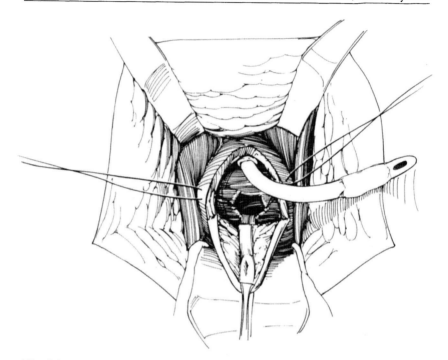

Fig. 24. Foley catheter insertion. A 24-Fr 30-mL catheter is inserted into the urethra and directed into the bladder utilizing a curved clamp. The balloon is then hyperinflated to 60–70 mL. This figure also depicts the placement of previously inserted hemostatic sutures through the prostatic capsule. These sutures are then snuggly tied to further obliterate dead space and optimize hemostasis. (Reprinted with permission from ref. *19.*)

A perineal binder should hold a fluffed-gauze dressing in place. In general, the Penrose drain can be removed in 1–2 d and the catheter in approx 1 wk (Fig. 25; *19*).

COMPLICATIONS OF OPEN PROSTATECTOMY

General Mortality and Morbidity Statistics

The information published in these sections is compromised by the paucity of published reports of current morbidity and mortality statistics for open prostatectomy. Based on an analysis of 21 studies involving more than 25,000 patients published in 1994, the mean perioperative mortality for open prostatectomy is about 2.4% (range 0–5%) *(21)*. The most commonly reported causes of death include myocardial infarction and pulmonary embolus *(22,23)*.

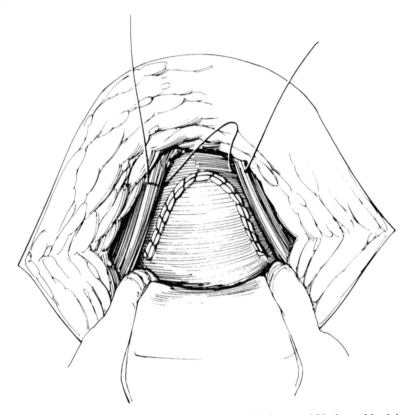

Fig. 25. Closure of the capsulotomy incision. The inverted U-shaped incision into the prostatic capsule can be closed with running or interrupted absorbable sutures. This figure also depicts the initial coaptation sutures used to reapproximate the levator muscles. A small Penrose drain will be placed before definitive wound closure and angled to one corner of the wound. The subcutaneous tissues are closed with interrupted or running absorbable sutures. The skin is closed with a subcuticular closure. (Reprinted with permission from ref. *19*.)

The incidence of nonlethal complications (perioperative morbidity) occurring within 90 d of surgery is approximately 21% (range 7–42%) *(2,22)*. The remainder of this section will highlight some of the more important complications encountered after open transvesical prostatectomy and simple perineal prostatectomy.

Bleeding

Significant perioperative bleeding has been observed, with frequencies ranging from 0.8 to 35% *(2)*. Reoperation to control persistent hemorrhage is exceedingly rare, with frequencies ranging from 0.8 to 1.5% in most series. Bleeding requiring a transfusion without operative intervention has occurred with a much higher anticipated frequency, ranging from 1.7 to 35.5% in three large representative series *(5,23,24).* It should be noted that in the study conducted by Nicoll et al., more than half of the patients undergoing transfusion received one unit of blood, which is an exceedingly unlikely occurrence today *(23).*

In general, preoperative transfusions are indicated in healthy patients with hemoglobin levels less than 8 g/dL. The preoperative transfusion threshold is hemoglobin level less than 10 g/dL for patients with underlying cardiopulmonary disease. Any intraoperative blood loss greater than 1000–1500 mL (20 mL/kg) must be replaced. In the absence of persistent bleeding, postoperative hemoglobin levels of 7–8 g/dL are well tolerated in patients with no other significant medical comorbidities *(4).*

The methods used to control persistent operative bleeding have already been discussed in detail. Persistent postoperative bleeding can usually be managed with conservative measures. The latter would include an attempt at evacuation of all clots from within the bladder followed by reapplication of gentle traction and the institution of continuous irrigation. If these maneuvers fail, control is usually best achieved by endoscopic means. This will entail complete evacuation of all clots and fulguration of bleeding vessels. The rollerball electrode can be used for this purpose. However, care must be taken to avoid injudicious fulguration in the region of the bladder neck. Very rarely, hypogastric artery embolization may be necessary *(2).*

Finally, delayed bleeding after open prostatectomy is exceedingly rare. Meier and associates observed this occurrence in one of 240 patients *(5).* In that instance, clot retention occurred 2 wk after suprapubic prostatectomy. Delayed bleeding of this type is generally managed with irrigation to evacuate all clots, gentle traction, continuous irrigation, and if this fails, endoscopic surgery to fulgurate bleeding vessels.

Incontinence

McConnell et al. observed that the median risk of stress incontinence was 1.5% after retropubic prostatectomy and about 2.6% after suprapubic prostatectomy *(21).* In that same analysis, total urinary incontinence occurred with a frequency of 0.5% after retropubic prostatectomy and only 0.3% using the suprapubic approach. Obviously, total incontinence can occur as a result of direct mechanical damage to the external sphincter or injury to sphincteric innervation. With respect to that latter, studies conducted by Ertekin and associates demonstrated that the somatosensory components of the pudendal nerve were not compromised after open prostatectomy *(25)*. Urge incontinence can occur more frequently after open prostatectomy. It has been observed in up to 7.7% of cases and generally results from detrusor instability *(24)*. This problem is self-limiting, and in most instances there is complete resolution within several months of surgery.

Erectile Dysfunction

Open prostatectomy can have an adverse impact on sexual performance. The review conducted by McConnell and associates revealed postoperative erectile dysfunction in 32%, 16%, and 18% in patients undergoing perineal, retropubic, and suprapubic prostatectomy, respectively *(21)*. In theory, leaving an intact and nonviolated prostatic capsule should mitigate against the development of either incontinence or erectile dysfunction. It has been assumed that preexisting erectile dysfunction may be more pervasive than previously suggested. However, the study conducted by Ertekin et al. documented postoperative erectile dysfunction in more than half of patients who claimed preoperative potency and subsequently underwent suprapubic prostatectomy *(25)*. In that study, however, there was no clear connection between surgical technique and development of erectile dysfunction. As anticipated, the incidence of retrograde ejaculation is very high, occurring in about 77% of all cases, a rate similar to that reported after TURP *(21)*.

Stricture and Bladder Neck Contracture

Complications usually, but not always, recognized with prolonged follow-up include urethral stricture, with a mean incidence of 2.6% and bladder neck contracture, with a mean incidence of 1.8% reported in the guideline review of open prostatectomy *(21)*. Both are reported to occur more frequently with a suprapubic than with a retropubic approach, but this may be more indicative of the period of data accumulation than of the procedures themselves *(1)*. Specifically, the incidence of contracture following suprapubic prostatectomy was about 3% vs 1% risk in patients undergoing retropubic prostatectomy *(21)*. In a study conducted by Roos and Ramsey, 6.9% of patients who underwent suprapubic prostatectomy required two or more dilations for treatment of bladder neck contracture *(26)*. In contrast, only 2.2% of the retropubic prostatectomy group required dilation. As stated previously, care during trigonalization of the prostatic fossa may mitigate against the development of contracture. In addition, avoiding injudicious fulguration in the vicinity of the bladder neck is also important. Other potential causes might include prolonged and excessive catheter traction with the hyperinflated Foley balloon. Most bladder neck contractures are easily managed with dilation or internal urethrotomy. A formal YV-plasty of the bladder neck is very infrequently required for the management of this problem.

Infection

The guidelines review indicated a mean incidence of epididymitis of 2.6% in patients undergoing open prostatectomy (21). Its occurrence was equivalent for all surgical approaches. It would appear that the presence of long-term indwelling catheters, chronic urinary tract infections, and a history of epididymitis predispose patients to this problem after open prostatectomy (6,27). This same guidelines review indicated a mean incidence of urinary tract infection of 13.4%, which appears to be related to antecedent instrumentation of the urinary tract and documented preoperative infections (2,21).

Osteitis Pubis

Osteitis pubis is an uncommon complication following prostatectomy. It can cause nagging to severe pain in the region of the symphysis, pelvis, or lower abdomen. Although it is most often associated with the retropubic approach, it has been observed after both suprapubic and transurethral prostatectomy. It has also been observed following simple urethral instrumentation (1). Symptoms usually begin within 6 wk of the operation. Typically, a low-grade fever develops, with limited adduction of the thighs and significant discomfort on bilateral medially directed pelvic pressure. Radiographic changes in the bone, although not universally observed, are generally recognizable 2–4 wk after the onset of symptoms (28). The disease is generally self-limiting and is most appropriately treated with antiinflammatory agents.

Urinary Fistula

Leakage from the suprapubic cystotomy or prostatic capsulotomy is not uncommon for approx 48 h. Beyond this point, the drainage is considered to be abnormal and persistent. The incidence of persistent urinary leakage following open prostatectomy is 1–2% (23). In most instances, the leakage can be attributed to high postoperative PVR, which occurs as a result of anatomic obstruction (clot, unremoved adenoma component, stricture) and/or detrusor hypocontractility. In most instances, the problem is easily managed with transurethral bladder drainage with or without concomitant urethral dilation. In most instances, the leakage will subside within 48–72 h. At that point, a voiding trial is generally successful. Patients with detrusor hypocontractility may benefit from the use of bethanechol in doses ranging from 10 to 50 mg three to four times per day. Generally, this problem is not attributable to a problem with technique as it relates to the creation of the cystotomy or closure of the capsulotomy. Stein et al. described using a third layer of closure of the cystotomy site after suprapubic prostatectomy (29). This involves the use of perivesical fat as the third layer of closure. They described a reduction in the incidence of leakage from 13.3 to 2.2% using this technique. The amount of leakage from the capsulotomy site can be influenced by the choice of operative drain. At times, the drain (either Penrose or sump drains) can be an impediment to healing if there is migration overlying the suture lines. When Penrose drains are used and a persistent leakage is encountered, the drains should be slightly advanced to eliminate their direct contact with the suture lines. In general, several advancement maneuvers will solve the problem. If sump drains have been used, they should be taken off suction. If this fails to solve the problem, they too can be sequentially advanced. In either case, the problem is generally easily remedied by simple drain management maneuvers.

Rectal Injury

Rectal perforation is generally a problem unique to simple perineal prostatectomy. This problem should be detected during surgery and is most often noted during the initial phases of the operative approach. When this occurs, the procedure should be terminated before the urethra is compromised. If the problem is detected during closure, it must be treated with a two-layer closure using absorbable sutures. In addition, the anal sphincter should be distended "3 fingers for 3 min" and a prolonged period of catheter drainage initiated, along with appropriate broad-spectrum antimicrobial therapy. The use of an elemental diet should be considered as well. If a fecal fistula develops, a diverting colostomy will be required. It is then reasonable to observe and hope for spontaneous closure. If the latter is not forthcoming, a formal closure will be required after the postoperative inflammatory reaction and associated infection have been completely resolved. In experienced hands, the frequency of this complication is exceedingly low (about 1%).

OPERATIVE RESULTS AND RETREATMENT RATES

Prostatectomy by any route is a significant surgical undertaking that attempts to achieve a satisfactory functional and symptomatic status in a complex multifunctional system (1). Undesirable results can occur because of inappropriate patient selection, unrecognized preexisting and imminent pathologic changes, and technical errors. Of the undesirable results, the most disturbing is inability to void.

In the cooperative evaluation of TURP, 6.5% of patients were unable to void when the catheter was removed, and 2.4% were sent home with an indwelling catheter. More than half of the latter had evidence of atonic bladder (30). Seaman et al. documented impaired detrusor contractility in 25% of 129 symptomatic men undergoing delayed postprostatectomy urodynamic evaluation (31). This perplexing voiding dysfunction may result from chronic severe obstruction and may be at least somewhat reversible with long-term catheter drainage. This problem clearly affects patients who have undergone open prostatectomy as well. For that reason, it is helpful to obtain preoperative pressure/flow urodynamic testing to identify patients with significant detrusor hypocontractility. If significant detrusor hypocontractility is documented, we favor the use of prolonged suprapubic catheter drainage to permit satisfactory symptomatic and objective voiding status.

Previous estimates of retreatment rates after surgical therapy of BPH have probably been underestimated. Taylor and Krakauer cited a 2.7% probability of repeat prostatectomy within 2 yr of TURP and a 1.8% probability within 2 yr of an open prostatectomy (32). Most of these repeated procedures resulted from technical errors, and others may represent unrecognized diagnostic errors. Roos and Ramsey assessed the re-operative rate at 17% for transurethral resection, 5% for suprapubic procedures, and 7% for retropubic procedures in an 8-yr data accumulation based on insurance claims information in Manitoba (26). Data from Denmark and the United Kingdom indicated a 12% re-operation rate, and data from Wisconsin showed a 16% re-operation rate after transurethral resection in 8- and 7-yr postoperation periods, respectively (33,34). The open prostatectomy re-operation rates at 8 yr were 5% for Denmark and 2% for the United Kingdom. The estimated re-operation rate at 5 yr cited in the BPH guidelines is 2% for open prostatectomy, 9% for TUIP, and 10% for TURP. These retreatment rates include treatment for complications of the surgical procedure and the removal of residual or recurrent BPH tissues (1).

More than 90% of men who undergo prostatectomy for the treatment of BPH benefit demonstrably from the procedure (1). More specifically, patient satisfaction and symptom improvement after suprapubic prostatectomy were evaluated by Hannappel and Krieger (24). In their study, 100% of patients had subjective improvement in the urinary stream; none exhibited unusual daytime frequency compared with 77% preoperatively, and only 7.7% complained of nocturia compared with 92.3% before surgery. Of importance, more than 90% reported that they were very satisfied with the outcome of surgery (2).

A variety of approaches have been used to assess the results achieved by prostatectomy, including subjective evaluation by the patient and objective assessments based on symptom scores, urodynamic evaluation, or both. Each of these approaches has inherent advantages and disadvantages. The varying indications for surgical intervention complicate the evaluation when rigid criteria are used, as does the knowledge that approx 45 and 40% of patients treated with placebo or watchful waiting report overall symptomatic improvement, respectively *(21)*.

The percentage of patients who judge their voiding symptoms to be better or much better after surgery varies from 75 to 93%, in part depending on the severity of the patient's initial symptoms and the duration of follow-up *(1)*. The BPH guidelines review indicates an overall symptomatic improvement of 98% for open prostatectomy, 88% for TURP, and 80% for TUIP. The guidelines data review indicates that the surgical procedures produced about an 80% improvement in symptom scores, which is appreciably higher than the 30–40% range for placebo and nonsurgical therapies. Although many have cautioned that patients with irritative as opposed to obstructive symptoms are at greater risk for poor results, evaluation by Jorgensen et al. and Lepor and Rigaud failed to confirm this finding *(35,36)*. Obviously, patients with predominantly irritative symptoms should be evaluated and selected carefully, which may have accounted for the good results (90%) reported in this latter group of patients.

Postprostatectomy urodynamic evaluation generally demonstrates a marked shift in the various urodynamic parameters, including an increase in maximum flow rate and voided volume and a decrease in residual urine and voiding pressure, which would be expected if a mechanical or functional outward obstruction had been diminished or relieved *(1)*. Indeed, the mean improvement in maximum flow rates in the BPH guidelines review was 14.4 mL/s after open prostatectomy and 9.8 mL/s after TURP, far greater than any other treatment analyzed except TUIP (about 7.3 mL/s).

Current assessments tend to interpret the initial and posttreatment PVR determinations with uncertainty and caution. Voiding is usually almost complete in normal individuals, and failure to approximate this normal state with treatment should be well documented. Even with the casual way in which the data analyzed were accumulated, the mean posttreatment PVR was less than 25 mL for TURP and open prostatectomy in the BPH guideline review *(21)*.

Finally, reversal of some of the preoperative urodynamic abnormalities is much less predictable. Normalization of or marked improvement in the preoperative urodynamic abnormalities does not necessarily correlate with a satisfactory clinical outcome. For that reason, the role of urodynamic evaluation and the routine monitoring of patients who undergo prostatectomy is not clearly established *(37)*.

CONCLUSIONS

Open prostatectomy (transvesical, retropubic, simple perineal) represents a durably effective low-risk procedure for properly selected patients with severe obstructive or irritative voiding symptoms caused by BPH.

ACKNOWLEDGMENTS

The authors would like to express their gratitude to Michael Mabaquiao and Beryl Schneiderman for their invaluable assistance in the preparation of this manuscript.

REFERENCES

1. Grayhack JT, McVary KT, Kozlowski JM. Benign prostatic hyperplasia. In: Gillenwater JY, Grayhack JT, Howards SS, Mitchell ME, eds., Adult and Pediatric Urology, 4th ed., Philadelphia: Lippincott Williams & Wilkens, 2002, pp. 1401–1470.
2. Miller EA, Ellis WJ. Complications of open prostatectomy. In: Taneja SS, Smith RB, Ehrlich RM, eds., Complications of Urologic Surgery: Prevention and Management, 3rd ed., Philadelphia: W. B. Saunders Co., 2001, pp. 399.
3. Weldon VE. Simple perineal prostatectomy. In: Hinman F Jr, ed., Atlas of Urologic Surgery, Philadelphia: W. B. Saunders Co., 1985, pp. 337.
4. Christou NV, Reiling RB. Non-emergency surgery: initial evaluation, preoperative planning, perioperative issues, and post-operative care. In: Wilmore DW, Chung LY, Harken AH, et al., eds., ACS Surgery Principles and Practice New York: WebMD Corp., 2002 pp. 535.
5. Meier DE, Tarpley JL, Imediegwu OO, et al. The outcome of superpubic prostatectomy: a contemporary series in the developing world. Urology 1995;46:40.
6. Kozlowski JM, Grayhack JT. Carcinoma of the prostate: In: Gillenwater JY, Grayhack JT, Howards SS, Mitchell ME, eds., Adult and Pediatric Urology, 4th ed., Philadelphia: Lippincott Williams & Wilkens, 2002, pp. 1471.
7. Foley SJ, Bailey DM. Microvessel density in prostatic hyperplasia. BJU Int 2000;85:70.
8. Hochberg DA, Basillote JB, Armenakas NA, et al. Decreased suburethral prostatic microvessel density in Finasteride treated prostates: a possible mechanism for reduced bleeding in benign prostatic hyperplasia. J Urol 2002;167:1731.
9. Hofer DR, Schaeffer AJ. Use of antimicrobials for patients undergoing prostatectomy. Urol Clin N Am 1990;71:595.
10. Morris MJ, Golovsky D, Guinness MDG, et al. The value of prophylactic antibiotics in transurethral prostatic resection: a controlled trial, with observations on the origin or post- operative infection. BJ Urol 1976;48:479.

11. Gorelick JI, Senterfit LB, Vaughn ED. Quantitative bacterial tissue cultures from 209 prostatectomy specimens: findings and interpretation. J Urol 1988;139:57.
12. Benizri E, Raucoules-Aime M, Amiel J, et al. Coagulation disorders after endoscopic resection of the prostate. J Urol 1994;100:299.
13. O'Conor VJ Jr. Superpubic and retropubic prostatectomy. In: Harrison JH, et al., Campbell's Urology, vol. 3, 4th ed., Philadelphia: W. B. Saunders, 1979.
14. Hinman F Jr. Superpubic prostatectomy. In: Hinman F Jr, ed., Atlas of Urologic Surgery, Philadelphia: W. B. Saunders Co., 1989, pp. 317.
15. Carson CC III, Malek RS. Transurethral prostatic resection: surgical anatomy of the prostate and prostatic hyperplasia. In: Greene LF, Segura JW, eds., Transurethral Surgery, Philadelphia: WB Saunders and Co., 1979.
16. O'Conor VJ Jr. Aid for hemostasis in open prostatectomy: capsular plication. J Urol 1982;127:448.
17. Waters WB. Superpubic and retropubic prostatectomy for benign prostatic hyperplasia. In: Fowler JE Jr, ed., Boston: Little, Brown and Co., 1992, pp. 369.
18. Grayhack JT, Sadlowski RW. Results of surgical treatment of benign prostatic hyperplasia. In: Grayhack JT, Wilson JD, Scherbenske MJ, eds., Benign Prostatic Hyperplasia, NIAMDD workshop proceedings on Feb. 20–21, 1975. US Department of Health, Education, and Welfare; Publication # (NIH) 76-1113, 1976, p. 125.
19. Hinman F Jr. Simple perineal prostatectomy. In: Hinman F Jr, ed., Atlas of Urologic Surgery, Philadelphia: WB Saunders Co., 1985, pp. 333.
20. Brendler H. Prostatic hypertrophy and perineal surgery. In: Glenn S, ed., Urologic Surgery, Hagerstown, MD: Harper & Row, 1975.
21. McConnell JD, Barry MS, Bruskewitz RC, et al. Benign prostatic hyperplasia: diagnosis and treatment. Clinical Practice Guideline, # 8. Rockville, Maryland: US Department of Health and Human Services, Public Health Service, Agency for Health Care Policy and Research, 1994.
22. Nanninga JB, O'Conor VJ. Superpubic prostatectomy: a review: 1966–1970. J Urol 1972;108:453.
23. Nicoll GA, Riffle GN, Anderson FO. Superpubic prostatectomy: the removable purse string: a continuing comparative analysis of 300 consecutive cases. J Urol 1978;120:702.
24. Hannappel J, Krieger S. Subjective and clinical results after transurethral resection and superpubic prostatectomy and benign prostatic hypertrophy. Eur Urol 1991;20:272.
25. Ertekin C, Yurtseven O, Reel F. Bulbocavernosus reflex in benign hypertrophy of the prostate. Int Urol Nephrol 1981;13:69.
26. Roos NP, Ramsey EW. A population-based study of prostatectomy: outcomes associated with differing surgical approaches. J Urol 1987;137:1184.
27. Graham JW, Grayhack JT. Epididymitis following unilateral vasectomy and prostatic surgery. J Urol 1962;87:582.
28. Witten DM, Myers GH, Utz DC. The plane film of the urinary tract (KUB) In: Witten DM, Myers GH, Utz DC, eds., Atlas and Textbook of Roentgenologic Diagnosis, Philadelphia: Sanders, 1977.
29. Stein A, Ratzkovitzki R, Lurie A. Perivesical fat closure during suprapubic prostatectomy. Does it prevent urinary leakage? A prospective randomized study. Tech Urol, 1996;2:99.
30. Mebust WK, Holtgrewe HL, Cockett ATK, et al. Transurethral prostatectomy: immediate and post-operative complications. A cooperative study of 13 participating institutions evaluating 3885 patients. J Urol 1989;141:243.

31. Seaman EK, Jacobs BZ, Blaivis JG, et al. Persistence of recurrence of symptoms after transurethral resection of prostate: urodynamic assessment. J Urol 1994; 152:935.
32. Taylor Z, Krakauer H. Mortality and reoperation following prostatectomy: outcomes in a Medicare population. Urology 1991;38(suppl 1):27.
33. Roos NP, Wennberg JE, Malenka DJ, et al. Mortality and reoperation after open and transurethral resection of the prostate for benign prostatic hyperplasia. N Engl J Med 1989;320:1120.
34. Nielsen KT, Christensen MM, Madsen PO, et al. Symptom analysis and uroflowmetry seven years after transurethral resection of the prostate. J Urol 1989;142:1251.
35. Jorgensen JB, Jensen KME, Morgensen P. Significance of predominantly irritative symptomatology prior to prostatic surgery. J Urol 1990;143:739.
36. Lepor H, Rigaud G. The efficacy of transurethral resection of the prostate in men with moderate symptoms of prostatism. J Urol 1990;143:533.
37. Dorflinger T, Frimodt-Moller PC, Bruskewitz RC, et al. The significance of uninhibited detrusor contraction in prostatism. J Urol 1985;133:819.

Index

A

α-Adrenergic receptor antagonists,
  alfuzosin, 71, 72
  comparative studies, 73, 74
  doxazosin, 68, 69
  efficacy and side effects, 67, 74
  history of use for benign
    prostatic hyperplasia, 62
  lower urinary tract symptom
    management in non-benign
    prostatic hyperplasia
    patients, 72, 73
  mechanism of action, 62, 63
  patient evaluation for treatment,
    65, 66
  phenoxybenzamine, 66, 68
  prazosin, 68
  receptor classification and signal
    transduction, 63, 65
  tamsulosin, 70, 71
  terazosin, 69, 70
  transurethral microwave
    thermotherapy
    comparative trials, 119
Alfuzosin, benign prostatic
  hyperplasia management,
  71, 72
American Urological Association
  symptom score, 23, 24

B

Benign prostatic hyperplasia (BPH),
  see also Lower urinary tract
  symptoms,
  causes, 12–14
  definition, 22, 30
  economic impact, 29, 30, 164
  epidemiology,
    aging, 27, 30
    diet, 28
    family history, 27, 28, 31
    insulin resistance, 29
    lifestyle factors, 28, 31
    male-pattern baldness, 29
    race, 27, 30, 31
  history of study, 8
  incidence, 8–10
  natural history, 10, 12, 22
  pathophysiology, 14–16, 21
  prevalence, 24–27
  symptom classification, 21, 61
  treatment, see α-Adrenergic
    receptor antagonists;
    Ethanol injection;
    High-intensity focused
    ultrasound; Interstitial
    laser coagulation;
    Prostatectomy; Prostatic
    stents; 5α-Reductase
    inhibitors; Transurethral
    incision of the prostate;
    Transurethral microwave
    thermotherapy;
    Transurethral needle
    ablation of the prostate;
    Transurethral resection of
    the prostate; Transurethral
    vaporization of the prostate;
    Water-induced
    thermotherapy
BPH, see Benign prostatic
  hyperplasia

C–D

Creatinine clearance,
        postobstructive diuresis, 42
Cystometry, lower urinary tract
        symptoms, 52
DHT, *see* Dihydrotestosterone
Dihydrotestosterone (DHT),
    androgen receptor affinity, 81
    benign prostatic hyperplasia
        etiology, 12, 14
    inhibition of synthesis, *see*
        5α-Reductase inhibitors
    prostate growth role, 80, 81
Doxazosin, benign prostatic
        hyperplasia management,
        68, 69

E–F

Embryonic reawakening hypothesis,
        benign prostatic hyperplasia
        etiology, 12, 14
Ethanol injection,
    efficacy studies, 212
    historical perspective, 211
    mechanism of action, 212
FeNa, *see* Fractional excretion
        of sodium
Finasteride,
    benign prostatic hyperplasia
        treatment,
        combination therapy, 93
        efficacy, 85, 86
        histologic effects, 90, 91
        magnetic resonance imaging
            study, 89, 90
        phase III clinical trials, 86, 87
        Proscar Long-Term Efficacy
            and Safety Study, 87–89
        prospects, 93
        prostate-specific antigen
            response, 87, 88, 92, 93

    Scandinavian Study
        on Reduction
        of the Prostate, 89
    urodynamic response, 91, 92
    pharmacology, 84, 85
    structure, 84
Fluid replacement, postobstructive
        diuresis, 44, 45
Fractional excretion of sodium
        (FeNa), postobstructive
        diuresis, 42

H

HIFU, *see* High-intensity focused
        ultrasound
High-intensity focused ultrasound
        (HIFU),
    efficacy studies in benign
        prostatic hyperplasia,
        156–160
    histologic studies, 155
    principles, 153–155
    prospects, 160
    technique, 155, 156

I

I-PSS, *see* International Prostate
        Symptom Score
ILC, *see* Interstitial laser coagulation
International Prostate Symptom
        Score (I-PSS), 24, 26, 65
Interstitial laser coagulation (ILC),
    anesthesis, 153
    complications, 151
    delivery systems, 142, 143
    efficacy studies, 146–151
    equipment, 143, 145
    medical therapy, 152, 153
    patient selection
        and preparation, 152
    safety, 151
    technique, 145, 146

L–N

Lower urinary tract symptoms
(LUTS),
American Urological Association
symptom score, 23, 24
causes, 23
evaluation, 23
International Prostate Symptom
Score, 24, 26
treatment, *see* α-Adrenergic
receptor antagonists;
Ethanol injection;
High-intensity focused
ultrasound; Interstitial
laser coagulation;
Prostatectomy; Prostatic
stents; 5α-Reductase
inhibitors; Transurethral
incision of the prostate;
Transurethral microwave
thermotherapy;
Transurethral needle
ablation of the prostate;
Transurethral resection
of the prostate;
Transurethral vaporization
of the prostate;
Water-induced
thermotherapy
urodynamic testing,
cystometry, 52
indications, 55, 56
predictive value, 53–55
pressure-flow studies, 49–51
symptoms and findings, 52, 53
uroflowmetry, 48, 49
videourodynamics, 51
LUTS, *see* Lower urinary tract
symptoms
Nonandrogenic testis secretory
factor hypothesis, benign
prostatic hyperplasia etiology,
12, 14

P

Phenoxybenzamine, benign
prostatic hyperplasia
management, 66, 68
POD, *see* Postobstructive diuresis
Postobstructive diuresis (POD),
case report, 35–38
diagnosis, 38, 39
laboratory findings, 40, 42, 43
treatment, 43, 44
Prazosin, benign prostatic
hyperplasia management, 68
Pressure-flow studies,
lower urinary tract symptoms,
49–51
treatment response studies, 54, 55
Prostate,
anatomy, 2–4
blood supply, 4
function, 1
growth and development, 7, 8,
80–83
innervation, 4
internal architecture, 4–7
Prostatectomy,
anesthesia, 227
antibiotic prophylaxis, 225, 226
complications,
bladder neck contracture,
255, 256
bleeding, 253, 254
erectile dysfunction, 255
incidence, 252, 253
incontinence, 254, 255, 258
infection, 256
osteitis pubis, 256
rectal injury, 257
urethral stricture, 255, 256
urinary fistula, 256, 257
efficacy in benign prostatic
hypertrophy management,
257–260
goals in benign prostatic
hypertrophy management,
221, 222

indications, 222, 223
mortality, 252
preoperative assessment,
    bowel preparation, 227
    comorbid status, 223, 224
    genitourinary evaluation, 227
    hematologic issues, 224, 225
    infection risk, 225, 226
    venous thromboembolism
        prevention, 226, 227
simple perineal prostatectomy,
    adenoma enucleation, 247, 250
    bleeding control, 250, 251
    closure, 251
    incisions, 243–247
    patient positioning, 243
    postoperative care, 252
    training, 243
suprapubic transvesical
        prostatectomy,
    adenoma enucleation,
        230–234
    bladder distension, 228
    bleeding control, 234–236
    closure, 237, 239–241
    incisions, 228–230
    patient positioning, 228
    postoperative care, 241–243
    urethra transection, 232, 233
Prostate specific antigen (PSA),
    finasteride long-term response,
    87, 88, 92, 93
Prostatic stents,
    balloon-expandable stent, 216
    classification, 214
    expandable stent studies, 215, 216
    historical perspective, 214, 215
    prospects, 218
    self-expandable stents, 216
    temporary stents,
        bioresorbable stents, 217, 218
        nonbioresorbable stents, 217
    thermosensitive nitinol stent,
        216, 217
PSA, *see* Prostate-specific antigen

R

5α-Reductase inhibitors,
    development, 83, 84
    enzyme functions, 81–83
    finasteride,
        benign prostatic hyperplasia
            treatment,
            combination therapy, 93
            efficacy, 85, 86
            histologic effects, 90, 91
            magnetic resonance
                imaging study, 89, 90
            phase III clinical trials,
                86, 87
            Proscar Long-Term
                Efficacy and Safety
                Study, 87–89
            prospects, 93
            prostate-specific antigen
                response, 87, 88, 92, 93
            Scandinavian Study on
                Reduction of the
                Prostate, 89
            urodynamic response, 91, 92
        pharmacology, 84, 85
        structure, 84
    isozymes, 81
    natural enzyme deficiency fea-
        tures, 81–83

S

Serum osmolarity, postobstructive
    diuresis, 40, 42
Simple perineal prostatectomy, *see*
    Prostatectomy
Spot urine electrolytes,
    postobstructive diuresis, 42
Stem cell hypothesis, benign
    prostatic hyperplasia etiology,
    12, 14
Suprapubic transvesical prostatec-
    tomy, *see* Prostatectomy

T

Tamsulosin, benign prostatic hyperplasia management, 70, 71
Terazosin, benign prostatic hyperplasia management, 69, 70
Testosterone,
    androgen receptor affinity, 81
    prostate growth role, 80, 81
Transurethral incision of the prostate (TUIP),
    complications,
        bladder neck contracture, 134
        blood transfusion, 134, 135
        re-operation rates, 134
        sexual dysfunction, 133, 134
    historical perspective, 126
    indications,
        trapped prostate, 127, 128
        urinary obstruction after brachytherapy, 128
    laser technique, 131
    one-incision technique, 129, 130
    outcomes,
        direct measures, 132, 133
        indirect measures, 133
        overview, 131, 132
    patient selection, 126, 127
    postoperative care, 130, 131
    preoperative preparation, 128, 129
    prospects, 135
    two-incision technique, 130
Transurethral microwave thermotherapy (TUMT),
    complications, 120, 121
    contraindications, 115
    efficacy trials,
        comparative trials,
            α-adrenergic receptor antagonists, 119
            transurethral resection of the prostate, 119–121
        overview, 118, 119
    urinary retention patients, 120
    histologic findings, 114, 115
    historical perspective, 110, 111
    indications, 112
    instrumentation, 116, 117
    mechanism of action, 111
    patient selection, 112
    postoperative care, 117, 118
    preoperative evaluation,
        imaging, 113
        laboratory studies, 113
        patient preparation, 115, 116
        symptom scores, 113, 114
    prospects, 121, 122
    technique, 116, 117
Transurethral needle ablation of the prostate (TUNA),
    anesthesia, 100, 101
    animal studies, 99
    clinical trials, 102–105
    complications, 105, 106
    instrumentation, 101
    patient selection, 100, 106
    principles, 98, 99
    rationale, 98
    safety, 99, 100
    technique, 101, 102
    urothelium preservation, 99, 100
Transurethral resection of the prostate (TURP),
    anesthesia, 167, 168
    complications,
        bladder neck contracture, 186, 187
        bleeding,
            intraoperative, 183
            long-term complications, 187
            perioperative, 185
        incontinence, 188
        overview, 97, 109, 182
        perforations, 184
        sexual dysfunction, 188, 189
        TUR syndrome, 184, 185, 205
        urethral stricture, 186, 187

urinary tract infection, 186
efficacy studies, 189, 190
historical perspective, 125, 126
instruments, 170, 171, 173
interstitial laser coagulation
    comparison, 151
irrigation fluid, 173
mortality, 186
patient selection and evaluation,
    164–167
preoperative preparation, 168, 169
pressure-flow studies of treatment
    response, 54
recommendations, 190, 191
technique, 169, 170, 175, 176,
    178, 179, 181, 182
transurethral
    electrovaporization
    of the prostate comparison
    study, 204
transurethral microwave
    thermotherapy comparative
    trials, 119–121
transurethral vapor resection
    of the prostate comparison
    study, 203
Transurethral vaporization
    of the prostate (TVP),
contraindications, 197
equipment,
    electrodes, 198–200
    electrosurgical generators,
        198
    overview, 195, 197
historical perspective, 196, 197
indications, 197
prospects, 208
transurethral
    electrovaporization
    of the prostate,
    complications,
        intraoperative, 205
        long-term, 206
        postoperative, 206

efficacy studies, 203, 204
technique, 202
transurethral resection
    of the prostate
    comparison study, 204
transurethral vapor resection
    of the prostate,
complications,
    intraoperative, 206, 207
    long-term, 207, 208
    postoperative, 207
efficacy, 202–204
technique, 200–202
transurethral resection
    of the prostate
    comparison study, 203
TUIP, *see* Transurethral incision
    of the prostate
TUMT, *see* Transurethral microwave
    thermotherapy
TUNA, *see* Transurethral needle
    ablation of the prostate
TURP, *see* Transurethral resection
    of the prostate
TVP, *see* Transurethral vaporization
    of the prostate

U

Urine osmolality, postobstructive
    diuresis, 40
Urodynamic testing, lower urinary
    tract symptoms,
cystometry, 52
finasteride response, 92, 93
indications, 55, 56
open prostatectomy outcomes,
    259, 260
predictive value, 53–55
pressure-flow studies, 49–51
symptoms and findings, 52, 53
uroflowmetry, 48, 49
videourodynamics, 51
Uroflowmetry, lower urinary tract
    symptoms, 48, 49

V–W

Videourodynamics, lower urinary
    tract symptoms, 51
Water-induced thermotherapy
    (WIT),
    efficacy studies, 213, 214

historical perspective, 212, 213
mechanism of action, 213
technique, 213
WIT, *see* Water-induced
    thermotherapy